MARKETING
HEALTH SERVICES

Second Edition

MARKETING
HEALTH SERVICES

Second Edition

RICHARD K. THOMAS

AUPHA

Your board, staff, or clients may also benefit from this book's insight. For more information on quantity discounts, contact the Health Administration Press Marketing Manager at (312) 424-9470.

Reprinting February 2011

Library of Congress Cataloging-in-Publication Data

Thomas, Richard K., 1944-
  Marketing health services / Richard K. Thomas. -- 2nd ed.
    p. cm.
  Includes bibliographical references and index.
  ISBN 978-1-56793-336-9 (alk. paper)
  1. Medical care--Marketing. I. Title.
  RA410.56.T48 2010
  362.1068'8--dc22

                          2009044461

The paper used in this publication meets the minimum requirements of American National Standard for Information Sciences—Permanence of Paper for Printed Library Materials, ANSI Z39.48-1984. ∞ ™

Acquisitions editor: Eileen Lynch; Project manager: Jennifer Seibert; Cover designer: Scott Miller; Layout: BookComp, Inc.

Found an error or a typo? We want to know! Please e-mail it to hap1@ache.org, and put "Book Error" in the subject line.

For photocopying and copyright information, please contact Copyright Clearance Center at www.copyright.com or (978) 750-8400.

Health Administration Press
A division of the Foundation
  of the American College of
  Healthcare Executives
One North Franklin Street
Suite 1700
Chicago, IL 60606
(312) 424-2800

Association of University Programs
  in Health Administration
2000 North 14th Street
Suite 780
Arlington, VA 22201
(703) 894-0940

CONTENTS

DETAILED CONTENTS

PART I: HEALTHCARE MARKETING: HISTORY AND CONCEPTS

PART V: THE FUTURE OF HEALTHCARE MARKETING

PREFACE TO THE SECOND EDITION

It seems like a lifetime since the first edition of this book was published in 2005. In the past five years, the world has changed significantly—and so have marketing and healthcare. One would think revising a textbook written five years ago would simply require noting the emergence of new marketing techniques, highlighting trends in marketing strategy preferences among healthcare organizations, and updating some of the hard numbers. Under ordinary circumstances in an ordinary industry, this would typically be the case.

The fact of the matter is that healthcare has been and is anything but ordinary. Since the 1980s, the healthcare industry has undergone a series of dramatic changes. Even to observers inured to the constant restructuring and shape shifting that characterize the field, recent developments reflect changes of such magnitude that seasoned professionals can hardly keep pace. By nature, healthcare is a dynamic enterprise that devotes massive resources to the creation of new devices, therapies, and drugs. Beyond advances in medical technology, the industry exhibits a constantly changing system of financing that makes short-term planning difficult and long-term planning impossible. Add to this the constant barrage of mergers and acquisitions affecting both the not-for-profit and the for-profit components of the industry.

Although health professionals have come to expect these types of changes, other forces have come into play that do not represent business as usual. In the past decade, the nation has experienced a dramatic increase in the number of people who lack health insurance. Add to the 47 million uninsured Americans the millions more who are underinsured, and we have the makings of a serious crisis not only in financial terms but also with regard to the health of the public. The uninsured are no longer simply the marginalized members of society who are unemployed, migrant, or too young to know better. They increasingly represent a cross-section of American society, reflected in the startling fact that, today, more than half of all personal bankruptcies are attributed to medical debts or loss of income associated with sickness. These developments have occurred against a backdrop of a failing medical safety net, health facilities overrun with nonpaying patients, financial setbacks for many providers, and shortfalls in Medicaid funding.

Since 2000, the vagaries of the political environment have had a particular impact on the healthcare industry. The arena has been dominated by free-market proponents who have promoted a laissez-faire approach to healthcare in an environment that has been dominated by vested interests—in particular the insurance and pharmaceutical industries. Major legislative action has been taken (e.g., the Medicare drug benefit) or not taken (e.g., expansion of the State Children's Health Insurance Program) in an arena that emphasized everyone's interests but the patient's. As this second edition goes to press, a new administration is in the White House and the political environment appears to be undergoing radical change. Almost overnight, a private-sector orientation to healthcare is being replaced with an approach that emphasizes much more governmental involvement and the resurrection of discussions on universal health coverage. Further, the economic stimulus package put forth by the Obama administration includes significant funding for medical research, information technology, and healthcare infrastructure development, and the first budget it submitted made healthcare reform a centerpiece. The extent to which the healthcare system will be transformed under the new administration remains to be seen, but it is clear that healthcare issues will be in the spotlight for the foreseeable future.

The changes occurring in the marketing field may appear less dramatic on the surface, and in many ways, current trends in healthcare marketing reflect the normal process of adapting marketing approaches to a constantly changing environment. Against this backdrop of evolutionary change, however, is evidence that a revolution has occurred in marketing. The Internet and other electronic forms of communication have created a paradigm shift in the method of information transfer that has far-reaching implications for marketing. Indeed, it has been argued that most of the old rules of marketing no longer apply and a set of new rules must be adopted. Although the healthcare field may be slower to join the revolution than some other industries, there is no doubt that the approach to marketing health services tomorrow will be much different than it is today.

One other development that sits at the intersection of healthcare and marketing relates to the changing role of marketing in healthcare, which has manifested itself in at least two important ways. First, marketing as a corporate function has shifted from the periphery of healthcare to the centers of power. Healthcare organizations have become much more market driven, and this development has placed marketers much closer to the decision-making process. Second, the marketing function has become much more integrated into the operations of many healthcare organizations. In fact, marketing is now often merged with strategic planning or business development operations and recognized for the pivotal role it can play beyond promotion. As such, the contribution that the marketing function is making in many healthcare organizations is more significant than the founders of the field could have ever envisioned.

This revision of *Marketing Health Services* is much more than an update of the first edition. It characterizes the forces that are changing healthcare and marketing and chronicles the transformation of the healthcare marketing enterprise. The turmoil in the healthcare industry at the time of publication of the first edition seems almost tame in comparison to today's events. With the developments poised just over the horizon, the future should be interesting for healthcare marketers.

INTRODUCTION TO THE SECOND EDITION

Most observers consider 1977 to be the year in which marketing as a component of healthcare was officially launched. In 1977, the American Hospital Association sponsored the first conference on healthcare marketing, and the first book on healthcare marketing was published. Although formal marketing activities became common early on among retail-oriented healthcare organizations, such as health insurance, pharmaceutical, and medical supply companies, health services providers resisted incorporating formal marketing activities into their operations. Hospitals and other healthcare organizations engaged in public relations, physician relationship development, community service, and other activities, but few health professionals equated these activities with marketing. To many, marketing meant advertising, and until the 1970s, advertising on the part of health services providers was considered inappropriate.

In the 1980s, healthcare reached an important milestone when it formally recognized marketing as an appropriate activity for health services providers. Once health professionals accepted marketing, a variety of new opportunities emerged. As a result of this newfound interest in marketing, many organizations established marketing budgets and created new positions, such as vice president for marketing. This development opened healthcare to an influx of concepts and methods from other industries and helped introduce modern business practices into the healthcare arena.

Although most would agree that, after years of grudging acceptance, marketing has become reasonably well established as a legitimate healthcare function, the process has not been without its fits and starts. In healthcare, surges of interest in marketing were often followed by cutbacks when marketing—and marketers—were considered unnecessary or inappropriate. Periods of marketing prosperity have alternated with periods of neglect. There have been periods of exuberant, almost reckless, marketing frenzy and periods of retrenchment. There has been ongoing tension between those who eagerly accept marketing as a function of the healthcare organization and those who doggedly resist its intrusion into their realm. With each revival of marketing in healthcare, new wrinkles have been added that have made available marketing approaches, if not better, at least different from previous approaches.

Once the dam broke and marketing made its initial incursion into healthcare, healthcare organizations, led by major hospitals, established aggressive marketing campaigns. Urged on by marketers recruited from other industries, hospitals and other healthcare organizations embarked on a whirlwind of marketing activity. The effectiveness of these initial marketing campaigns did not match their proponents' enthusiasm, however, and organizations soon realized that marketing healthcare was not the same as marketing hamburgers. The approaches required for the healthcare arena were not easily adapted from other industries, and much of what was effective elsewhere was not necessarily effective in the healthcare industry.

Today, healthcare is still struggling to find the appropriate role for marketing, and healthcare marketers continue to strive to find their niche. The industry still suffers from a lack of standardization when it comes to marketing, which has not been helped by the fact that few academic marketing programs offer coursework in healthcare marketing. Healthcare marketing appears poised to play a greater role in the new healthcare environment, but it is likely to be different from that envisioned in the mid-1970s.

Before the 1980s, marketing campaigns targeting healthcare consumers were relatively rare. Most of the marketing activity at the time was undertaken by industry segments that were not involved in patient care (e.g., pharmaceutical and insurance companies), whose targets were not patients but other players in the healthcare arena (e.g., physicians and employers). Healthcare organizations did not need to market their services. The industry was product driven, and most service providers operated in semi-monopolistic environments. They enjoyed an almost unlimited flow of customers (patients), and their revenues were essentially guaranteed by third-party payers.

This situation began to change in the early 1980s. Along with a number of other important changes in healthcare, competition was introduced for the first time. To survive in this new healthcare world, organizations began to realize that they would have to adopt business practices long established in other industries. Embracing these practices involved, among other things, a shift from a product orientation to a service orientation. For the first time, the market became a factor in the healthcare industry. As a result, marketing came to be perceived as a legitimate function in healthcare.

By the mid-1980s, most large healthcare organizations had established marketing departments. Once introduced to each other, marketing and healthcare passed through a tentative getting-to-know-you period. By the mid-1980s, however, it was a romance in full bloom, and the two were seen together everywhere. Healthcare organizations were spending feverishly on their newfound partner, and marketers rushed to take advantage of the sudden burst of interest. Those without formal marketing departments developed marketing functions through other mechanisms, such as outsourcing.

By the early 1990s, healthcare executives realized that marketing did not consist of spending truckloads of money on mass media advertising. Progressive healthcare organizations began to reassess their marketing objectives. Much like their counterparts in other industries, healthcare organizations sought to understand the market, their customers, and their customers' motivations. Now that marketing was a legitimate function, these organizations created high-level positions for their marketing professionals, including vice president of marketing and chief marketing officer.

Today, healthcare marketers have a much better understanding of the markets in which they operate and the customers who reside in those markets. Sophisticated techniques have been developed specifically for the healthcare market, and a large cadre of professional healthcare marketers has emerged.

This book is devoted to helping readers develop an understanding of marketing as a field and its application to healthcare. The chapters introduce readers to the concepts, methods, and data used in healthcare marketing; describe the role of marketing in healthcare; and provide the tools needed to plan and implement a marketing initiative.

The Audience

This book is designed as a comprehensive guide for students of healthcare administration and marketing. Today, most healthcare administration programs include a component on healthcare marketing. This text provides the core information necessary for such a course. Many business administration programs offer healthcare marketing as a component of their marketing concentrations. This text could serve that audience as well. It could also serve as a reference work for academicians who teach or conduct research in healthcare administration or marketing but are not directly involved in the practice of marketing.

Healthcare practitioners also should find this book useful as a reference work. Healthcare administrators who require an understanding of the marketing process, health planners, and others directly involved in marketing activities should benefit from its contents as well. Most health professionals in today's environment are expected to be familiar with marketing concepts, not only to support the organization's marketing efforts but to be able to "market" their departments to those who establish the budget. This book would also introduce marketing firms and advertising agencies with an interest in healthcare to the unique aspects of health services marketing.

Organization of the Book

The text surveys the field of healthcare marketing by presenting the perspectives, concepts, techniques, and data common to the field. It takes the reader through the entire process of marketing, from a perceived need for a marketing campaign through final evaluation of a project.

Part I provides an overview of marketing and its applications to healthcare. Chapter 1 addresses the history of marketing and recent marketing developments in healthcare. This chapter also addresses the unique aspects of healthcare that create challenges for marketers. Chapter 2 describes the changing context of healthcare and provides a glimpse of the volatile nature of the contemporary healthcare arena. Chapter 3 introduces and defines the basic marketing concepts that will be used throughout the text and exposes readers to the language of marketing as a prerequisite to further study. Chapter 4 describes the current status of marketing in healthcare and identifies the contexts in which marketing is presently taking place.

Part II introduces readers to the nature of healthcare markets, the consumers who populate them, and the factors that influence the demand for health services. Chapter 5 provides an overview of the market for health services and describes the ways in which healthcare differs from other industries in this regard. Chapter 6 focuses on healthcare consumers and the variety of constituents healthcare organizations serve. It notes the unique characteristics of the end users of health services and the manner in which healthcare decision making differs from decision making in other industries. Chapter 7 describes healthcare services and products and distinguishes them from the services and products marketers promote in other fields. Chapter 8 introduces the concepts of healthcare needs, wants, and utilization and describes the factors that influence the demand for health services and the ultimate level of utilization.

Part III, which focuses on the practical aspects of healthcare marketing, describes both traditional and cutting-edge marketing strategies and marketing techniques as they relate to healthcare. Chapter 9 discusses marketing strategy, from the strategy development process to means of strategy implementation. Chapter 10 distinguishes between public relations, advertising, and other traditional marketing activities. Chapter 11 describes contemporary marketing techniques, often adapted from other industries, and discusses the potential applications of these techniques to healthcare. Chapter 12, new to this edition, examines healthcare marketing from an international perspective and reflects on the increasing globalization of healthcare and the emergence of such new concepts as medical tourism.

Part IV is a practical guide to managing the marketing process in healthcare. Chapter 13 provides an overview of the marketing process, tying together components discussed earlier in the text, and presents the issues involved in managing and evaluating marketing initiatives. Chapter 14 presents an overview of the marketing research process, describes how marketers use research, and reviews how basic research techniques are applied to the healthcare field. Chapter 15 introduces the concept of marketing planning. Notwithstanding its late introduction in this text, marketing planning should be an early and constant consideration in the marketing process. Chapter 16 describes the categories of data used for marketing research and planning and indicates the manner in which these data are generated and the sources from which they can be obtained.

Part V includes a single chapter (Chapter 17) on the future of healthcare marketing. Chapter 17 summarizes the current status of the field and offers prospects for the future. It also proposes factors likely to influence the future course of marketing and speculates on the future characteristics of healthcare marketing—and marketers.

I

HEALTHCARE MARKETING: HISTORY AND CONCEPTS

Part I places the field of marketing and its applications to healthcare in a historical context. One cannot understand where the field is going unless one knows where it has been.

Chapter 1 presents an overview of the history of marketing, from its introduction to healthcare to its contemporary iteration. It outlines the stages of development through which healthcare marketing has progressed and notes changes that occurred in the field in each stage. In addition, Chapter 1 reviews the factors that have contributed to periods of healthcare marketing success and setback over the past 30 years. This chapter also describes the ways in which healthcare is different from other industries and the ways in which healthcare marketing is different from other types of marketing. Last, Chapter 1 identifies the factors that have helped marketing become accepted in healthcare and the contribution marketing can make to the industry.

Chapter 2 reviews recent developments in healthcare and describes their implications for marketing. In particular, the transformation of the healthcare field in the 1980s was an important factor in the emergence of marketing as a function in healthcare organizations. The chapter also discusses the halting evolution of marketing as a legitimate healthcare endeavor.

Chapter 3 defines key terms and concepts basic to the marketing endeavor and reviews how these terms and concepts are applied to the healthcare field. In particular, the chapter discusses how the four Ps of marketing have been modified for the healthcare arena. The challenge of adapting marketing concepts and techniques from other industries to healthcare is also examined.

Chapter 4 examines the current status of marketing in healthcare and identifies the types of organizations most actively involved in promotional activities. It discusses the healthcare industry's perspective on marketing today and reviews current trends in the application of marketing techniques in healthcare.

THE ORIGIN AND EVOLUTION OF MARKETING IN HEALTHCARE

Since the notion of marketing was introduced to healthcare providers during the 1970s, the field has gone through periods of growth, decline, retrenchment, and renewed growth. This chapter reviews the history of marketing in the U.S. economy in general and traces its evolution in healthcare over the last quarter of the twentieth century. The chapter then turns to the challenges marketers have faced in their efforts to gain a foothold in healthcare.

The History of Marketing

Marketing, as the term is used today, is a modern concept. The term was first used around 1910 to refer to what would now be called *sales* in the contemporary sense. Marketing is a uniquely American concept; the English word *marketing* has been adopted into the vocabulary of other languages that lack a word for this activity. Although the 1950s mark the beginning of the marketing era in the United States, the marketing function within the U.S. economy took several decades to establish, and marketers had to overcome a number of factors that slowed the field's development.

Many of these factors reflected characteristics of the U.S. economy carried over from the World War II period. In the 1950s, America was still in the Industrial Age, and the U.S. economy was production oriented until well after the war. Because essentially all aspects of the U.S. economy were geared to production, the prevailing mind-set emphasized the producer's interests over the consumer's. This production orientation assumed that producers already knew what consumers needed. Products were produced to the manufacturer's specification and then customers were sought. A "here is our product—take it or leave it" approach characterized most industries during this period. The stages through which marketing subsequently progressed are described in the following sections.

Phase One: Product Differentiation and the Rise of the Consumer

A wide variety of new products and services emerged during the postwar period, particularly in the consumer goods industries. Newly empowered consumers demanded a growing array of goods and services (even if existing goods and services had adequately served previous generations). This development contributed to the emergence of marketing for two primary reasons. First, consumers had to be introduced to and educated about these new goods and services. Second, the entry of new producers into the market introduced a level of competition that was unknown in the prewar period. Mechanisms had to be developed to make the public aware of a new product and to distinguish that product in the eyes of potential customers from the products of competitors. Consumers had to be made aware of purchase opportunities and then persuaded to buy a certain brand.

The standardization of existing products during this period further contributed to the need to convince newly empowered consumers to purchase one good or service over another. Where few differences existed between the products in a market, the role of marketing became crucial. Marketers were enlisted to highlight and, if necessary, create differences between similar products.

As a result of these developments, the seller's market transformed into a buyer's market. Once the consumer market began to be tapped, the highly elastic demand for many types of goods became evident. The prewar mentality had emphasized meeting consumer *needs* and assumed that a population could purchase only a finite amount of goods and services. With the increase in discretionary income and the introduction of consumer credit after World War II, consumers began to satisfy *wants*. Fledging marketers discovered they could not only influence consumers' decision-making processes but also *create* demand for certain goods and services.

The emergence of marketing was aided and abetted by changes in U.S. culture. The postwar period was marked by a growing emphasis on consumption and acquisition. The frugality of the Depression era gave way to a degree of materialism that shocked older generations. The availability of consumer credit and a mind-set that emphasized "keeping up with the Joneses" generated demand for a growing range of goods and services. America had given rise to the first generation of citizens with a consumer mentality.

By the 1970s, there was a growing emphasis on self-actualization in American culture, which many observers felt was often carried to the point of narcissism. This development called for additional goods and services and even created a fledgling market for consumer health services (e.g., psychotherapy and cosmetic surgery). A growing consumer market with expanding needs, coupled with a proliferation of products, created a fertile field for marketing activity.

Underlying these developments was the growing emphasis on change itself. As society continued to undergo major transformations, not only had change become accepted as inevitable, but it also began to take on a positive connotation. Newly empowered consumers demanded a growing array of goods and services. The future orientation emerging within U.S. society further underscored the importance of change in forging a path to a better future. People began changing jobs, residences, and even spouses at a rate unheard of to their forebears. The social and economic advancement of each generation over the previous became a maxim—a part of the American dream.

Phase Two: The Role of Sales

The second stage of marketing evolution focused on sales. Many U.S. producers had enjoyed regional monopolies (or at least oligopolies) since the dawn of the Industrial Age. Under these conditions, sales representatives took orders from what were essentially captive audiences. Marketing would have been considered an unnecessary expense under this scenario. However, as competition increased in most industries after World War II, these regional monopolies began to weaken.

The emphasis on sales that characterized the U.S. economy during the last third of the twentieth century continued to reflect the production aspects of society. Sales representatives eventually served as a bridge between the production economy and the service economy as they developed and maintained relationships. They progressed from their roles as "order takers" to become consultants to their clients, sending information from customers back to producers and facilitating the emergence of a market orientation in American business.

Phase Three: The Rise of the Customer

By the last third of the twentieth century, the industrial economy had given way to a service economy, and the remaining production industries became increasingly standardized. This shift from a product orientation to a service orientation was a sea change in relation to marketing. Service industries tend to be market driven, and American corporations began abandoning their father-knows-best mind-set in favor of a market orientation. For the first time, progressive managers in a wide range of industries sought to determine what consumers wanted and then strived to fulfill those needs. This shift opened the door to market research and to exploitation of consumer desires by professional marketers. The new market-driven firms adopted an outside-in way of thinking that viewed service delivery from the customer's point of view.

The emergence of a service economy had important implications for both marketing and healthcare. Services are distinguished from products because they are generally produced as they are consumed and cannot be stored or taken away. The marketing of services is different from the marketing of goods and thus challenging for marketers in any field. A new mind-set and new promotional approaches to the marketing of services had to be developed as the United States became a service-oriented economy.

Marketing in Healthcare

Healthcare did not adopt marketing approaches to any significant extent until the 1980s, although some healthcare organizations in the retail and supplier sectors had long employed marketing techniques to promote their products. Well after other industries had adopted marketing, these activities were still uncommon among organizations involved in patient care.

Nevertheless, some precursors to marketing were well established in the industry. Every hospital and many other healthcare organizations had long-standing public relations functions that disseminated information about the organization and announced new developments (e.g., new staff, equipment purchases). The public relations staff worked mainly with the media—disseminating press releases, responding to requests for information, and dealing with the press when a negative event occurred.

Most large provider organizations also had communications functions (often under the auspices of the public relations department). Communications staff would develop materials to disseminate to the public and to the employees of the organization, such as internal (and, later, patient-oriented) newsletters and patient education materials.

Some of the larger healthcare organizations also established government relations offices. Government relations staff was responsible for tracking regulatory and legislative activities that might affect the organization, served as an interface with government officials, and acted as lobbyists when necessary. Government relations offices frequently became involved in addressing the requirements of regulatory agencies.

Healthcare organizations of all types were involved in informal promotional activities to an extent. Hospitals sponsored health education seminars, held open houses at new facilities, or supported community events. Hospitals marketed themselves by making their facilities available to the community for public meetings and otherwise attempting to be good corporate citizens. Physicians marketed themselves through such activities as networking with colleagues at the country club, sending letters of appreciation to referring physicians, and providing services to high school athletic teams. See Exhibit 1.1 for a discussion of some of the pioneers of healthcare marketing.

EXHIBIT 1.1
Pioneers in Healthcare Marketing

Although the 1970s marked the formal emergence of marketing in the health services industry, few healthcare organizations—as organizations—had yet bought into marketing. For-profit hospital chains like Columbia and HCA may have had more of a marketing orientation, and Evanston (Indiana) Hospital had a vice president of marketing in 1976. However, many observers of the field would cite the publication of Philip Kotler's *Marketing for Nonprofit Organizations* (1975) as the event that legitimized marketing in the not-for-profit healthcare sector.

The emergence of marketing in healthcare was not driven at the corporate level, however. Ultimately, it came down to a handful of assertive and creative people who took the initiative and, often against great odds, established marketing programs. True, organizations like the Mayo Clinic and Cleveland Clinic developed permanent marketing programs, but the inroads marketing made were a result of the tenacity of a handful of true believers. A few practitioners were instrumental in developing marketing at their institutions, but few marketing initiatives were able to survive once they lost their "champion."

To the extent that marketing was incorporated into healthcare in the 1970s and 1980s, it was a result of the hard work of people like Kent Seltman at the Mayo Clinic and William Gombeski at Cleveland Clinic rather than any commitment on the part of their organizations. Seltman entered the healthcare field in 1984 when marketing was in its infancy. He began his career in marketing in Florida—where the hospital marketing department was thought of in the same category as the maintenance department at that time—and went on to develop innovative marketing programs at Loma Linda University Medical Center and the Mayo Clinic. Gombeski guided the early development of marketing initiatives at Cleveland Clinic and established that organization as a textbook example of successful marketing.

Other pioneers included Ann Fyfe and Judith S. Neiman, who often carried the marketing banner in the face of strong resistance. Fyfe served as a top marketing and strategy administrator for several healthcare systems and, later, as an executive with a healthcare Internet consulting firm. She served as a board member of the American Marketing Association and helped the American Marketing Association

(continued)

EXHIBIT 1.1 (*continued*)

form a healthcare section, the Academy of Health Services Marketing. Among marketing practitioners were pioneers like Dan Beckham, who played an early role in establishing organizations for healthcare marketing professionals.

Neiman served as the executive director of the Society for Healthcare Strategy and Market Development of the American Hospital Association (AHA), the director of AHA's Division of Strategic Planning and Marketing, and the program director of the nationally recognized Foster G. McGaw Prize for excellence in hospital community service.

Scott MacStravic's pioneering marketing activities can be traced to the mid-1970s, and his 1977 book on healthcare marketing, *Marketing Health Care*, is considered the first of its kind. MacStravic served as a marketing executive for hospitals and health systems all over the country and pioneered some of the early healthcare marketing initiatives. He served as an officer in various professional organizations for healthcare marketers and strategists and helped establish healthcare marketing as a separate profession.

In the academic arena, Eric Berkowitz, a long-time professor of marketing at the University of Massachusetts, built on the early work of Philip Kotler. Berkowitz helped establish healthcare marketing as a legitimate component of academic marketing through numerous books and articles on the topic. Other academics who contributed to the establishment of healthcare marketing were Steven W. Brown, who contributed numerous publications in the 1980s, and Roberta Clark, who collaborated with Philip Kotler in applying marketing principles to healthcare.

This brief discussion cannot include all of those who contributed to the development of healthcare marketing as a separate field, but it does pay tribute to a few of the pioneers who, often in the face of great odds, advanced the cause of healthcare marketing in its early days.

Stages of Healthcare Marketing

The stages through which marketing has evolved in the healthcare setting are outlined in the following section. Exhibit 1.2 summarizes the implications of this evolution on the hospital industry.

The 1950s

Although the 1950s are often viewed as the "age of marketing," marketing was not on the radar screen in healthcare until much later, even though

EXHIBIT 1.2
The Evolution of Marketing

Business Orientation	Manufacturer	Hospital
Production	Produce quality product	Deliver quality care
Sales	Generate volume	Fill hospital beds
Marketing	Satisfy needs/wants	Satisfy needs/wants

the emerging pharmaceutical industry was beginning to market to physicians and the fledging insurance industry was beginning to market health plans to consumers. In the healthcare trenches, healthcare providers were light-years away from formal marketing activities. Hospitals and physicians, for the most part, considered marketing (read: advertising) to be inappropriate and even unethical. This stance, however, did not preclude hospitals from offering free educational programs or implementing public relations campaigns, nor did it prevent physicians from cozying up to potential referring physicians and networking with colleagues at the country club. At the time, these activities were not considered marketing.

As the hospital industry came of age and many new facilities were established, the industry continued to reflect the production orientation that was by then waning throughout the rest of the U.S. economy. The demand for physician and hospital services was considered inelastic, and little attention was paid to the characteristics of either current patients or prospective customers. The emphasis was on providing quality care, and most providers held monopolies or oligopolies that shielded them from competition in their markets.

The 1960s

As the health services sector expanded during the 1960s, the role of public relations was enhanced. Although the developments that would force hospitals and other healthcare organizations to embrace marketing were at least a decade away, the public relations field was flourishing. This relatively basic marketing function was the healthcare organization's primary means of keeping in touch with its various publics.

The publics of this period were primarily the physicians who admitted or referred patients to healthcare facilities and the donors who made charitable contributions to the organization. Consumers were not considered an important constituency because they did not directly choose hospitals but were referred by their physicians. The use of media to advance strategic marketing objectives had not evolved, and media relations in this era often consisted of answering reporters' questions about patients' conditions.

Print was the medium of choice for communications throughout the 1960s, despite the increasingly influential role the electronic media were playing for marketers in other industries. This era was marked by polished annual reports, informational brochures, and publications targeted to the community. Healthcare communications became a well-developed function, and hospitals continued to expand the role of public relations.

Some segments of the healthcare industry not involved in patient care entered the sales stage during this decade. For example, pharmaceutical companies and insurance plans established sales forces to promote their drugs to physicians and market insurance plans to employers and individuals, respectively.

The 1970s

During the 1970s, urgency began to grow among hospitals with regard to promoting their services within the community. The desire for greater market presence was reinforced by the growing conviction that, in the future, healthcare organizations were going to have to be able to attract patients. Many organizations expanded their public relations functions to include a broader marketing mandate. These types of activities appeared to be particularly common in parts of the country where health maintenance organizations (HMOs) were emerging.

The for-profit hospital sector also grew in importance during the 1970s. With few limits on reimbursement, both nonprofit and for-profit hospitals expanded their services. Continued high demand for health services and the stable payment system created by Medicare made the industry attractive to investor-owned companies. Numerous national for-profit hospital and nursing home chains emerged during this period.

Some early attempts at advertising health services were made, and interest in marketing research was beginning to emerge. Marketing by the healthcare establishment was officially recognized in a conference on the topic during the mid-1970s, sponsored by AHA. The marketing movement in healthcare was given impetus by rulings that relaxed restrictions on advertising on the part of healthcare providers. (More on these restrictions appears later in the chapter.)

For hospitals, the sales era began in the mid-1970s with the changes that occurred in reimbursement. Under cost-based reimbursement (e.g., Medicare), competition with other hospitals had not been a major concern. Hospitals had ample patients, and occupancy rates were high. The top priority was to attract as many customers as possible by enticing physicians to admit their patients. To this end, hospitals developed physician relations programs and offered other enticements to encourage physician loyalty.

When hospitals recognized that patients might play a role in the hospital selection decision, a second strategy for selling to the public emerged. In the mid-1970s, some hospitals adopted mass advertising strategies to promote their programs, including billboard displays and television and radio commercials touting a particular service. The goal of the marketer was to convince prospective patients to use his hospital when presented with a choice between competing hospitals.

Marketing as we know it today still had not taken root in hospitals by the end of the decade. Competition for patients was increasing, and hospitals and other providers turned to the familiar function of public relations for their promotional efforts. Communication efforts were beginning to be targeted toward patients, and patient satisfaction research grew in importance. Even so, most healthcare organizations did not recognize marketing in the sense of managing the flow of services between an organization and its customers. See Exhibit 1.3 for a chronology of the development of healthcare marketing.

The 1980s

If healthcare marketing was born in the 1970s, it came of age in the 1980s. The healthcare industry had evolved from a seller's market to a buyer's market, a change that was to have a profound effect on the marketing of health services. Employers and consumers had become purchasers of healthcare, and the physician's role in referring patients for hospital services was beginning to diminish. The hospital industry continued to grow during the 1980s as centrally managed health systems (both for-profit and not-for-profit) expanded during this period. National chains of hospitals, nursing homes, and home health agencies were emerging—another development that had a profound effect on marketing.

Marketers had to begin looking at target audiences in an entirely different way, and the importance of consumers was heightened by changes in insurance reimbursement patterns. Hospitals began to think of medical care in terms of product or service lines, a development that had major consequences for the marketing of health services. Hospitals realized that marketing directly to consumers for such services as obstetrics, cosmetic surgery, and outpatient care could generate revenue and enhance market share.

Although marketing was beginning to be accepted in healthcare, the industry suffered from a lack of professional marketing personnel. Few marketers had experience with healthcare, and attempts at importing marketing techniques from other industries were generally unsuccessful. Many healthcare administrators still saw marketing as an expensive gimmick and considered marketers to be outsiders with no place in healthcare.

The rise of service-line marketing launched the great hospital advertising wars of the 1980s. Barely a blip on the healthcare marketing radar screen

EXHIBIT 1.3
Healthcare Marketing Timeline

	1950	1960	1970	1980	1990	2000	2010
Stage:	Premarketing ——————————→			Introduction ——→	Growth ——→	Maturity	
Primary techniques:	Public relations Communication	Government relations		Advertising Marketing research Direct marketing Personal sales	Direct-to-consumer Relationship marketing Social marketing Internet marketing		Social media
Main theme:	Publicity Information management	Regulatory influence Consumer research		Sales Technology applications	Relationship management	Consumer engagement	
Marketing target:*	General public	Government agencies Health plans		Physicians Employers	Referral agents Businesses	Consumers Market segments	

*Patient care organizations

a decade earlier, advertising grew dramatically during this decade. In 1983, hospitals spent $50 million on advertising; by 1986, that figure had risen to $500 million, a tenfold increase in three years (Bashe and Hicks 2000). Once a medium of dubious respectability, advertising was now hailed as a marketing panacea for hospitals.

A growing number of health professionals who suddenly found themselves in competition for patients came to see marketing as a key to competitive success. This perception brought about a surge in advertising activity on the part of large healthcare organizations. Unfortunately, much of the advertising of the mid- to late 1980s was ineffectual at best and disastrous at worst. Many campaigns were poorly conceived and wasted an enormous amount of money. Ad copy tended to be institutionally focused, and healthcare marketing initiatives lacked the impact of the advertising produced in other industries, in large part because of the conservative, risk-averse culture of hospitals.

Advertising came to be the activity that epitomized marketing for many in healthcare during this period. Marketers themselves perpetuated this notion, and even today, many healthcare executives equate marketing with advertising. Ultimately, the surge in advertising was both a blessing and a curse. On the one hand, advertising campaigns were something relatively concrete; an organization could invest in them and reasonably expect to incur some benefit as a result. On the other hand, the ineffectiveness of much healthcare advertising and the negative fallout it often generated were setbacks for the proponents of healthcare marketing. After experiencing the initial rush of seeing their billboards and television commercials, hospital administrators began to question the expense and, more important, the effectiveness of the marketing initiatives they were funding.

Healthcare organizations faced serious financial retrenchment during the 1980s. Hospitals were looking for cuts wherever they could find them, and marketing expenditures were easy targets. Budgets were cut and marketing staff were laid off. Although the marketing function was not entirely eliminated, it was often incorporated under the umbrella of business development or strategic planning. In many organizations, marketing was squeezed out of the budget and kept alive by just a few dedicated marketing professionals. In some healthcare organizations, marketing disappeared as a corporate function and was never reinstated. On the positive side, this retrenchment allowed healthcare marketers to reassess the field and concentrate on developing baseline data that could be used when a marketing revival occurred.

Consumer research in healthcare came into its own during this decade. Most hospitals had conducted patient satisfaction research for some time, but consumer research was virtually unknown until the 1970s. By the mid-1980s, a majority of hospitals were conducting physician and consumer research.

The latter was crucial in developing advertising messages and monitoring the success of marketing programs.

The 1990s

Healthcare became more market driven in the 1990s, and the marketing function grew in importance in healthcare organizations. The institutional perspective that had long driven decision making gave way to market-driven decision making. Every hospital was trying to win the hearts and minds of healthcare consumers.

Advertising on the part of healthcare organizations resurged during the mid-1990s, spurred by the massive wave of hospital mergers. The consolidation of healthcare organizations into ever-larger systems resulted in the creation of larger organizations with expanded resources and more sophisticated management. Many executives entered the field from outside of healthcare, bringing a more businesslike atmosphere with them.

The consumer was rediscovered during this process, and the direct-to-consumer movement was initiated. The popularity of guest relations programs during the 1990s solidified the transformation of patients into customers. As consumers gained influence, marketing became increasingly integrated into the operations of healthcare organizations. The consumers of the 1990s were better educated and more assertive about their healthcare needs than were consumers of the previous generation. The emergence of the Internet as a source of health information further contributed to the rise of consumerism. Newly empowered consumers were taking on an increasingly influential (if informal) role in reshaping the U.S. healthcare system.

A more qualified corps of marketing professionals emerged who brought ambitious but realistic expectations to the industry. Pharmaceutical companies began advertising directly to consumers, which made everyone in the industry more aware of marketing's potential. In addition, everyone in healthcare was becoming more consumer sensitive, and new data gave healthcare professionals a better understanding of the healthcare customer.

Marketing research grew in importance during this decade. The need for information on consumers, customers, competitors, and the market demanded an expanded research function. Patient and consumer research was augmented, and newly developed technologies brought the research capabilities of other industries to healthcare.

Business practices in general came to be more accepted in healthcare during this period, and marketing was an inevitable beneficiary. Marketing was repackaged in a more professional guise, and the shift away from advertising was noticeable. Marketing ended the decade as a more mature discipline, emphasizing market research and sensitivity to the needs of the consumer. Healthcare had finally reached the third stage in the evolution

EXHIBIT 1.4
Average Hospital Marketing Budgets and
Staffing by Hospital Size, 2007

	Bed Size				
	All	<101	101–200	201–400	401+
Marketing budget (000s)	$1,194	$431	$802	$1,655	$2,788
Staff size	4.9	2.4	3.2	5.7	10.0

Source: Society for Healthcare Strategy and Market Development (2008).

of the marketing function. (Exhibit 1.4 presents recent statistics on hospital marketing expenditures and budgets.)

By the end of the twentieth century, healthcare marketing had changed substantially. In the 1990s, the emphasis shifted from sick people to well people in response to the emergence of managed care and capitated payments. There was a new focus on patient satisfaction and increased efforts at generating consumer data. The baby boomers who were coming to dominate the healthcare landscape viewed marketing as a source of valuable information rather than hucksterism and were disinclined to use an organization that did not cater to their interests.

Image advertising was deemphasized in favor of targeted promotions for specific services, making for more content and less fluff. Techniques from other industries, like customer relationship marketing, began to be explored. The new generation of healthcare administrators seemed to be more comfortable with marketing and considered this function an inherent aspect of healthcare operations.

With the repackaging and maturation of marketing in the 1990s, the field became more sophisticated overall. The market was in many ways more competitive, and even the managed care environment held opportunities for promotional activities. In addition, mergers not only created more potential marketing clout but often involved for-profit healthcare organizations that were inherently more marketing oriented.

Healthcare Marketing's Next Phase

By the end of the 1990s, a new cohort of healthcare administrators had begun exhibiting a greater acceptance of business practices, including marketing. The industry had witnessed a massive turnover in hospital administrators, through retirement, mergers, and downsizing. Many of the new wave of administrators came from other, often more profit-oriented, industries where marketing was considered a normal corporate function. These administrators instilled a marketing mind-set in keeping with the more strategic orientation they brought to the industry.

Although some still focus primarily on advertising and sales, marketing executives today are expanding their toolbox with a renewed emphasis on research, measurement, planning, analysis, forecasting, targeting, segmentation, and strategy. Reliable and effective public, media, and community relations, customer service, and reputation and relationship management are making a comeback, demonstrating the effectiveness of carefully designed low-cost methods in reaching audiences and swaying public opinion.

Why Healthcare Is Different from Other Industries

Healthcare as an industry is set apart from the other sectors of the economy because of its unique characteristics. In particular, healthcare providers behave in a manner often inconsistent with that of organizations in other industries. Health professionals, especially clinicians, fall into a special category, and the fact that clinicians—not administrators or businesspeople—make most of the decisions with regard to patient care creates a dynamic unique to healthcare. The nature of healthcare goods and services sets them apart from the goods and services offered in other industries. Further, significant differences exist between healthcare consumers and the consumers of virtually any other good or service. These differences are particularly apparent with regard to the consumer decision-making process. The factors that make healthcare different are discussed in the following sections.

The Healthcare Industry

The development of a marketing culture in any industry is predicated on certain assumptions about that industry and the marketing enterprise, including the existence of a rational market for the goods and services proffered by the organizations in that industry. The market is presumed to involve organized groups of sellers, informed buyers, an orderly mechanism for carrying out transactions between sellers and buyers, and a straightforward process for transferring payment for products between buyers and sellers.

The existence of a true healthcare market in an economic sense has been much debated. In addition to involving the elements named in the previous paragraph, markets operate under the assumption that consumers have adequate, if not perfect, knowledge about the available goods and services, that a rational system of pricing exists, and that the laws of supply and demand apply.

Further, the existence of a market is predicated on assumptions about the motives and activities of buyers and sellers in the market. For example, the assumption that buyers are driven primarily, if not exclusively, by economic motives does not fit well with what is known about the behavior of healthcare consumers. Another assumption from economic theory, that buyers seek to maximize their benefits from the exchange, is also an uncomfortable fit. In healthcare a number of factors operate to prevent the buyers and sellers of health services from interacting in the same manner as buyers and sellers in other industries.

The existence of a market also presumes that there are sellers competing for the consumer's resources and that this competition determines the price of the goods and services offered. In healthcare, however, providers commonly maintain monopolies over particular services in particular markets. Even more common is domination of certain markets by oligopolies of healthcare organizations. Thus, buyers of health services are often limited in their choice of medical personnel or facilities.

In view of these prerequisites for the existence of a market, one could argue that, to the extent that any type of market for health services exists, it is not "rational" in the way that the markets for other goods and services are.

As an industry, healthcare also differs from other sectors of the economy in terms of the diverse goals of its key organizations. The packaged goods industry, for example, has the unitary goal of producing, marketing, and distributing products directly to consumers. The goals are straightforward whether the product is detergent, cereal, or office supplies. The intent is to sell as many units as possible while extracting the maximum profit from the transactions. While these industries provide employment for their employees, profits for their shareholders, and benefits to their communities, these activities are secondary to their single-minded goal of selling consumer products.

In other industries, potential buyers who do not have the ability to pay or who, for some other reason, are considered to be undesirable customers can be refused service. Most healthcare organizations, on the other hand, are obligated to accept clients whether or not they can pay for the services and whether or not they are deemed desirable customers. Hospitals are bound by law in most cases to accept patients regardless of their ability to pay. Although providers may have some discretion in accepting patients with stable, routine conditions, emergency departments cannot turn away any patient needing emergency care until the patient has at least been stabilized. Physician offices may require some payment up front from patients who do not have insurance, but there are ethical considerations associated with turning a clearly symptomatic patient away.

This situation means healthcare organizations often provide services that are not profitable. In some cases, this reflects the fact that certain services (e.g., emergency departments at hospitals) may be legally mandated or otherwise controlled through regulation; in others, it reflects the fact that hospitals and, to a lesser degree, physicians must offer the comprehensive services the community requires if they are to remain competitive. Thus, the economic considerations that apply to other industries may be compromised as a result of factors unique to healthcare.

The healthcare industry also tends to be much less organized than other industries in the United States. Often referred to as a "nonsystem," healthcare lacks the coordination and centralized (albeit often informal) systems of control found in other industries. Even industries characterized by cutthroat competition typically have a central clearinghouse of industry data and mechanisms for cooperating for the benefit of the industry overall. In contrast, the healthcare industry is characterized by fragmentation, discontinuity, and a lack of coordination. It is also characterized by a dismaying lack of information on the industry and its key players. As a result, healthcare lacks the organization that is typically characteristic of an established market.

Also unlike other industries, healthcare lacks a straightforward means of financing the purchase of goods and services, particularly patient care services. Consumers in other industries typically pay directly for the goods and services they consume, either out of pocket or through some form of credit. While healthcare consumers may pay some small portion of the cost out of pocket, most fees are paid by a third party, whether a private insurance plan or a government-sponsored plan such as Medicare or Medicaid. The seller may have to deal with thousands of different insurance plans, and the cost of health services is reimbursed using a combination of different payment mechanisms. Thus, it would not be unusual for an elderly patient to have the costs of one hospital visit paid for with Medicare reimbursement, supplementary private insurance reimbursement, and out-of-pocket payments. This arrangement is not found in any other industry and creates a more complicated financial picture for healthcare.

Finally, healthcare is different from other industries in that the normal rules of supply and demand seldom apply. An increase in the supply of health services, for example, does not necessarily result in a decrease in prices, nor does increased demand invariably drive up prices. For one thing, the availability (supply) of services dictates, to a certain extent, the demand for these services. In fact, the historical maxim was: "A bed built is a bed filled." Pent-up demand for health services often surfaces when more facilities become available. As a result, neither the increased supply of beds nor the increase in demand has a significant impact on prices.

The factors that govern supply, demand, and price in healthcare are complex and unique to this industry. The supply of health services is affected by the vagaries of health professional training programs, restrictions enforced by regulatory agencies, and even fads. The level of demand, arguably the most problematic of the three, is typically not controlled by the end user. Except for elective procedures for which the consumer pays out of pocket, most decisions that affect the demand for health services are made by gatekeepers, such as physicians and health plans. Thus, the level of demand is more often a function of such factors as insurance plan provisions, the availability of resources, and physician practice patterns than it is a function of the level of sickness in the population.

Healthcare Organizations

Healthcare organizations have a number of characteristics that set them apart from the service providers in other industries. Many healthcare organizations (particularly hospitals) still linger in the production stage of their evolution. Such organizations may contend that their goal is to provide high-quality medical care. By providing state-of-the-art technology and the physicians, nurses, and allied health personnel to support it, they believe they will be able to attract customers.

As with the early industrialists, many healthcare organizations once maintained oligopolistic or even monopolistic control over their markets. Because of their dominance in the market and/or arrangements with competitors, health services providers were often able to ensure a steady flow of patients without having to solicit them. Today, however, few organizations can command that type of loyalty. Nearly all healthcare organizations face some serious competition, and innovations like telemedicine have broadened the scope of would-be competitors.

Healthcare organizations tend to be multipurpose organizations. Although some purveyors of healthcare goods or services are single-minded in their intent, large healthcare organizations like hospitals are likely to pursue a number of goals simultaneously. Indeed, the main goal of an academic medical center may not be to provide patient care at all. It may be education, research, or community service, with direct patient care as a secondary concern. Even large specialty practices are likely to be involved in teaching and research, and although they are not likely to neglect their core activity, they often have a more diffuse orientation than organizations in other industries.

Not-for-profit organizations have historically played a major role in healthcare, and even today, not-for-profits continue to control a large share of the hospital bed inventory. Although physician groups are usually incorporated as for-profit professional corporations, many community-based clinics, faith-based clinics, and government-supported programs operate on a nonprofit basis. This "charitable" orientation creates an environment that differs from that of other industries. The financial support that the government provides to some health facilities and programs also creates a different dynamic. For some organizations, the unpredictability of government subsidy is an unsettling factor. For others, the assurance of government support means they may not be as vulnerable to the vagaries of the market.

Another factor that sets healthcare organizations apart from their counterparts in other industries is the emphasis on referral relationships. Hospitals depend on admissions from their medical staffs, and staff members in turn depend on referrals from other physicians. Indeed, except in emergency situations, patients can gain hospital admission only through a physician referral. Many specialists will not accept self-referred patients at their clinics; rather, they rely on other physicians to refer patients to them. The same types of referral relationships exist with regard to other services (e.g., home health care, nursing homes).

This situation has become more complicated because health plans may also exert some level of influence over the referral process. Not only do health plans determine which healthcare providers can be used under a particular coverage plan; they may also attempt to control the referral process. In no other industry do parties who are not the end users exert such an influence on the process. Exhibit 1.5 discusses the importance of referral relationships.

EXHIBIT 1.5
The Importance of Referral Relationships

Healthcare is distinguished from other industries in terms of its reliance on referral relationships. "Referral relationships" is used here in the broad sense of any mechanism that exists for a third party to steer consumers into the distribution channels of a healthcare organization or for an intermediary to promote goods and services to healthcare consumers. The importance of such relationships in healthcare is reflected by the fact that the end users of health services frequently do not make consumption decisions themselves. The purchase decision may be made by a physician, a health plan, or some party other than the actual patient. In these cases a marketer is more likely to target physicians, provider networks, health plans, and other gatekeepers who might influence the referral process, rather than the end user.

The end user is targeted in some healthcare situations, but referral relationships account for the bulk of healthcare encounters. The most entrenched example of this is the situation wherein a physician referral is required for hospital admission. Patients cannot present themselves directly to a hospital for admission; they must have an admitting physician. Even emergency cases require a physician to take responsibility before a patient will be admitted to the hospital. If a physician does not have admitting privileges at a particular hospital, he or she cannot admit a patient there or treat patients hospitalized by other physicians.

Other institutions, such as nursing homes and hospices, may also depend on referrals from physicians or other referral agents.

Physicians often depend on referrals from other physicians and, in some cases, health or social service agencies for their patient volume. Medical and surgical specialists, for example, may be unwilling to accept a patient without a referral from another physician. With most contemporary health insurance arrangements, a referral from a primary care physician to a specialist is required before the insurer will cover the treatment episode. Nonphysician providers, such as psychologists, optometrists, and chiropractors, may make referrals to psychiatrists, ophthalmologists, and neurosurgeons, respectively, if the treatment requirements exceed their capabilities. Mental health centers and social service agencies may be major sources of patients for some specialists, as these agencies represent the front line of contact with many potential patients.

Prescription drugs are becoming an increasingly important aspect of patient care, and this area also involves indirect access to the end user. A patient must have a prescription written by a physician to obtain a drug from a pharmacist, and numerous safeguards are in place to prevent unauthorized access to prescription drugs. Pharmaceutical companies rely on physicians to recommend their drugs.

A final example of the referral process involves the way health insurance plans steer patients. Typically, a health plan will have an arrangement with a network of providers, and the plan enrollee will be channeled to one of these providers rather than an out-of-network provider. Thus, the choice of physician, hospital, home health agency, and other provider is likely to be essentially outside the control of the end user. In these cases, it is more important for the provider to develop relationships with various health plans than it is to market directly to patients.

The importance of referrals in healthcare is further emphasized by the sources of information on health services that consumers use. When asked how they selected a particular provider, patients usually report that they based their decision on the recommendations of friends, relatives, or associates; the recommendations of a physician or other clinician; or a referral through their health plan. Whether the referral was informal or formal, it is obvious that many parties other than the patient play a part in determining where the patient ultimately ends up for care. For this reason, the marketing of health services (and, to a certain extent, healthcare goods) is more often directed toward referral agents, intermediaries, and gatekeepers than it is to the ultimate end user.

Healthcare Products

The goods and services that constitute healthcare products are also unique. Although many healthcare consumer goods (e.g., adhesive bandages, fitness equipment, and over-the-counter drugs) may be marketed like any other product, most healthcare products do not fall into this category. Even the most common consumer-oriented healthcare products—pharmaceuticals—must be prescribed by an intermediary before they can be acquired and consumed.

Healthcare providers are generally concerned with promoting a service, yet the nature of their services is difficult to describe. A physician might break down services by procedure code (e.g., CPT codes), but few services stand alone. Services come in bundles, such as the group of services that surrounds a surgical procedure. Although clinicians (and their billing clerks) may see them as discrete services, the patient perceives them as a complex mix of services related to a heart attack, diabetes management, or cancer treatment, for example.

As will be seen in the discussion of healthcare products in a later chapter, the products generated by a healthcare organization are difficult to conceptualize. The things providers think they provide (e.g., quality care, prolonged life, elimination of pathology) are often hard to define or measure. The difficulty in specifying the services provided becomes obvious when a marketer asks a hospital department head what services the department provides.

Healthcare products are also characterized by a lack of substitutability. A substitute is a good or service that can be used in place of another good or service. Although one form of transportation might be substituted for another, for example, a surgical procedure can seldom be substituted for another. Unlike other industries, healthcare often provides only one solution for a particular need.

Health Professionals

Historically, the healthcare industry has been dominated by professionals rather than by administrators. Clinical personnel (usually physicians, but other clinicians as well) define much of the demand for health services and are directly or indirectly responsible for most healthcare expenditures. This setup is comparable to the systems in other industries, in which technicians rather than administrators run the organization. The situation in healthcare is complicated by the fact that clinicians and administrators may not share the same goals.

The medical ethics that drive the behavior of health professionals exist independently of system operations. Clinicians are bound by oath to do what is medically appropriate, whether or not it is cost-effective or contributes to the organization's efficiency. Decisions made in the best interests of the patient may not reflect the best interests of the organization. Although health professionals have had to become more realistic with regard to indiscriminate use of resources, clinical interests continue to outweigh financial considerations in most cases. Conflict between the goals of clinicians and administrators is an inherent feature of the healthcare organization, and no comparable situation can be found in any other industry.

The conflict between the clinical and business sides of the healthcare operation is augmented by the antibusiness orientation of many health professionals. Most healthcare workers entered the field because they wanted to be in a profession, not a business, and physicians and other clinicians often have a distorted perception of the business world. If health professionals cannot appreciate the business side of the operation, they are not likely to appreciate the importance of marketing. Even among nonclinicians, many common business practices may be considered inappropriate for the not-for-profit healthcare world.

Healthcare Consumers

The term *consumers* refers to persons with the potential to consume a good or service. In other words, anyone who has a want or need for (and presumably the ability to pay for) a product could be considered a potential consumer. The good news for healthcare is that virtually everyone is a potential health services consumer. Everyone is likely to use healthcare goods or services at some time and be involved in the healthcare system. From this perspective, the entire U.S. population (approximately 300 million) is a market for some type of healthcare good or service. In contrast, many people in the United States do not own a lawnmower, a computer, or an automobile, and many people will never take a cruise vacation, hire an accountant, or attend a rock concert; large segments of the population are not potential customers for these goods and services.

Despite this unique attribute of healthcare consumers, healthcare organizations historically failed to perceive consumers in this manner. Until recently, the assumption was that a person was not a prospect for health services *until* he or she became sick. Thus, healthcare providers made no attempt in the past to develop relationships with non-patients. People were not considered paying customers until they presented themselves for treatment. Today, however, numerous parties cater to non-patients. Major industries have developed around prevention, fitness, and lifestyle management. Much of the social marketing that takes place in U.S. society is geared toward non-patients.

Most healthcare organizations' historical perception of consumers starkly contrasts with that of the consumer goods industries. Marketers of food products and household goods assume that there must be a need (or at least a want) they could exploit. Arguably, however, healthy people do not need health services. Wouldn't it be a waste of marketing resources to solicit business from people who don't need the goods or services? How do you convince someone to undergo heart surgery if he or she doesn't have a heart problem?

These questions reflect some misconceptions about healthcare that need to be addressed. First, there is a misconception about what constitutes health services. One immediately thinks of surgical procedures, trauma care, and other life-saving efforts—situations that usually occur unexpectedly, require an immediate response, and demand extensive resources on the part of the healthcare system.

Ultimately, however, many healthcare purchases are not made in response to a health *need* (and certainly not an urgent need) but in response to a *want*. The trendy areas of health services today make this behavior evident. Business is booming for cosmetic surgery, laser eye surgery, skin care, and medically supervised weight-loss programs. The conditions these procedures address are not life threatening or even medically necessary. The fact that few of these services are covered by standard insurance plans reflects their elective nature. Astute marketers recognize a want when they see one and realize that waiting until a need is discovered is not necessary.

Healthcare consumers are perhaps most distinguished from consumers of other goods and services by their insulation from the price of the products they consume. Because of healthcare's unusual financing arrangements and lack of access to pricing information, healthcare consumers seldom know the price of the services they are consuming until after they have consumed them. In typical cases, the physician or clinician providing the service is also not likely to know the price of the service being provided. Because third-party payers, not end users, usually pay for the service provided, healthcare consumers may not even notice how much their care costs.

As a result, clinicians are likely to provide or recommend the services they believe to be medically necessary, regardless of price. However, there are at least two problematic consequences of this situation. First, consumers are not likely to willingly limit resource utilization. If they do not know the amount of the fees being charged and, further, do not have to pay them anyway, there is no incentive to consider the cost. Similarly, there is no incentive for providers to provide services efficiently if cost is not a consideration. In fact, under traditional fee-for-service arrangements, the incentives available to physicians have actually encouraged greater use of resources in that physicians receive an additional fee for each additional service performed.

The second implication is that few healthcare providers are able to use price as a means of competition or as a basis for marketing. With the exception of organizations that provide elective services or serve a retail market, there is no way to compete on the basis of price. Few healthcare organizations make their fee schedules public, and even when they do, they are likely to employ varying mechanisms for determining the price of a service. For example, the per diem rates for a hospital room may be determined on the basis of different factors by two competing hospitals, thereby making comparisons meaningless.

Healthcare consumers not only are hampered by a lack of knowledge about the cost of care but lack knowledge on other issues as well. Few consumers know how the healthcare system operates or have direct experience with its delivery mechanisms. Consumers typically have no basis for evaluating the quality of services provided by health facilities or practitioners and thus no way of making meaningful distinctions. Consumers must make judgments on the basis of the provider's reputation or on superficial factors, such as the appearance of the facility, the available amenities, and the tastiness of the hospital's food. In turn, the marketer struggles to find a basis for differentiation.

Another factor setting healthcare consumers apart from other consumers is the personal nature of the services involved. Most healthcare encounters involve an emotional component that is absent in other consumer transactions. Every diagnostic test is fraught with the possibility of a "positive" finding, and every surgery, no matter how minor, carries the potential for complications. Today's well-informed consumers are aware of the severity of medical errors made during the provision of hospital care and the rate of system-induced morbidity associated with healthcare settings. Even if people can remain stoic with regard to their own care, they are likely to exhibit an emotional dimension when the care concerns a parent, a child, or some other loved one. Whether this emotionally charged, personal aspect of the healthcare episode prevents the affected individual from seeking care, colors the choice of provider or therapy, or leads to additional symptoms, the choices made by the patient or other decision makers are likely to be affected. The fact that many consumers cannot bring themselves to even say the word *cancer* demonstrates this influence, and emotions like fear, pride, and vanity often come into play.

Why No Healthcare Marketing?

Given the pervasiveness of marketing in the United States, how can one explain the relative lack of marketing in an industry that accounts for 15 percent of the gross national product? The following sections discuss some of the barriers that have slowed the acceptance of marketing in the healthcare arena.

No (Real or Perceived) Need

Until the 1980s, most healthcare organizations thought they had no competitors. They had plenty of patients, and revenues were essentially guaranteed by third-party payers. Competition had been minimized through unwritten agreements among various healthcare providers. If providers did not overtly collude among themselves to carve up the patient market, they respected informal boundaries that were set to reduce competition. They often maintained monopolies or oligopolies in their market areas and evinced a product orientation. Even today, many providers remain at the production stage of their development, expecting patients to seek them out because of the services they provide, whether they market them or not.

These factors contributed to the perception (and, in many cases, the reality) that marketing was an unnecessary activity for healthcare organizations. From the perspective of mainstream providers, physicians referred their patients to the hospital and insurance plans steered their enrollees to the facility. Why market to end users who were not going to make the decision anyway? This mind-set perpetuated the impression that marketing was not needed and overlooked such important marketing tasks as physician relationship development and health plan contract negotiation.

No Knowledge of Marketing

In the past, few healthcare administrators were schooled in the business aspects of healthcare, and fewer still had training in or experience with marketing. Many senior healthcare administrators were not exposed to marketing courses during their training, and those entering the field before 1980 were unlikely to have any exposure to healthcare marketing.

Even if a healthcare administrator had some interest in marketing, there were, until recently, few sources of information related to the topic. In contrast to the wealth of information on marketing in other fields, few texts have been written on the topic of healthcare marketing, and a limited number of models could be held up for emulation. Few administrators were inclined to develop an initiative from scratch, and, as a result, few took the initiative to become knowledgeable about the topic.

Resistance to Business Aspects of Healthcare

Much of the resistance to marketing reflected misconceptions about the nature of business and marketing. For health professionals, business practices carried an unfavorable connotation that implied the subjugation of clinical concerns to business needs. A similar misperception existed with regard to the nature of marketing. "Marketing equals advertising" was the dominant perception early in the history of healthcare marketing, and even today, many health professionals retain that narrow (and negative) perception of marketing. The concern over contaminating a helping profession with business principles led to the enactment of various provisions against advertising on the part of healthcare organizations. (Case Study 1.1 describes how a hospital departed from its core philosophy to pursue a business opportunity.)

CASE STUDY 1.1
An Early Attempt at Healthcare Marketing

In the late 1970s, healthcare providers rarely discussed marketing. Indeed, early pioneers in the field of healthcare marketing were just emerging. Ann Fyfe was an aggressive 28-year-old owner of a small advertising agency in Colorado. Her clients included a western clothing manufacturer, an irrigation system company, and an international food distributor. Fyfe subscribed to Philip Kotler's marketing formula based on the four Ps: product, price, promotion, and place. This approach had worked pretty well for her; once she figured out who the customers were, what they wanted, and all the mechanics of how to get the message to them, she could pretty much count on positive results.

In 1978, Fyfe was enticed by a visionary chief executive officer (CEO) at a major hospital in San Francisco to bring her marketing formula and suitcase of implementation strategies to a hospital setting. Fyfe jumped at the opportunity to bring what appeared to be a virtually bulletproof system for generating revenue into a field that seemed to be rich with possibility and amazingly untouched by the whole notion of marketing. Hospitals weren't convinced that they had "customers." Health food stores may have customers, it was argued, but doctors had patients.

At that time, hospitals were still being reimbursed for providing whatever services a doctor said a patient needed. However, margins were tight, and many consumers were turning to innovative nonhospital sources of care for their healthcare needs. The combination of a perceived need and ample resources appeared to be a perfect opportunity for an enterprising marketer.

Fyfe and her colleagues rolled up their sleeves and got to work. They surveyed consumers using both qualitative and quantitative methods. They found out what consumers wanted and what approaches they would respond to. They designed innovative programs built around customer-friendly products, including an executive physicals program called "Vital," an urgent care center in the hospital called "CliniCare," and one of the first sports medicine programs in the nation.

In the area of promotions, no expense was spared. A sales force was established and a major ad agency was engaged to develop clever collateral materials and radio spots. They used direct mail and radio for public service announcements and paid advertising. They also

(continued)

CASE STUDY 1.1 (*continued*)

implemented a full program of community services, from dinners for seniors to wellness programs at health clubs to educational seminars. The marketing initiative was so impressive that it boasted Charles Schwab as the chair of the board's marketing committee and was considered newsworthy enough to be featured on the *Today Show*.

All of their innovative programs had very respectable returns on investment, despite (or maybe because of) the fact that they spared no expense on promotions. Corporations were eager to offer a suite of health services to their executives, consumers loved the urgent care clinic, and sports medicine boomed along with the wellness craze of the 1970s.

Despite the apparent success of the hospital's aggressive marketing program, the process soon experienced an ironic twist. Within two years of pulling off this marketing miracle, one which nearly every other hospital in the country was eager to copy, Ann Fyfe and the hospital's CEO were summarily fired by the physician-dominated hospital board.

As a fledging healthcare marketer, Fyfe had not heard anything about physicians. She was busy listening to customers, and they loved what the hospital was doing. However, the medical staff was an entirely different type of hospital customer. To some physicians, the hospital represented direct competition, in that physicals and urgent care patients were being diverted away from their practices. For most staff doctors, however, it was a more visceral reaction: This slick marketing approach felt sleazy, commercial, and inappropriate, and the culture of medicine was simply not ready for it.

Meanwhile, of course, hospitals everywhere were lining up to learn how to replicate this organization's success. In response to overwhelming demand, Fyfe helped the American Marketing Association form a healthcare section. She also formed and became president of the Northern California Health Care Marketing Association. Fyfe received one of the first *Modern Healthcare* "Up and Comer" awards and was presented with a cash prize by the HealthCare Forum for her article on CliniCare. (Unfortunately, a hospital CEO in the audience at the award ceremony actually stood up and reminded Fyfe's enthusiastic fan club that her activities had managed to get her CEO fired.)

Fyfe is still active in her field and believes she has helped shape a profession and contributed to a more mature approach to healthcare marketing. Over time her contributions have made healthcare organizations smarter about their business decisions, more cautious about advertising, and more sensitive to the needs of their customers. And the experience has made Fyfe smarter, too. Today, she works closely with her primary strategic partner in the marketing enterprise—the physician.

Discussion Questions

- Why did the healthcare environment of the 1970s appear attractive to energetic young marketing professionals?
- What were some of the innovative programs introduced during this period?
- What forms of marketing were used to promote hospitals' services?
- What unintended consequence developed as a result of marketing, and what fallout ensued?

Concern over Marketing Costs

Concerns related to the cost of marketing also played a role in the slow incorporation of marketing practices by healthcare organizations. Marketing (again, primarily advertising) was seen as an expensive proposition. While more commercial operations like pharmaceutical companies saw marketing expenses as a normal cost of doing business, hospitals and physicians with no previous experience in this regard suffered sticker shock at the marketing price tag. This lack of experience with marketing also caused them to overlook numerous aspects of marketing that involved little or no expense.

There was—and still is—concern in healthcare over the return on investment that marketing can generate. Most industries have well-developed mechanisms for measuring the return on their marketing investments, but healthcare does not. Healthcare organizations are seldom able to measure the cost of providing a service, making cost-benefit analyses difficult to perform. Further, so many factors come into play (e.g., referral patterns, consumer attitudes) in determining the use of services that it is hard to isolate the impact of marketing activities.

Given a chronic shortage of resources, many health professionals question the appropriateness of expending scarce resources on an activity perceived to have limited benefit. These concerns have been reinforced by disgruntled patients who linked their high hospital bills to excessive spending on expensive advertising. Even if the spending does not affect the patient's bill, the negative fallout from highly visible marketing efforts could affect the public image of many healthcare organizations.

Unlike other industries, healthcare has viewed marketing as an expense—not an investment. Health professionals' lack of knowledge about marketing—and its potential impact—has led them to consider marketing as, at best, a necessary evil. Further, there is widespread concern that marketing can do little to alter practice patterns, market shares, or any other indicator of importance to the provider.

Ethical and Legal Constraints

Ethical and legal constraints have also posed a major barrier to the incorporation of marketing into healthcare. The nature of health-related goods and services has made them the target of restrictions not found in other industries. As stated earlier, until recent years, it was considered unethical for physicians and many other clinicians to advertise. Although other types of marketing were generally accepted, overt advertising initiatives were discouraged, if not prohibited. Physicians were restrained by professional considerations, and hospitals often imposed internal constraints on their marketing activities. Exhibit 1.6 presents additional issues related to the ethics of healthcare marketing.

EXHIBIT 1.6
Ethical Issues in Healthcare Marketing

Since the advent of the marketing era in the United States after World War II, ethical issues have nagged the healthcare industry. Concerns over the marketing practices for various medical remedies can be traced back 200 years—to the days of patent medicines sold on street corners, at carnivals, and by traveling salesmen. The claims made for such potions were often exaggerated or clearly false. Eventually, government regulations were put into place to control the claims of purveyors of such products and, with the support of the American Medical Association (AMA), the first medicine labeling laws were passed in 1938. Today, in the United States the federal Food and Drug Administration (FDA) and the Federal Trade Commission (FTC) serve as watchdogs over health-related products and medical devices.

In the post–World War II period, physicians commonly endorsed various products in exchange for payment from the manufacturer. Physicians were paid to endorse various pharmaceutical products, for example, by indicating that one drug was superior to its competitors. During this period, physicians sometimes strayed from their areas of expertise and endorsed other products as well. The most controversial of these actions involved physicians who endorsed various cigarette brands. Doctors were paid to attest that Brand X was healthier for consumers to smoke than Brand Y. The influence of the AMA and other forces was eventually brought to bear, and such practices were eliminated.

These experiences led the AMA to enforce a virtual prohibition of marketing on the part of physicians. In 1947, the AMA forbade physicians from advertising for self-promotion. This prohibition continued through 1957, when it was modified to only restrict physicians from soliciting patients. These restrictions did not affect such traditional marketing activities as networking and entertaining would-be referrals, and it was even customary at that time for doctors to provide kickbacks (referred to as "fee splitting") to referring physicians.

By the 1960s, the strict injunction against advertising had been eased somewhat and physicians were allowed to cite their name, address, and specialty in telephone directories and similar publications as a means of demonstrating their professionalism and distinguishing themselves from other health professionals. The AMA eventually back-pedaled from its strong stance against physician advertising, and in the 1990s many physicians initiated aggressive marketing campaigns. Even so, such physicians are often perceived in a bad light by their colleagues.

Although hospitals were not constrained to the same extent, many hospital administrators also had ethical qualms concerning marketing (or at least advertising). These qualms did not restrict marketing activities such as public relations, educational activities, and communication strategies, but they did discourage many hospitals from overt media advertising. Ultimately, the combined effect of increasing competition, reduced revenues, and a more demanding consumer overcame any lingering reluctance related to marketing on the part of hospitals and health systems.

Much of the controversy surrounding marketing in healthcare has involved the pharmaceutical industry. The marketing of over-the-counter drugs, of course, is covered by federal regulations that control the claims that can be made with regard to their efficacy. The marketing of prescription drugs directly to consumers is tightly controlled by federal regulation, and until the end of the twentieth century, pharmaceutical companies were prohibited from marketing directly to consumers. Even with relaxed rules concerning pharmaceutical marketing, there are still strict limits on the claims that can be made in drug advertisements.

Drug manufacturers have stirred up the most controversy by focusing their marketing activities almost exclusively on the physicians

(continued)

EXHIBIT 1.6 (*continued*)

who prescribe drugs to their patients. Pharmaceutical companies spend up to 25 percent of their budgets on marketing and sales activities, and the bulk of this has historically been allocated to advertising in medical journals, supporting educational programs for potential subscribers, and making sales calls on physicians.

The pharmaceutical companies' long-standing practice of providing free samples of drugs to physicians eventually came under fire and is facing restrictions. More controversial, however, have been the blatant attempts to "buy" physician support for particular pharmaceuticals by providing gifts, free trips, and other incentives designed to encourage physicians to endorse a particular drug through their prescribing practices. Congress eventually reacted to the perceived excesses on the part of pharmaceutical companies attempting to influence the decision making of physicians, and legislation was enacted that severely limited the ability of drug companies to provide incentives to physicians.

Although the marketing activities of health professionals will continue to be guided by self-imposed ethical standards, regulations governing the marketing of health-related products are not likely to disappear. Because of the nature of healthcare products and services, continued oversight on the part of various regulatory agencies can be expected. As marketing activities expand in healthcare, they will continue to be affected by a combination of ethical restraints and legal regulations.

In some cases, legal restraints have been put in place to prohibit advertising and other overt forms of marketing. The Federal Trade Commission (FTC), for example, limits the types of advertising and the advertising content pharmaceutical companies and other healthcare consumer products companies can provide. Congressional legislation also has been enacted to limit the marketing activities of providers reimbursed under the Medicare and Medicaid programs.

Why Healthcare Marketing Is Different

Because marketing philosophies and techniques cannot be readily transferred from other industries to healthcare, healthcare marketing requires its own unique approach and takes on characteristics unlike those of marketing in other industries. Marketing in healthcare is different for the following reasons:

- The demand for many health services is relatively rare and highly unpredictable.
- The end user may not be the target for the marketing campaign.
- The product being marketed may be highly complex and may not lend itself to easy categorization.
- Not all prospective customers for a health service are considered desirable.
- It is difficult to measure the outcome of the provision of health services.
- It is difficult to quantify the differences between healthcare organizations and the services they deliver.
- It is more of a challenge to market services than goods.

Developments Encouraging Healthcare Marketing

Despite the barriers to incorporating marketing into healthcare already noted in the previous paragraphs, significant progress was made during the 1980s and 1990s toward establishing marketing as an integral function of healthcare organizations. Marketing was finally accepted as a legitimate healthcare function as a result of a number of developments that reflected changes in society overall, trends in the healthcare industry, and changes in the nature of consumers. The following list includes some of these important developments:

- *Introduction of competition*. Until the 1980s, true competition was unknown in healthcare. Most healthcare organizations had operated since the 1960s in monopolistic or oligopolistic environments. Suddenly, healthcare organizations were faced with competition from many sources for what had become in many ways a shrinking market.
- *Overcapacity in the hospital industry*. The hospital-building binge that spanned three decades following World War II, coupled with the trend toward lower admission rates, created an oversupply of hospital beds. Suddenly, hospitals that had once scrambled to find beds were faced with the prospect of closing nursing units. Given an essentially flat market for hospital services, additional patients were going to have to be acquired from competitors.
- *Rise of the consumer*. The traditional customers (i.e., patients) of healthcare organizations historically had little say in the care they received and their choice of providers. As a result, healthcare providers, especially hospitals, paid little attention to their patients' characteristics. Consumerism surged in the 1970s, 1980s, and 1990s and into the new millennium, and healthcare organizations were forced to research the characteristics of customers and potential customers and to determine their needs and wants.

- *Introduction of new services.* Since the 1960s, the healthcare industry has witnessed the continuous creation of new services and programs. Innovative services were introduced and existing services were repackaged. New "boutique" initiatives, such as seniors' and women's programs, were developed. The public had to be educated about these new services and encouraged to obtain them from a particular provider.

- *Growth of elective procedures.* Healthcare had always been characterized by certain procedures that were not considered medically necessary. Procedures to improve quality of life or enhance appearance were offered by a relatively small number of providers to patients who could pay for them out of pocket. As consumer wants became as important as consumer needs, the variety of elective procedures increased dramatically, and heated competition developed among practitioners providing elective procedures.

- *Introduction of a retail component.* By the late 1980s, a strong retail component had emerged in the healthcare industry. Although different observers may view this development in different ways, a variety of services (mostly elective) and goods were added to the inventories of healthcare organizations. Fitness centers, weight management programs, and hair replacement were among the retail-type services offered. Nutritional supplements, cosmeceuticals, and self-help products also found their way into practitioners' offices.

- *Entry of entrepreneurs.* One reason for the surge in competition was the entry of entrepreneurs from other industries into healthcare. By the 1970s, the healthcare industry was seen as a lucrative field for businesspeople with no healthcare background. These new entrants were used to competing, observed sound business principles, and were accustomed to marketing. Not only did they set an example with regard to marketing, but they also helped to create an environment in which marketing became a survival factor.

- *Service-line development.* During the 1980s, hospitals adopted an approach from other industries that emphasized vertical service lines in the health system. Service lines were established around cardiology, oncology, women's services, orthopedics, and other clinical areas as self-contained business units that had to survive on available resources. Organization of marketing at the service-line level became common because each service line had a distinct target market.

- *Mergers and acquisitions.* By the 1980s, consolidation was well under way in the healthcare industry. Both for-profit and not-for-profit chains of hospitals, specialty facilities, and nursing homes were emerging and building regional or national networks through aggressive acquisitions.

Physician practices were being consolidated as a result of the short-lived surge of physician practice management organizations. Each merger and acquisition provided more resources for marketing, and the image issues that resulted from such actions also led to an increased need to market corporate identities.

- *Need for social marketing.* Public-sector organizations were faced with a need to communicate their message to consumers but had limited means of doing so. The concept of social marketing emerged as public health agencies developed campaigns to inform the public about the dangers of smoking and drinking, methods of reducing the spread of sexually transmitted diseases, and the importance of prenatal care. Where past methods of delivering information had failed, marketing provided a channel through which information could be disseminated in a wholesale fashion.

Reasons Healthcare Should Be Marketed

By the late 1970s, the arguments against investing in marketing in healthcare were being stripped away one by one. Although marketing was still a long way from being enthusiastically embraced, the reasons for incorporating marketing as a corporate function were beginning to mount. Not all reasons were conceded by all healthcare organizations at the same time, but different reasons were cited under varying circumstances. Marketing efforts during this period began to be supported by the following justifications:

- *Building awareness.* With the introduction of new products and the emergence of an informed consumer, healthcare organizations needed to build an awareness of their services and expose target audiences to their capabilities.
- *Enhancing visibility or image.* With the increasing standardization of healthcare services and a growing appreciation of reputation, healthcare organizations needed to initiate marketing campaigns that would improve top-of-mind awareness and distinguish them from their competitors.
- *Improving market penetration.* Healthcare organizations were faced with growing competition, and marketing was a means for increasing patient volumes, growing revenues, and gaining market share. With few new patients in many markets, marketing was critical for retaining existing customers and attracting customers from competitors.
- *Increasing prestige.* Many healthcare organizations, especially hospitals, believed success hinged on being able to surpass competitors in terms

of prestige. If prestige could be gained through having the best doctors, the latest equipment, and the nicest facilities, these factors needed to be conveyed to the general public.

- *Attracting medical staff and employees.* As the healthcare industry expanded, competition for skilled workers increased. Hospitals and other healthcare providers needed to promote themselves to potential employees by marketing the superior benefits they offered to recruits.
- *Serving as an information resource.* As healthcare became more complex and the array of services offered by healthcare organizations grew, these organizations needed to constantly inform the general public and the medical community about the products they had to offer. Whether through press releases or recorded telephone announcements, there was growing pressure to get the word out.
- *Influencing consumer decision making.* Once healthcare organizations realized that consumers had a role to play in healthcare decision making, the role of marketing in influencing this process became recognized. Whether it involved convincing consumers to decide on a particular organization's services or to speed up the decision-making process, marketing was becoming increasingly important.
- *Offsetting competitive marketing.* Once healthcare organizations realized their competitors were adopting aggressive marketing approaches, they began to adopt a stance of defensive marketing. They felt compelled to respond to the gambits of competitors by out-marketing them.

Healthcare Marketing Comes of Age

What evidence exists today that the healthcare industry has accepted marketing as a legitimate function? Beyond the traditional marketing-oriented sectors (e.g., pharmaceuticals, consumer products, health plans), have healthcare organizations embraced marketing? A number of indicators attest to this acceptance.

The industry has witnessed a continuous, if unsteady, advance in the role and status of marketing over the past 25 years. During the period after World War II, the concept of marketing was unknown in healthcare. The public relations role was expanded over time, and communications and government relations functions were added. By the late 1970s, formal marketing activities were being initiated, and advertising on the part of healthcare providers was becoming common. Even during the 1980s, however, many still saw marketing as an external function—not something inherent to healthcare, but a supportive service that was used when needed.

By the end of the 1980s, marketing was being incorporated into the structure of healthcare organizations. Marketing departments were being established, and marketing expenses were being factored into organizational budgets. Marketers were being promoted and became managers, directors, and, ultimately, vice presidents. Marketing was moving from the periphery of the organization to the boardroom. Once technical resources who were consulted as needed, marketers were becoming full partners in the corporate decision-making process. The most progressive healthcare organizations developed a marketing mind-set to ensure that marketing was a consideration in every initiative and that marketers provided input on the direction of the enterprise.

A 2007 Society for Healthcare Strategy and Market Development (SHSMD) survey of nearly 300 hospitals found that hospital marketing departments averaged 4.9 staff members and budgets of $1.2 million. Larger hospitals reported an average of 10 staff members and budgets near $3 million. Most marketing executives were at the director or vice president level of the organization, with over one-third of marketing managers holding the title of vice president or senior vice president (SHSMD 2008). Another SHSMD study of 833 marketing, communications, and strategy staff reported that marketing executives earned an average annual salary of $149,575 in 2008. This figure compares favorably to the compensation of healthcare executives in other departments (SHSMD 2009).

The importance of marketing in healthcare is also reflected in the emergence of publications devoted to the topic, including *Marketing Health Services*, the healthcare journal of the American Marketing Association, and *Health Marketing Quarterly*. Articles on healthcare marketing regularly appear in other marketing journals as well. Numerous newsletters are devoted to healthcare marketing or some component of it, such as health communications or public relations.

Associations devoted to healthcare marketing have been established, such as SHSMD. The American Marketing Association has an active healthcare marketing division, and one of its eight special interest groups is devoted to healthcare.

Textbooks on healthcare marketing began appearing in the 1980s, and healthcare marketing courses are part of the marketing curriculum in many U.S. universities. Courses on the topic are now standard in healthcare administration programs. Numerous universities and other training programs offer specialized training programs on various aspects of healthcare marketing.

These developments reflect the growing importance of marketing in the healthcare arena and its changing role. The ways in which marketing is being transformed as it matures in the healthcare industry will be discussed throughout this book.

Summary

Since the concept of marketing was introduced to healthcare providers in the 1970s, the field has undergone periods of growth, decline, retrenchment, and renewed growth. Initial resistance to healthcare marketing had to be overcome by an industry that was primarily not-for-profit and averse to self-promotion. The healthcare industry is unique in a number of ways, and numerous barriers prevented the immediate acceptance of marketing as an essential function.

Healthcare organizations slowly adopted marketing concepts and techniques from other industries and eventually developed approaches more suited to the unique nature of healthcare. Early on, marketing was often equated with advertising, so many healthcare organizations mounted major advertising campaigns during the 1980s. Realizing the limitations of advertising in a service industry, healthcare organizations added direct-sales capabilities and technology-based marketing approaches to supplement the more traditional public relations and communication marketing techniques.

Over time, a new generation of health professionals more oriented to business principles emerged. Marketing departments were established, positions were carved out for marketing directors and vice presidents, and marketing became an accepted part of healthcare administration. By the 1990s, most healthcare organizations had active marketing programs, and marketers were brought into the inner circle, converting marketing from an external activity to a core function of a progressive healthcare organization.

Key Points

- Although American industry accepted marketing in the 1950s, a number of factors prevented the healthcare industry from adopting marketing initially.
- The pioneers in healthcare marketing can be traced back to the 1970s, but marketing was not widely accepted as a legitimate function for healthcare organizations until much later.
- Early on, there were no experienced healthcare marketers, and marketing experts had to be imported from other industries.
- Changes in the healthcare arena during the 1980s (particularly the increase in competition) resulted in a surge of interest in marketing.
- Once health professionals accepted marketing, the field underwent various stages of growth and contraction in response to market developments.

- Initially, marketing was often equated with advertising, and organizations underwent considerable trial and error before accepting other promotional techniques.
- By the 1990s, healthcare marketing was maturing as a field, and a new generation of hospital administrators and healthcare marketers was on board.
- By the turn of the twenty-first century, healthcare organizations had come to consider marketing an essential function for healthcare organizations, and marketing resources were increasingly wed to strategic planning and development efforts.

Discussion Questions

- Why didn't healthcare professionals consider marketing to be important until the 1980s?
- What factors mitigated against the introduction of marketing into healthcare?
- Why do health professionals view marketing in a different way than their counterparts in other industries do?
- How do ethical and legal constraints affect marketing in healthcare more than in other industries?
- What factors ultimately forced the incorporation of marketing into healthcare?
- Why is today's healthcare environment more hospitable to marketing and marketers than past environments were?
- What indicators attest that marketing has matured as a legitimate function in the healthcare field?

Additional Resources

American Marketing Association website: www.marketingpower.com
Health Marketing Quarterly (periodical): Published by The Haworth Press
Marketing Health Services (periodical): Published by the American Marketing Association
Society for Healthcare Strategy and Market Development website: www.shsmd.org

THE EVOLVING SOCIETAL AND HEALTHCARE CONTEXT

Several developments in U.S. society and in healthcare over the last quarter of the twentieth century laid the foundation for the emergence of healthcare marketing. Current trends in healthcare have now brought marketing to center stage. Changes in demographic characteristics, lifestyles, and other population attributes have all contributed to the growing importance of healthcare marketing. Trends in the healthcare arena that are anticipated to continue for the foreseeable future indicate that the role of marketing in healthcare is growing. This chapter reviews recent developments in U.S. society and the healthcare system and discusses the implications for healthcare marketing.

The Emergence of Healthcare as an Institution

No two healthcare delivery systems are exactly alike. A healthcare system can be understood only within the sociocultural context of the society in which it exists. Differences between healthcare systems are primarily a function of this context. The social structure of a society, along with its cultural values, establishes the parameters for the healthcare system. In this sense, the form and function of the healthcare system reflect the form and function of the society in which it resides. Ultimately, the development of marketing in healthcare (or any industry) reflects the characteristics of both that industry and that society.

Social Context and Governance

American society (or any society for that matter) can be viewed as a system, or an assemblage of parts combined in a complex whole. Each part is interconnected directly or indirectly, and, thus, all are interdependent. These parts, working in concert, create a dynamic, self-sustaining system that maintains a state of equilibrium. The parts perform their respective functions, and each component must work in synchronization with the others if the system is to function efficiently and remain viable. These major components can be thought of as institutions, the intangible structures involving patterns of behavior directed toward accomplishing societal goals.

The goals of society reflect the needs every social system must address. Every society must perform certain functions: reproduce new society members, socialize the new members, distribute resources, maintain internal order, provide for defense, deal with spiritual/religious issues, and provide for the health and well-being of the population. Organizational structures (institutions) evolve to meet each of these needs. Some form of family evolves to manage reproduction, some form of educational system develops to deal with socialization, some form of economic system emerges to deal with the allocation of resources, and so forth. Likewise, a healthcare/social services system of some type evolves to ensure the health and welfare of the population. Because healthcare was dependent on a certain level of knowledge and technological progress to be able to fully develop, it was one of the slowest U.S. institutions to be formally established.

Like other institutions, healthcare sets forth rules that guide the behavior of individuals in the institutional context. For example, there are guidelines for living a long, healthy life. If citizens don't follow these rules, they risk sickness and early death. These guidelines are often codified in the form of doctor's orders. Because individuals in a free society cannot be forced to live a healthy lifestyle, the healthcare institution invokes legal and regulatory contrivances to enforce its requirements. Thus, people are generally required to obtain certain childhood immunizations, addicts may be required to enter rehabilitation, and patients with contagious diseases can be isolated from the rest of the population.

On another level, there are rules stating that patients must have insurance before being treated by certain healthcare providers, that health plan members must meet certain requirements in order to reduce their insurance premiums, and that people involved in risky activities must pay higher prices for insurance. Although there is no systematic plan for encouraging or discouraging health-related behaviors, various parties, appearing to act in their self-interest, work toward the goals of the healthcare institution by promulgating such rules.

Adaptability and Change

Despite the permanence institutions achieve in society, they must also have the flexibility to adjust to changing conditions. No other institution has undergone the rapid changes that healthcare experienced during the twentieth century. At the start of that century, healthcare was a rudimentary institution with limited visibility and little credibility. Hospitals were perceived as places where people went to die, and doctors were to be avoided at all costs. Indeed, there was little doctors could do for patients anyway. There was no agreement on the nature of health and illness, and scientists were only beginning to understand the effects of various therapeutic approaches. Healthcare was not even on the national radar screen for the first half of the twentieth century, and it accounted for a negligible amount of the gross national product.

By the end of the twentieth century, however, not only had the institution become well established in the United States, but it had also come to play a dominant role in U.S. society. The importance of the institution was such that sociologists often referred to the *medicalization* of American society. Few members of contemporary U.S. society are not under some type of medical management. In the last half of the twentieth century, the institution came to be accorded high prestige and to exert a major influence over other institutions. At the beginning of the twenty-first century, the healthcare institution claimed approximately 11 percent of the nation's workforce and 15 percent of the gross national product, a share that is expected to continue to grow (AAHC 2006).

Formal Organization and Scope of Influence

The ascendancy of the healthcare institution in the twentieth century was given impetus by the growing dependence on formal organizations of all types. The industrialization and urbanization of the United States reflected a transformation from a traditional, agrarian society to a complex, modern society in which change, not tradition, was the central theme. In such a society, formal solutions to societal needs take precedence over informal responses.

Healthcare provides possibly the best example of this emergent dependence on formal solutions because it is an institution whose very development was a result of this transformation. People in the nineteenth century would have considered formal healthcare to be the last resort when faced with sickness and disability. Few of them ever entered a hospital or regularly saw a physician. Today, in contrast, the healthcare system is often seen as the first resort when health problems arise. Traditional, informal responses to health problems have given way to complex, institutionalized responses. Healthcare has become entrenched in the fabric of American life to the point that Americans turn to it not only for clear-cut health problems but also for a broad range of psychological, social, interpersonal, and spiritual problems.

By any measure, healthcare could be considered a dominant institution in contemporary American society. Other institutions, such as the political institution, the military, and the arts, receive comparatively fewer resources. Further, Americans have become increasingly obsessed with their health. On public opinion polls, respondents frequently cite health as one of their most pressing personal concerns and healthcare as a leading national concern. Exhibit 2.1 displays trends in healthcare as a proportion of the nation's gross national product.

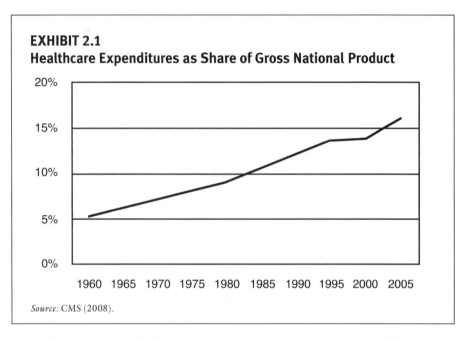

EXHIBIT 2.1
Healthcare Expenditures as Share of Gross National Product

Source: CMS (2008).

The size of the healthcare institution has attracted substantial resources from other industrial sectors, and healthcare is an unavoidable issue in political campaigns. The pharmaceutical industry, insurance industry, American Medical Association, and American Hospital Association are major political lobbying groups. Further, much of the educational system is devoted to training health personnel. The fact that the federal government has become responsible for 60 percent of personal healthcare expenditures attests to the influence of healthcare on the central government.

Americans increasingly turned to the healthcare institution in the late twentieth century as the solution for a wide range of social, psychological, and even spiritual issues, and physicians came to be regarded as experts on virtually any human problem. This expansion of scope is evidenced by the fact that less than half of the people in a general practitioner's waiting room suffer from a clear-cut medical problem. They are there because of emotional disorders, sexual dysfunction, social adjustment issues, nutritional problems, or some other nonclinical threat to their well-being. Even though physicians are generally not trained to deal with these conditions, the healthcare system is seen as an appropriate place to seek solutions to these and other nonmedical maladies.

Media Coverage

Another indicator of healthcare's dominance is the amount of media airtime devoted to health-related topics. Americans continue to be deluged by advertisements for all kinds of consumer goods, and over the past 20 years, there has been an explosion of advertisements and paid programming related to health, beauty, and fitness. Television commercials for health products and services are ubiquitous. Paid programming featuring fitness training and cable television channels devoted solely to health issues indicate the extent to which the healthcare institution has gained ascendancy. In a few short years, health-care marketing in the media has grown from a nonentity to a major presence in both print and electronic media.

The rise of healthcare marketing in the media has been accompanied by the enormous growth of healthcare information on the Internet. According to some estimates, there are more sites devoted to healthcare than to any other topic. More and more healthcare consumers are turning to the Internet for their healthcare information, and the health-related content of the Internet is playing an increasing role in consumer decision making. Consumer interest in cyber-information has been accompanied by increased use of Internet-based marketing on the part of healthcare organizations. Once considered a mecha-nism only for providing information about hospitals, health plans, pharma-ceutical companies, and consumer products companies, the Internet has now become a medium for aggressive marketing of healthcare goods and services.

All things considered, healthcare was the up-and-coming institution of the second half of the twentieth century. The growing significance of health for consumers' personal lives and healthcare's growing role in the public arena cannot be denied. Indeed, many corporations have indicated that health ben-efits are one of their single largest costs. The increasing involvement of U.S. citizens in the use of health services and the annual per capita expenditures on healthcare set the United States apart from other countries and are reflected in the growing importance of healthcare marketing.

The Cultural Revolution and Healthcare

The restructuring of U.S. institutions during the twentieth century was accom-panied by a cultural revolution that resulted in an extensive value reorientation in American society. The values associated with traditional societies, such as kinship, community, authority, and primary relationships, were overshadowed by the values of modern industrialized societies, such as secularism, urbanism, and self-actualization. Ultimately, the restructuring of American values was instrumental in the emergence of healthcare as an important institution.

The modern values that emerged in the United States after World War II supported the development of an institutional structure that would subsequently spawn the development of modern Western medicine. These values shifted the emphasis in American society to economic success, educa-tional achievement, and scientific and technological advancement and sup-ported the ascendancy of healthcare as a dominant institution.

Implicit throughout the evolution of the U.S. healthcare system has been the importance of economic success, as the U.S. healthcare system has emerged as the only for-profit healthcare system in the world. Today, the profit motive remains strong as for-profit national chains have absorbed much of the nation's health services delivery capacity. This free-enterprise aspect of healthcare is intrinsically linked to other American values, such as freedom of choice and individualism.

Other values became important as American culture evolved in the twentieth century. Change became recognized as a value in its own right, and Americans eagerly embraced changes in residences, jobs, partners, and lifestyles. At the same time, an activist orientation emerged that called for a proactive approach to all issues, and the aggressive approach taken by Americans faced with health problems reflects this activist orientation.

The conceptualization of health as a distinct value in U.S. society represented a major development in the emergence of the healthcare institution. Before World War II, health was generally not recognized as a value by Americans but was vaguely tied to other notions of well-being. Public opinion polls before the war did not identify personal health as an issue for the U.S. populace, nor was healthcare delivery considered a societal concern. By the 1960s, however, personal health had climbed to the top of public opinion polls as an issue, and the adequate provision of health services became an important issue in the mind of the American public (Thomas 2003b). By the last third of the twentieth century, Americans had become obsessed with health as a value and with the importance of institutional solutions to health problems.

Once health became established as a value, it was a short step to establishing a formal healthcare system as the institutional means of achieving that value. An environment was created that encouraged the emergence of a powerful institution that supported many other contemporary American values. Some values, like the value placed on human life, were considered immutable. The ethos promoted by the emerging scientific, technological, and research communities contributed to the growth of the industry. The value that Americans came to place on youth, beauty, and self-actualization further contributed to the expanded role of healthcare. The ability of the nascent healthcare system to capitalize on emerging U.S. values and garner support from the economic, political, and educational institutions ensured the emergence of an increasingly influential healthcare system.

The Changing Societal Context

The twentieth century spawned a dependence on formal institutions of all types, and this created a favorable environment for the rise of a strong healthcare system. Just as Americans had turned to formal educational, political, and economic systems for meeting their social needs, they began to turn to a formal healthcare system to meet their health-related needs. The transformation of American society in the twentieth century clearly affected the provision of healthcare, as the traditional managers of sickness and death—the family and the church—gave way to more formal responses to health problems. The health of the population became the responsibility of the economic, educational, and political systems and, eventually, of a fully developed and powerful healthcare system. Traditional, informal responses to health problems gave way to complex, institutional responses. Home remedies, with their high-touch nature, could not compete in an environment that valued high-tech (and subsequently high-status) responses to health problems.

Demographic Trends

The U.S. population experienced a number of dramatic demographic trends during the last half of the twentieth century that contributed to changes in its composition. This demographic transformation may have been a major determinant of the needs the healthcare system had to address. The impact did not end simply with a different age distribution or racial composition but was reflected in the radically changed attitudes of healthcare consumers.

These demographic trends also triggered the epidemiologic transition that took place in the United States in the second half of the twentieth century. Throughout recorded history, acute health conditions were major health threats and the leading causes of death. Communicable, infectious, and parasitic conditions; accidents; complications of childbirth; and other acute conditions were ubiquitous in human society. At the beginning of the twentieth century, the leading causes of death were tuberculosis, influenza, and other communicable diseases.

As a result of the demographic transformation of the second half of the twentieth century, chronic conditions superseded acute conditions as the predominant form of health problem. Improved living conditions, better nutrition, and higher standards of living, accompanied by advances in medical science, reduced or eliminated the burden of disease from acute conditions. This void was filled, however, by the emergence of chronic conditions as the leading health problems and leading causes of death. People were living longer, but this older population was plagued by hypertension, arthritis, and diabetes, as well as numerous conditions that reflected the lifestyles that emerged in the American population in the postwar period.

The following sections focus on key demographic trends that helped drive changes in the healthcare environment and their likely implications for healthcare marketing.

The Changing Age Structure

The first and perhaps most important demographic trend is the U.S. population's changing age distribution. The aging of America has been one of the most publicized demographic trends in history, and the implications of this trend on the demand for health services are especially significant.

Population growth in the older age cohorts (aged 55 or older), particularly among the oldest-old (aged 85 or older), is currently faster than that in the younger cohorts. The total population increased by an estimated 6.2 percent between 2000 and 2006, but the population aged 85 or over increased by more than 21 percent. As baby boomers enter middle age, the largest age cohort in the first decade of the twenty-first century is those aged 45 to 65. Several younger cohorts (e.g., those aged 25 to 34) have experienced virtually no growth since 2000 (U.S. Census Bureau 2009).

Among age-related factors, the movement of the huge baby boom cohort into middle age has the most significant implications for future healthcare demand. The first of some 77 million baby boomers turned 60 during the first decade of the twenty-first century. This cohort grew up in affluence and comfort, and baby boomers are used to having things, including their health, in working order. Now having to contend with the onset of chronic disease and the natural deterioration that comes with aging, their impact on the healthcare system is being increasingly felt. This cohort grew up during the marketing era and is more comfortable than any previous generation with healthcare marketing. Because baby boomers are savvy consumers, healthcare marketers will have to give them special consideration.

The nature of the future senior population will be determined to a great extent by the characteristics of the baby boomers. In fact, boomers have already influenced the healthcare delivery system in significant ways. This group is primarily responsible for the success of health maintenance organizations, birthing centers, urgent care centers, and outpatient surgery centers. Now it is driving the demand for a wide range of new services, such as laser eye surgery, skin rejuvenation, and menopause management. Because the golden years are a context for new and different lifestyles, boomers are determined to reinvent retirement. The changing age distribution also has important implications for the population's ratio of males to females. Generally speaking, the older the population is, the greater the "excess" of females. Except for the youngest age groups, females outnumber males in every age cohort. Among seniors, females outnumber males two to one, and, at the oldest ages, there may be four times as many women as men. In 2006, the median age for women was 37.8 years, compared to 35.2 years for men. Further, 25.1 percent of the female population was aged 55 or older, compared to 21.0 percent of the male population. In 2006, there were an estimated 4.5

million more women than men in the U.S. population (U.S. Census Bureau 2009).

These statistics on the female population have important implications for healthcare marketers. For one, the female healthcare market is considerably larger than the male market. Further, women are more aggressive users of health services than are men. Perhaps even more important, women bear much of the burden for healthcare decision making, not only for themselves but also for their families. They are also more likely to influence the health behavior of their peers.

Growing Racial and Ethnic Diversity

Another demographic trend that characterized American society during the last half of the twentieth century was increasing racial and ethnic diversity. The number of newcomers who immigrated to the United States from foreign countries during the 1990s broke century-old records. In addition, long-established ethnic and racial minorities are growing at faster rates than are native-born whites. The cumulative effect of the trends of the past several years has been a shrinking of the relative size of the white population (especially the non-Hispanic white population) and the growth of the African American, Asian, and Hispanic components of U.S. society. More important, by 2001, according to the U.S. Census Bureau, Hispanics had surpassed African Americans as a percentage of the U.S. population. As most population growth for the foreseeable future will be a function of immigration, the proportion of non-Hispanic whites in the population will continue to decline. A telling statistic is the fact that, in 2000, minorities accounted for more than 46 percent of children under five years old but accounted for only 37 percent of the total population (U.S. Census Bureau 2009).

Given that the U.S. healthcare system has historically been geared to the needs of the mainstream white population, the trend toward greater racial and ethnic diversity has major implications for the healthcare operations. Marketing activities must take into consideration the changing racial and ethnic characteristics of the population and the demands these changes will make on the system. Indeed, a subfield of healthcare marketing has developed that is devoted to marketing to ethnic groups and minorities.

Changing Household and Family Structure

The changing household and family structure is another demographic development characterizing U.S. society. This trend is no surprise to demographers, although it has seldom been linked to health issues. For decades, the family has been undergoing change. First it was high divorce rates, then it was fewer people marrying (and those who did marry were marrying at a later age), and then it was fewer people having children (and those who did have children had fewer of them and at a later age).

In 2006, an estimated 50.1 percent of the U.S. population over age 15 years was married—a low figure by historical standards, and four points lower than the figure for 2000. Some 30.6 percent had never married, 12.7 percent were separated or divorced, and 6.4 percent were widowed. These figures for the unmarried all represent record highs (U.S. Census Bureau 2009).

These changes in marital status have had major implications for the structure of U.S. households. What is popularly considered the typical American family (i.e., 2 parents and 2.5 children) has become a rarity, accounting for only 24 percent of households in 2000. Today, the most common household form is married couples without children. Even so, this type of household accounts for less than 28 percent of the total. Nontraditional households have become the norm, and an unprecedented proportion of households are one-person households (U.S. Census Bureau 2009).

Changing patterns of marital status and household structure have important implications for health status and health behavior. Two-parent families, single-parent families, and elderly people living alone place different demands on, and require different responses from, the healthcare system. The continued diversification of U.S. household types for the foreseeable future is likely to require commensurate modifications to the healthcare delivery system. To a great extent, health services have been historically geared to the needs of traditional households involving two parents and one or more children. This orientation was encouraged by the extensive provision of employer-sponsored insurance that focused on the wage-earning head of household. In addition, traditional marketing approaches in other industries have focused on the family life cycle as a guide for the appropriate marketing approach. Future marketing initiatives must take into consideration the growing complexity of the U.S. household structure.

Changing Consumer Attitudes

Although patterns of consumer attitudes in U.S. society tend to be complex, a new orientation toward healthcare clearly emerged during the second half of the twentieth century. The "patient" was transformed into a "customer," creating a new entity who had the combined expectations of a traditional patient and a contemporary customer. This consumer was more knowledgeable about the healthcare system, more open to innovative approaches, and more intent on playing an active role in the diagnostic, therapeutic, and health maintenance processes than any previous generation had been.

These new attitudes were fostered by the baby boomers, a cohort that is now facing the chronic conditions associated with middle age. This group has been influential in limiting the discretion and control of physicians and hospitals and has provided the impetus for the rise of alternative therapy as a competitor to mainstream allopathic medicine.

The baby boom population favors a more patient-centered approach to healthcare and is more likely to emphasize its nonmedical aspects. In general, baby boomers are less trusting of professionals and institutions and are control oriented to the point of stubbornness. This group is more self-reliant than previous generations, places greater value on self-care and home care, and is outcome oriented and cost sensitive. This generation prides itself in getting results and extracting value for its expenditures. Although baby boomers began influencing the healthcare system by "voting with their feet" (i.e., switching to new types of providers) during the 1980s, they are increasingly assuming positions of power that allow them to influence the shape of the healthcare landscape.

To a certain extent, these new attitudes toward healthcare reflect the rise of consumerism that is affecting all segments of society. Seeing themselves as customers rather than patients, these new consumers expect to receive adequate information, demand to participate in healthcare decisions that directly affect them, and insist that they receive the highest-quality care possible. These consumers want to receive their healthcare close to their homes, with minimal interruption to their family life and work schedules. They also want to maximize the value they receive for their healthcare expenditures. The transformation of baby boomers from patients to consumers clearly has significant implications for healthcare marketing.

Healthcare Developments

The trends affecting U.S. society during the second half of the twentieth century were accompanied by a number of significant healthcare developments. During the 1980s and 1990s, America experienced a major transformation in the delivery and financing of healthcare. A new generation of therapeutic techniques and pharmaceuticals was introduced. The delivery of healthcare shifted to a great extent from inpatient settings to outpatient settings, and the manner of financing healthcare was modified as managed care became a dominant feature of the healthcare landscape.

At the same time, the healthcare institution experienced shifting power relationships. The unfettered influence of the physician was challenged by other competing providers, and third-party payers increasingly set the parameters for reimbursement and, hence, the delivery of care. Employers, who were bearing most of the cost of private insurance, began to play a more active role and brought numerous changes to care delivery.

The physician's high and unassailable status had come into question by the end of the twentieth century as evidence of the fallibility and limitations of medical care mounted. The increasing number of women and foreign-trained physicians in the medical profession also changed the image of the physician. Baby boomers, armed with information from the Internet, influenced the shift away from the dependent patient to an aggressive consumer-patient who demanded a role in the therapeutic process.

The changes in healthcare in the 1980s and 1990s were numerous and dramatic and transformed the healthcare industry of the early 1980s into a different creature. These changes also had significant implications for healthcare marketing. Space does not allow a review of all of the changes that occurred during this time, but some of the more important ones are described in the following sections, along with their significance for healthcare marketing.

Growing Competition

During the 1980s, healthcare providers were exposed to unprecedented competition on a number of fronts. For the first time, healthcare providers were forced to profile their customers so they would be able to determine their needs. They also had to understand their competition and develop a level of market intelligence never dreamed of in the past. Most observers would agree that the emergence of competition has been a major driver of healthcare marketing.

A Shift of Emphasis from Inpatient Care to Outpatient Care

At one time, medical care was synonymous with inpatient care, and hospitalization was often a prerequisite before insurance coverage would kick in. By the 1980s, however, numerous factors were discouraging the use of inpatient care. Hospitals had to rapidly understand changing market conditions and position themselves to capture the growing outpatient market. Hospitals had to think in terms of a different approach to marketing as the traditional patterns of physician referral for inpatient care were deemphasized and consumerism emerged as a force in the system.

A Shift of Emphasis from Specialty Care to Primary Care

Historically, hospitals have relied on the medical specialists on their staffs to admit patients and generate their revenue. By the late 1980s, industry forces were encouraging the use of primary care physicians rather than specialists. Hospital systems had to examine their referral patterns and revise their thinking with regard to primary care physicians. Hospitals began to actively court family practitioners, internists, and pediatricians; marketers had to develop a means of showcasing the primary care capabilities of hospitals to consumers and health plans. Although reimbursement still favors specialists, primary physicians are expected to play a greater role in the future healthcare system.

The Emergence of Employers as Major Players in the Industry

After World War II, employers began offering health insurance to their employees and passively footed the bill for their medical expenses. By the mid-1980s, however, employers were taking a more active role in managing their employees' health benefits. Suddenly, healthcare providers found they had a new customer with a set of needs that was different from that of their traditional customers. Business coalitions emerged to negotiate with healthcare providers from a position of strength, and the health benefit costs borne by employers became a major driver of healthcare reform.

An Increasingly Market-Driven Industry

Until the healthcare industry became market driven in the 1980s, patients' opinions were seldom considered important. All of a sudden, however, healthcare providers needed to know what the patient liked and did not like about the services provided. Patient satisfaction surveys became commonplace, and patients started rating the performance of providers and health plans with report cards. Marketers were called on not only to identify the wants and needs of the market but also to provide consultation on ways to improve customer satisfaction.

The Emergence of Managed Care as a Dominant Force

The emergence of managed care as a major force essentially changed the ground rules for healthcare providers. The patient had been transformed into an enrollee or a plan member. Instead of searching for sick patients who would require health services, marketers were encouraged to identify healthy persons who would not run up costs by using a lot of services. Healthcare providers participating in managed care plans had to shift their focus from treatment and cure to health maintenance. Managed care plans developed marketing expertise to capture the employer market, and managed care negotiations came to be considered a marketing function by many health systems.

The Changed Nature of the Decision Maker

Before the marketing era in healthcare, physicians made most decisions, and consumers had limited control over their medical episodes. Later, health plans began exercising inordinate influence over the use of health services as their enrollees were directed to specific provider networks. During the 1990s, consumers began to wield considerable influence as consumer choice began to characterize the industry, and changes in the nature of health benefits brought a new perspective to healthcare marketing. Each of these developments had implications for marketers as the focus shifted from physician to health plan to consumer. Pharmaceutical companies and health plans, which had traditionally marketed to intermediaries, began focusing on consumers.

The Redefinition of Medical Care as Healthcare

Most observers of the healthcare scene contend that the overarching development in healthcare of the 1980s and 1990s was the paradigm shift from an emphasis on medical care to an emphasis on healthcare (see Exhibit 2.2). The broader concept of "healthcare" was replacing the narrower concept of "medical care." The latter focused almost exclusively on the clinical aspects of care, while the former also considers social and psychological factors. As health and healthcare took on broader connotations, the role of the marketer increased in importance.

EXHIBIT 2.2
From Medical Care to Healthcare

Since the 1970s, there has been a movement away from medical care toward healthcare. The growing awareness of the connection between health status and lifestyle and the realization that medical care is limited in its ability to control the disorders of modern society have prompted a move away from a strictly medical model of health and illness to one that incorporates more of a social and psychological perspective. Originally noted by Engel (1977), this paradigm shift in which "medical care" was redefined as "healthcare" gained momentum during the 1980s and 1990s.

Medical care is narrowly defined in terms of the formal services provided by the healthcare system and refers primarily to those activities that are under the control of a physician. This concept focuses on the clinical or treatment aspects of care and excludes the nonmedical dimension. *Healthcare* refers to any function that might be directly or indirectly related to preserving, maintaining, and/or enhancing health status. This concept includes not only formal activities (such as visiting a health professional) but also such informal activities as preventive care (e.g., brushing teeth), exercise, proper diet, and other health maintenance activities.

Since the beginning of the twentieth century, the dominant paradigm in Western medical science has been the medical model of disease. Built on the germ theory formulated late in the nineteenth century, the medical model provided an appropriate framework within

---

which to address and respond to the acute health conditions prevalent well into the twentieth century. By the 1970s, however, enough anomalies had been identified to bring the prevailing paradigm into question. Despite the ever-increasing sophistication of medical technology, the importance of the nonmedical aspects of care was increasingly recognized.

Clearly, the epidemiologic transition, by which acute conditions were displaced by chronic disorders, has played a major role. As acute conditions waned in importance and chronic and degenerative conditions came to the forefront, the medical model began to lose some of its salience. Once the cause of most health conditions ceased to be environmental microorganisms and became aspects of lifestyle, a new model of health and illness was required. The chronic conditions that had come to account for most health problems did not respond well to the treatment-and-cure approach of the medical model. Chronic conditions could not be cured but had to be managed over a lifetime, and this called for a quite different approach.

Independent of this trend, patients had been expressing growing dissatisfaction with the operation of the healthcare system. The traditional approach to care was not a comfortable fit with the attitudes baby boomers were bringing to the doctor's office. This population, more than any other group in U.S. society, has led the movement toward the changing emphasis in healthcare. This cohort emphasizes convenience, value, responsiveness, patient participation, and other attributes not traditionally incorporated into the medical model. Further, the runaway costs of the system have led all observers to question the wisdom of pursuing the one-size-fits-all approach to solving health problems that is traditional in medical care.

The transition from medical care to healthcare has affected every aspect of care from the standard definitions of health and illness to the manner in which healthcare is delivered. Health status is now defined as a continuous process rather than in terms of a specific episode of care. Causes of ill health are now sought in the environment and the patient's social context as often as under the microscope. The importance of the nonmedical component of therapy has come to be recognized to the point that fathers are now allowed to participate in childbirth and families are encouraged to participate in the treatment of cancer patients. This paradigm shift calls for a significant change in the manner in which healthcare organizations structure their marketing activities.

The Redefinition of the "Patient"

Of all the developments in healthcare during the 1980s and 1990s, perhaps the one with the most implications for healthcare marketing was the reconceptualization of the patient. By the end of the twentieth century, fewer health professionals were using the term *patient* because of its narrow connotation. Patients came to be referred to as *clients, customers, consumers,* or *enrollees.* The major consideration, regardless of the label applied, was the fact that clients, customers, consumers, and enrollees all had different characteristics from patients. While the term *patient* implies a dependent, submissive status, each of the other terms implies proactive involvement in the therapeutic process. Ultimately, this development made healthcare marketing more similar to the marketing activities of other industries, as the consumer of the product became, for the first time, the focus of the healthcare marketer. The emphasis healthcare marketers placed on "consumer engagement" in the early part of the twenty-first century reflects the growing need for marketing expertise. Case Study 2.1 describes a marketing approach to the new consumer-patient.

CASE STUDY 2.1
Capturing an Emerging Market

The growing racial and ethnic diversity of the U.S. population seems to overwhelm some healthcare providers. A system that is used to providing one-size-fits-all care is now faced with a patient population that is increasingly heterogeneous and whose members often have different perspectives on healthcare than do the providers of care. However, if a provider can adapt to the needs of this growing market, a lot of opportunities will present themselves.

For example, the challenge of engaging a community in the opening of a birthing center is always significant, and it becomes even more daunting when community members speak 40 different languages. One hospital in an urban Midwestern community not only took on this challenge but also turned it into one of its greatest marketing successes.

Thirteen hospitals within a ten-mile radius of the primary service area provided obstetrics services to the community. An estimated 24,274 women of childbearing age lived in the primary service area. Another 134,055 women of childbearing age lived in the secondary service area. A service area analysis identified the following ethnic breakdown for the population: 72.2 percent white (including 18.9 percent Hispanic), 11.2 percent Asian or Pacific Islander, 9.1 percent other, 7.0 percent

African American, and 0.5 percent American Indian. The percentage of Asians in the service area was quadruple state and national averages, and the percentage of Hispanics was double state and national figures. The racial and ethnic breakdown, however, failed to convey the unique features of the service area. Among the white population, recent immigrants from the Middle East and Eastern Europe supplemented the Hispanic population. The Asian immigrants came predominantly from Korea, Pakistan, India, and the Philippines.

To more narrowly define the major ethnic breakdown of the childbearing market, obstetrics discharge data by physician were reviewed, and physicians were asked to identify the major ethnic and cultural groups of their patients. The following major groups using obstetrics services were identified using this technique: Indian, Pakistani, and Middle Eastern (29 percent); Korean (23 percent); Hispanic (13 percent); and Assyrian (6 percent). Research into cultural considerations for these groups identified a significant subgroup of Indian, Pakistani, and Middle Eastern patients who were Muslim. On the basis of this information, four target ethnic markets were defined: Korean, Middle Eastern, Muslim (Middle Eastern, Pakistani, and Indian), and Hispanic (Mexican, Puerto Rican, and Cuban).

To increase market share for obstetrics services at the hospital, marketing strategies were developed to raise awareness of the new family birthing center in these ethnic communities. To achieve this goal in a highly competitive market, the following objectives were adopted:

- Differentiate services from those of competitors by means of
  - ○ graphic images and color coding for directional signage in the facility;
  - ○ multilingual and multicultural physicians (men and women), nursing staff, cultural liaisons, and interpreters;
  - ○ culturally diverse artwork throughout the facility;
  - ○ large state-of-the-art labor/delivery/recovery/postpartum rooms with hot tubs and space for family members;
  - ○ ethnic menus along with microwaves and refrigerators for patient use;
  - ○ childbirth preparation classes taught in Spanish, Korean, Arabic, and Hindi by native speakers;
  - ○ a family-centered program of care; and
  - ○ superior quality measures.

(continued)

CASE STUDY 2.1 (*continued*)

- Enhance the hospital's marketing presence through
  - ○ creating a new maternity services brand for the hospital, featuring the graphic image of infant footprints;
  - ○ aggressively marketing and promoting the new features and benefits of the hospital's maternity services; and
  - ○ reinforcing the hospital's unique positioning as a provider of culturally sensitive, family-centered maternity care.

On the basis of these objectives, the following marketing initiatives were identified for the hospital:

- Tailor market research to build knowledge and understanding of each ethnic group.
- Implement culturally appropriate advertising campaigns for each targeted group, including native-language posters/fliers, newspaper ads, billboards, and radio ads.
- Develop a comprehensive guide to hospital services in Spanish, Arabic, Hindi, and Korean.
- Launch aggressive media relations efforts to promote the hospital's unique commitment to meeting the needs of its "neighborhood of nations."
- Implement a comprehensive community relations program.
- Tailor a series of grand opening events to each ethnic market, with ethnic menus, appropriate dignitaries, and entertainment.
- Develop a strong community presence for customized ethnic maternity services. Include photos of the physical space and amenities in the hospital newsletter distributed to 125,000 households in the primary and secondary service areas.
- Distribute fliers to the religious institutions in the target market.

Source: Adapted from Noonan and Savolaine (2001).

Discussion Questions
- What changes taking place in American society make a one-size-fits-all healthcare system obsolete?
- What particular challenge did the community hospital face?
- What marketing techniques were utilized to address the needs of a diverse population?

- In what ways did the hospital disseminate its message to the community (rather than relying on impersonal advertising)?
- What indicators could the hospital have used to evaluate the impact of these marketing efforts?

Anticipated Future Trends

Most of the trends described in this chapter are expected to continue for the foreseeable future. The healthcare institution will remain a dominant institution, and its share of the gross national product is expected to continue to grow. Healthcare delivery will continue to be influenced by the major demographic trends affecting U.S. society, particularly the continued aging of the population and its increasing diversity. Various parties will continue to vie for influence within the system, and recent political developments have raised the prospect of healthcare reform. The growing numbers of uninsured and underinsured citizens will continue to be a concern because of the implications of this situation on the viability of the system and the health status of the population. The paradigm shift from medical care to healthcare will continue as chronic disease becomes more common than acute conditions.

Nearly all trends point to the growing importance of marketing in the healthcare system. Competition is expected to remain intense as more providers vie for fewer patients. The redefinition of the patient as consumer means healthcare organizations must become increasingly market driven. The growing role of the consumer means healthcare organizations must be more knowledgeable about their current and prospective customers than they were in the past. The growing emphasis on consumer engagement opens the door to a wide range of marketing activities.

Summary

Changes in demographic characteristics, lifestyles, and other population attributes are all contributing to the growing importance of healthcare marketing. A number of trends in the healthcare arena are expected to continue for the foreseeable future and portend a growing role for marketing professionals. Just as the form and function of the healthcare system reflect the form and function of society, the attributes of healthcare marketing reflect the nature of both the industry and the society in which it resides.

Healthcare, like any other social institution, has evolved to meet the needs of an increasingly medicalized society and has become a dominant industry as a result of that growing emphasis. The fact that healthcare now accounts for more than 15 percent of the gross national product reflects, among other trends, the growing concern of Americans for their health.

The cultural revolution in the second half of the twentieth century laid the groundwork for the emergence of a powerful healthcare system. The growing emphasis on economic success, educational achievement, and technological advancement, along with the emphasis traditionally placed on human life, humanitarian efforts, and personal autonomy, all contributed to its rise and growth. Americans' obsession with youth and beauty and a growing emphasis on self-actualization further spurred its expansion. Several demographic trends affecting the United States during the last quarter of the twentieth century also had a major impact on the nature of the healthcare institution.

Within healthcare, growing competition, the shift from inpatient care to outpatient care, the growing influence of employers, the emergence of managed care, and other developments led to a major transformation of the industry. Of particular significance was the growing appreciation of the market's role in driving demand for health services and the newfound recognition of the consumer's impact on healthcare delivery. Not only has medical care been redefined as healthcare, but the nature of the patient has also been transformed. All of these trends have contributed to the growing importance of marketing in healthcare.

Key Points

- In any society, the healthcare institution reflects the values that are important to that society.
- At the same time, the healthcare institution can exert a powerful influence on other aspects of society.
- In the United States, healthcare evolved from a cottage industry at the time of World War II to become one of the society's most powerful institutions.
- Social and cultural changes, coupled with advances in the efficacy of medical care, contributed to the ascendancy of the healthcare institution.
- During the 1980s, a number of trends emerged (most of which continue today) that resulted in the dramatic transformation of the healthcare system.
- The emergence of competition in the industry was a major factor in the introduction of healthcare marketing.

- As a result of changing consumer needs (and a shift in major health problems), the system's emphasis evolved from medical care to healthcare.
- Over time, the healthcare system became more market driven and more consumer oriented.
- Almost every trend affecting healthcare in recent years has highlighted the importance of marketing for the industry.

Discussion Questions

- Before World War II, what factors constrained the development of healthcare as a distinct institution?
- After World War II, what social and cultural developments contributed to the emergence of healthcare as a modern institution?
- What are implications of the emergence of health as a distinct value in U.S. society?
- What evidence can be offered for the medicalization of U.S. society?
- How has the "epidemiologic transition" contributed to the changing nature of U.S. healthcare?
- What factors led to the redefinition of the patient as consumer in the late twentieth century?
- What developments led to the paradigm shift from medical care to healthcare, and what were the implications of this shift for healthcare marketing?

Additional Resources

Omran, A. R. 1971. "The Epidemiologic Transition: A Theory of the Epidemiology of Population Change." *Milbank Memorial Fund Quarterly* 49: 509–38.

Thomas, R. K. 2003. *Society and Health: Sociology for Health Professionals.* New York: Springer.

BASIC MARKETING CONCEPTS

This chapter introduces the basic marketing concepts used in healthcare and other industries. Standard marketing terminology is presented, and relationships between the various concepts are outlined. Many of these concepts are foreign to healthcare, and some are problematic in the healthcare setting. However, these definitions lay the groundwork for an understanding of the marketing endeavor and help health professionals understand the language marketers use. Most of the concepts considered in this chapter are addressed in more detail in later chapters.

Marketing Concepts

Far too often, authors of textbooks dive straight into the intricacies of their subject matter without clearly defining the concepts with which they are working. They assume that the reader already has an appreciation of the basics. This assumption is often not the case and not likely to be true for those approaching healthcare marketing for the first time. For this reason, the fundamentals discussed in this text are presented here, along with a discussion of their applications in the healthcare arena.

Marketing

Marketing can be defined in a variety of ways. According to the American Marketing Association, marketing is "the process of planning and executing the conception, pricing, promotion, and distribution of ideas, goods, and services to create exchanges that satisfy individual and organizational objectives" (Bennett 1995). Another definition depicts marketing as a management process that identifies, anticipates, and supplies customer requirements efficiently and profitably. Philip Kotler, one of the early proponents of marketing in healthcare, defines marketing as a social and managerial process by which individuals and groups obtain what they need and want by creating and exchanging products and value with others (Kotler 1999).

A parsing of the first definition provides some important information about marketing. First, marketing is a process, which implies that the marketing operation involves several systematic steps. The definition specifies planning as part of the process. In other words, marketing should not be done impulsively; the execution of a marketing campaign should be well thought out. This definition notes four components of the marketing process (elsewhere referred to as the four Ps): product conception, pricing, promotion, and the distribution channels (or "place") through which the products are distributed.

Products include the ideas, goods, and/or services the organization is promoting. Ideas may involve such concepts as a hospital's image or the notion that pregnant women should receive prenatal care. Goods and services combined are thought of as products, and in healthcare, products include tangible goods, such as crutches, hospital beds, and adhesive bandages, and intangible services, such as physical examinations, immunizations, and cardiac catheterization.

The economic aspect of the marketing transaction is demonstrated by the fact that an exchange is seen as the end result of the marketing process. Thus, a physician offers medical services in exchange for money (directly from the patient or from a third party), a hospital offers physicians staff privileges in exchange for their admissions, and an insurance plan offers healthcare coverage in exchange for the insured's premiums. All of these exchanges are facilitated through marketing at some level. Ultimately, the intent of marketing is to meet the goals of the organization (as the seller) while, at the same time, meeting the goals of the customer (as the buyer). Unless the goals of both parties are met, the marketing process is considered unsuccessful.

Healthcare Marketing

When marketing is extended to the healthcare field, not all components of the original definition fit comfortably, and the process must often be modified for application to the healthcare environment. For example, providers may have limited ability to use pricing as a marketing tool because third-party payers are willing to pay only a specified amount, regardless of the provider's fee. Or, hospitals may be limited in their ability to change their locations in response to consumer demand. Thus, one challenge for healthcare marketers is to adapt marketing principles to the unique characteristics of the healthcare industry. Exhibit 3.1 moves beyond the standard definitions and talks about what marketing really is.

Market

The concept of marketing implies the existence of a market. In its original premarketing form, a market referred to a real or virtual setting in which potential buyers and potential sellers of a good or service came together for the

---

EXHIBIT 3.1
What Marketing Really Is

Most health professionals tend to think of marketing in terms of advertising, public relations, direct mail, or any number of other promotional techniques. All too often in healthcare, the term *marketing* is used to reference one of these specific functions, masking the range of activities carried out under the banner of marketing and the extent to which marketing should pervade an organization.

Marketing has been defined as any activity related to the development, packaging, pricing, and distribution of healthcare products along with any mechanisms used for promoting these products. This definition, however, does not capture the essence of marketing. Marketing is a multifaceted process that involves a wide range of activities of which the promotional piece (i.e., advertising) is a small—albeit highly visible—part. Marketing involves research, planning, strategy formulation, and a number of activities that have little to do with promotion. (Indeed, promotion is only one of the four Ps that constitute the marketing mix.)

Looked at in a less pecuniary light, marketing serves the healthcare consumer as a force for health education, an information resource, a guide to decision making, and an opportunity to make his or her perspective known. From the organization's perspective, the marketing program can provide input into strategic direction, coordinate a wide range of corporate activities, and support the development of a customer service organization. Marketing can make or break the organization's reputation and serve as the driving force in relationship development efforts.

Marketing—and marketers—are often looked at in a less than favorable light, not only in healthcare but in other industries as well. However, if one understands the true functions of marketing, marketing clearly can make a more significant contribution to the success of the organization than is generally acknowledged.

---

purpose of exchange. In this sense, it refers to both function (as in the system for exchange) and form (as in a marketplace). The notion of a market *place* has been modified to refer to the individuals or organizations in that market that are potential customers. Thus, to marketers, a market is a set of people (or organizations) who have an actual or a potential interest in a good or service or, according to Kotler (1999), a set of actual and potential buyers of a product. Alternatively, a market is defined as a group of consumers who share some characteristic that affects their needs or wants and makes them potential customers for a good or service.

Markets are often thought of in terms of a "market area"—that is, a geographical area containing the customers of a particular organization for specific goods or services. Markets may also be defined in nongeographical terms and may refer to segments of the population independent of geography. The market, however defined, is thought to generate a measurable level of "market demand," which represents the total volume of a product or service likely to be consumed by specific groups of customers in a specified market area during a specified period. (Demand is a problematic concept in healthcare. A later chapter is devoted to this topic.)

The Functions of Marketing

Now that the base definitions are out of the way, it may be worthwhile to consider what the functions of marketing in healthcare (or any other industry) actually are. The functions of marketing form a hierarchy with the broad, big-picture functions at the top and the narrow, focused functions at the bottom. The sections that follow describe the types of marketing functions at the various levels of the hierarchy.

Enterprise-Wide Functions

The most expansive marketing operations carried out by a healthcare organization affect the entire enterprise (i.e., the hospital, health system, or health plan). At this level, marketers have the following functions:

- *Conceptualizing the market.* From the perspective of the organization, a marketer's primary function may be to conceptualize the market in which the organization operates. Conceptualization means profiling the organization in terms of its attributes, determining the market it serves (and the characteristics of the market area population), assessing the environment in which healthcare functions, and otherwise determining where the organization fits into the overall scheme of things.
- *Determining strategic direction.* The marketer's functions include identifying the organization's strategic thrust (if one has been stated), examining the organization's position in the market, and identifying opportunities that might exist in the marketplace. The marketer considers various strategic options and chooses the approach that best fits the organization and the market it seeks to cultivate.

- *Supporting business goals.* The marketer supports the organization's business development by identifying segments of the market on which to focus, clarifying opportunities that exist in the marketplace, revealing the organization's position in relation to its competitors, and otherwise determining the nature of the services the market desires. A range of promotional techniques can be used to support this function.
- *Establishing a reputation.* Some marketers would argue that the essence of marketing is building and enhancing an organization's reputation. All organizations are assigned a reputation by the consuming public, whether they want one or not. Marketers are responsible for proactively creating a positive reputation, enhancing it through an integrated marketing approach, and protecting it against the efforts of competitors.

Operational Functions

Enterprise-wide marketing addresses the needs of the organization through strategy development and reputation management. Marketing also supports the narrower concerns related to the operations of the organization, as indicated by the following functions:

- *Performing marketing research.* Marketing research provides the foundation for all other marketing functions. On an ongoing basis, the marketer should delineate the service area for the organization, specify the service area's characteristics and population, and analyze the competition. Marketing research should identify opportunities that exist in the market in terms of growing demand, underserved populations, and/or new product potential.
- *Developing a marketing plan.* Health professionals often neglect to develop systematic plans for accomplishing their goals, and in marketing, there is a tendency to rush into a marketing campaign without an overarching plan. The marketing plan should reflect the goals and objectives established by the organization, not just for marketing but also for overall organizational advancement. The marketer's primary responsibility is to ensure that a well-conceived marketing plan is in place before any promotional activities are implemented.
- *Coordinating enterprise-wide promotional efforts.* One of the first things any marketer should do is to identify all existing promotional efforts that are under way on the part of the organization. Existing marketing efforts should be evaluated and standards developed to ensure a consistent message across all promotional activities. The marketer should coordinate the marketing efforts of the various entities in the

organization and serve as a liaison between internal marketing efforts and external marketing resources.

- *Developing relationships.* Many would argue that the primary goal of marketing is to develop relationships, which is also an area of emphasis in contemporary healthcare. Relationships may involve patients and other customers, referring physicians, health plans, business partners, government representatives, and a host of other entities with whom the healthcare organization needs to maintain relationships. The marketer has a key role in most aspects of developing and maintaining relationships.

- *Creating a marketing organization.* Organizations' marketing efforts often overlook their own employees. Healthcare organizations can establish a marketing mind-set among their employees via internal marketing, thereby turning every associate into a salesperson and creating a marketing organization. Ideally, every employee should have some marketing skills, and every decision should be made with marketing implications in mind. The marketer is responsible for ensuring that marketing is incorporated into the organization's DNA.

Educational Functions

An important but sometimes overlooked function of marketing is educating the public. As indicated in the following list, providing information to existing and prospective customers, referring physicians, potential donors, and other constituent groups is a major responsibility of marketing professionals.

- *Educating patients and the general public.* With the introduction of new products and the emergence of informed consumers, healthcare organizations must build awareness of their services and expose target audiences to their capabilities. Healthcare consumers have short attention spans, and the public must be continuously reminded of the organization's availability. For some, the educational function of marketing takes precedence over all other functions.

- *Providing information and referral resources.* Healthcare organizations are considered an important resource for the community. Not only does marketing make consumers aware of the organization's services; it also fulfills the organization's responsibility to educate the community with regard to positive health behavior. In community after community, the most trusted healthcare organizations are those that are perceived as reliable sources of health information.

- *Enhancing visibility and corporate image.* With the increasing standardization of healthcare services and a growing appreciation of reputation, healthcare organizations find it necessary to initiate marketing campaigns that improve top-of-mind awareness and distinguish them from their competitors. Consumers are bombarded by ever-increasing message "clutter," and marketers must be able to communicate the organization's message effectively to maintain a high level of visibility and promote a positive corporate image.

- *Differentiating the organization and its services.* At a time when it is increasingly difficult for healthcare consumers to distinguish one healthcare organization from another, a marketer needs to impress upon the target audience how his or her organization is different from its competitors and why consumers should care about the difference. In the unlikely case that little or no differences exist, the marketer must make a creative case that establishes a competitive advantage.

Promotional Functions

Promotional activities are generally the first things that come to mind when the topic of marketing comes up. The functions described in the following list relate to the day-to-day activities of marketers in a healthcare setting.

- *Influencing consumer decision making.* With consumers now taking a more active role in healthcare decision making, marketers have an unprecedented opportunity to make a case for their organization. After building awareness on the part of consumers, the marketer's next responsibility is to influence consumer behavior. Marketers should be sensitive to the stage of readiness of various customer groups and implement marketing techniques accordingly.
- *Improving market penetration.* Healthcare organizations faced with growing competition can use marketing as a means of increasing patient volumes and growing market share. With few new patients in many markets, marketing becomes critical to retaining existing customers and attracting competitors' customers. Marketers are well positioned to identify opportunities in the marketplace and implement programs that will attract customers and increase market penetration. If the organization cannot establish a favorable position in the market, its competitors will dictate its position.
- *Increasing profit.* On the surface, we might assume that the raison d'être for healthcare marketing should be to increase profits and, hence, should be first among marketing functions. The obvious conclusion may not be the most appropriate conclusion in healthcare, given the high proportion of not-for-profit organizations in the industry and the need to satisfy other goals in addition to bottom-line profits. More important, perhaps, is the need to perform a wide range of other functions before the profit motive can even be considered.

- *Winning awards versus being effective.* Note that the previous statements say nothing about winning awards for marketing campaigns. For many marketing professionals who entered healthcare from other industries, the goal was to sponsor award-winning media campaigns that involved flashy promotional materials or award-winning television spots. Unfortunately, there appears to be little correlation between receiving accolades for marketing campaigns and the success of the organization being promoted. For whatever reason, decision makers and those paying for services in healthcare are less influenced by slick advertising campaigns than they are by the actual substance offered by the healthcare organization.

Marketing Techniques

The action dimension of marketing is embodied in the techniques marketers use to support the functions outlined in the previous lists. On a day-to-day basis, marketers are likely to pay less attention to the lofty goals of the marketing endeavor than they are to concrete marketing activities. The techniques marketers use to achieve their objectives are summarized here and described in more detail in a later chapter.

Public Relations

Public relations (often called *PR*) is a form of communication management that uses publicity and other nonpaid forms of promotion and information to influence feelings, opinions, or beliefs about an organization and its products. The PR function is carried out through press releases, press conferences, distribution of feature stories to the media, public service announcements, and other publicity-oriented activities. In the past, healthcare organizations have used PR to manage crises and control damage, justify questionable actions, explain negative events, and so forth. Over time, however, PR has been cast in a more proactive light as healthcare organizations have come to appreciate the benefits of a strong PR program.

Communications

Large healthcare organizations typically establish mechanisms for communicating with their publics (internal and external). Communications staff develops materials to disseminate to the public and to the employees of the organization, generates internal newsletters and publications geared to relevant customer groups (e.g., patients, enrollees), and develops patient education materials. Separate communications departments may be established, or this function may overlap with the public relations or community outreach functions. Marketers expend a great deal of effort in determining the best approaches to communication. Exhibit 3.2 discusses communication concepts applied to healthcare marketing.

EXHIBIT 3.2
Communication Theories in Marketing

Communication refers to the transmission or exchange of information and implies the sharing of meaning among those who are communicating. Students of marketing have expended considerable effort in specifying models of communication that relate to the marketing process. Communication in marketing may be directed at (1) initiating actions; (2) making needs and requirements known; (3) exchanging information, ideas, attitudes, and beliefs; (4) establishing understanding; and/or (5) establishing and maintaining relations.

Communications in marketing can occur in a variety of ways:

- *Face-to-face communication* includes formal meetings, interviews, and informal contact.
- *Oral communication* includes telephone contact, public address systems, and video conferencing systems.
- *Written communication* includes letters (external), memoranda (internal), e-mail, reports, forms, notice boards, journals, bulletins, newsletters, and manuals.
- *Visual communication* includes charts, films, slides, video, and video conferencing.
- *Electronic communication* includes Internet chat, voice mail, and electronic data interchange.

A number of communication models have been developed for application to marketing, and Berkowitz (2006) has adapted one of these models for healthcare. According to Berkowitz, this marketing communication model has the following nine components in healthcare. An understanding of each of these components is important for effective marketing communication.

1. *Sender.* The sender is the party sending the message to the other party. Also referred to as the communicator or the source, the sender is the "who" of the process and takes the form of a person, company, or spokesperson for someone else.

(continued)

EXHIBIT 3.2 (*continued*)

2. *Message.* The message is the combination of symbols and words the sender wishes to transmit to the receiver. The message is the "what" of the process and indicates the content the sender wants to convey.

3. *Encoding.* Encoding is the process of translating the meaning of the message into symbolic form (e.g., words, signs, sounds). At this point, a concept is converted into something transmittable.

4. *Channel.* The channel is the means used to deliver a marketing message from sender to receiver. The channel is the "how" of the process and connects the sender to the receiver.

5. *Receiver.* The receiver is the party receiving the message, also known as the audience or the destination. Marketing efforts are directed toward a receiver.

6. *Decoding.* Decoding refers to the process carried out when the receiver converts the "symbols" transmitted by the sender into a form that makes sense to him or her. This process works under the assumption that the receiver is using the same basis for decoding that the sender used for encoding.

7. *Response.* Response refers to the receiver's reaction to the message. At this point, the effect of the message is gauged in terms of the meaning the receiver attaches to it.

8. *Feedback.* Feedback refers to the aspect of the receiver's response that the receiver communicates back to the sender. The type of feedback depends on the channel, and the effectiveness of the effort is gauged in terms of the feedback.

9. *Noise.* Noise refers to any factor that prevents the receiver from decoding a message in the way the sender intended. Noise can be generated by the sender, the receiver, the message, the channel, the environment, and so forth.

   The marketing communication process could be unsuccessful for any number of reasons. Factors that might influence this process include selective attention on the part of the receiver, selective distortion on the part of the receiver (e.g., changing the message to fit preconceptions), selective recall (i.e., the receiver absorbs only part of the message), and message rehearsal (i.e., the message reminds the receiver of related issues that tend to distract from the point of the message).

Communication experts indicate that effective communication requires certain attributes: It must contain value for the receiver; be meaningful, relevant, and understandable; and be transmittable in a few seconds. Further, the communication must lend itself to visual presentation, if possible; be relevant to the lives of everyday people; and stimulate the receiver emotionally. Marketing communication must also be interesting, entertaining, and stimulating.

Source: Adapted from Berkowitz (2006).

Community Outreach

Community outreach is a form of marketing that seeks to present the organization's programs to the community and establish relationships with community organizations. Community outreach may involve episodic activities, such as health fairs or educational programs for community residents, or it may involve ongoing initiatives carried out by outreach workers who are visible in the community. This aspect of marketing emphasizes the organization's commitment to the community and its support of local organizations. Community outreach initiatives seek to generate word-of-mouth communication concerning the organization and/or its services.

Government Relations

Long before most healthcare organizations considered incorporating a formal marketing function, they were involved in government relations activities. Healthcare organizations are typically regulated by state and federal government agencies. Decisions related to adding, eliminating, or changing a service may be constrained by government regulations, and the reimbursement available to healthcare providers may be controlled by government agencies. Not-for-profit organizations must continuously demonstrate that they deserve their tax-exempt status. For these reasons, healthcare organizations must maintain discourse with a variety of government agencies, cultivate relationships with politicians and other policymakers, and often initiate lobbying activities directed toward various levels of government.

Networking

Networking involves developing and nurturing relationships with individuals and organizations with which mutually beneficial transactions can be carried out. Physicians and other clinicians who, until recently, would never deign to advertise actively network among their colleagues. Networking may take the form of a specialist casually running into potential referring physicians at the country club or a hospital administrator attending meetings that might involve potential clients, partners, or referral agents. Networking is particularly effective when dealing with parties who are reluctant to provide "face time" or when one prefers an informal setting involving personal interaction when getting to know prospective business associates.

Sales Promotion

Sales promotion involves any activities or materials that act as a direct inducement to customers by offering added value to a product. Sales promotions are more likely to be associated with the sale of consumer health products (e.g., rebates) or business-to-business healthcare sales (e.g., low-interest financing) than with the provision of health services. The sales promotion mix might involve health fairs and trade shows, exhibits, demonstrations, contests and games, premiums and gifts, rebates, low-interest financing, and trade-in allowances. Sales promotion is separate from, but often an adjunct to, personal sales.

Advertising

Advertising refers to any paid form of nonpersonal presentation or promotion of ideas, goods, or services by an identifiable sponsor transmitted via mass media for purposes of achieving marketing objectives. The advertising mix might include print advertisements, electronic advertisements, mailings, catalogs, brochures, posters, directories, outdoor advertisements, and displays. These activities are organized in the form of an advertising campaign that involves designing a series of advertisements and placing them in various advertising media to reach a target market.

Personal Sales

Personal sales involve the oral presentation of promotional material in a conversation with one or more prospective purchasers for the purpose of making sales. The salesperson attempts to foster a mutually profitable economic exchange between buyer and seller through interpersonal contact. The success of personal sales depends on the seller's ability to communicate the product's qualities and its benefits for the buyer. The personal selling mix might include sales presentations, sales meetings, incentive programs, distribution of samples, and participation in health fairs and trade shows.

Database Marketing

Database marketing involves establishing and exploiting data on past and current customers and future prospects in a way that allows effective marketing

strategies to be implemented. Database marketing can be used for any purpose that can benefit from access to customer information. These functions
may include evaluating new prospects, cross-selling related products, launching new products to potential prospects, identifying new distribution channels, building customer loyalty, converting occasional users to regular users,
generating inquiries and follow-up sales, and establishing niche marketing
initiatives. The database established for this purpose often provides the basis
for customer relationship management and may be an integral part of an
organization's call center.

Direct Marketing

Direct marketing targets groups or individuals with specific characteristics, and
promotional messages are transmitted directly to them. These promotional
activities may take the form of direct mail or telemarketing, as well as other approaches aimed at specific individuals. Increasingly, the Internet is being used
for direct marketing. An advantage of direct marketing is that the message can
be customized to meet the needs of target populations.

Customer Relationship Management

Customer relationship management (CRM) is a business strategy designed
to optimize profitability, revenue, and customer satisfaction by focusing on
customer relationships rather than transactions. Although long used in other
industries, CRM is relatively new to healthcare. The industry's lack of focus
on customer characteristics and its limited data management capabilities have
slowed the acceptance of CRM in healthcare. However, the new market-driven
environment is encouraging healthcare organizations to develop and use customer databases.

Social Marketing

In healthcare, social marketing involves applying commercial marketing techniques to influence the attitudes, knowledge, and behavior of target audiences
related to the improvement of individual and community health status. Social
marketing differs from other types of marketing only with respect to the objectives of marketers and their organizations. Social marketers seek to influence
social behaviors for the benefit of their target audience and general society, not
for the benefit of the marketing organization. In contrast to the top-down approach of traditional marketing, social marketers listen to the needs and desires
of the target audience and build the marketing campaign from the bottom up.

Case Study 3.1 describes a marketing campaign that uses a variety of
marketing techniques.

CASE STUDY 3.1
Capturing the "Older Adult" Market

Many healthcare organizations came to see the aging of the baby boom generation as an opportunity to expand their services. Regional Medical Center* responded to this opportunity by establishing a service line devoted to "older adults." The intent was to capture the business—and the loyalty—of this large, relatively affluent, and increasingly needy segment of the population. The service line was designed to meet the emerging needs of this population for specialty services such as cardiology, orthopedics, ophthalmology, and urology in a manner that was appealing to this relatively demanding consumer population.

Because this service was considered innovative in the community served by Regional Medical Center, an aggressive promotional campaign was undertaken. The Center's marketing department considered a wide range of marketing options and decided on a multipronged campaign to approach the target population from a variety of directions. The first phase of the promotional campaign focused on internal marketing. It was important that the Center's employees be familiar with this new program and be able to articulate its merits to potential customers. Many of the customers for the new program were likely to be existing patients of Regional Medical Center.

Well before the new program was scheduled to open, an aggressive PR campaign was initiated. Press releases were distributed, articles were prepared for local publications and professional journals, and celebrity spokespersons were lined up. Simple yet attractive collateral materials were developed for distribution to prospective customers and to referral agents who might channel customers to the Center. Information was distributed to other providers and organizations that might serve other needs of the target population, and the community's major insurance plans were made aware of the new program and its benefits. Tours of the facility housing the new program were provided to key constituents such as referring physicians and health plan representatives, and open houses were scheduled for both medical professionals and the general public.

The marketing initiative also involved direct solicitation of members of the target population. The Center extracted data from its internal database on existing customers and purchased mailing lists of households that included members aged 50–65. Using the findings from previous research on the "buttons to push" in this age cohort, materials were prepared that would appeal to the particular needs of this population. The address lists were then used to mail materials directly to the target population.

While the Center did not want to rely on expensive media advertising for attracting customers, its marketers felt that some media presence was necessary, not only to attract customers who might be missed through the direct-mail campaign but also to make the general public aware of this new program. In some cases, other family members might be making decisions for the older adult population, and awareness of this program on the part of the general public was considered important. After careful research on the communication attributes of the target population, a series of newspaper, radio, and television advertisements were produced. These advertisements were placed in the sections of the local newspaper that members of this age group read, aired on the radio stations they preferred, and presented on the television channels they viewed most often. For the electronic media, particular attention was paid to the time of day and day of the week members of the target population were expected to be engaged.

The success of the new older adult service line offered by Regional Medical Center during the first year exceeded the expectations of the Center's administrators. While it is difficult to determine which of the various promotional techniques had the most impact on the program's early success, the Center's marketing staff concluded on the basis of its evaluation of the campaign that it was the integrated approach—a variety of coordinated activities—that led to the successful program launch.

*"Regional Medical Center" is a fictional name for the organization on which this case study is based.

Discussion Questions

- Why did Regional Medical Center think that this population presented enough of an opportunity to establish an entirely new program?
- What information did the Center need to gather about this target population before the program could be established?
- What information did the Center need to gather about this target population before the marketing campaign could be planned?
- What were the different paths through which the Center attempted to reach the target audience?
- Which marketing techniques did the Center use to reach the target population?
- Why was internal marketing an important first step in marketing this new program?

Levels of Marketing

Marketers employ marketing strategies that reflect the audience they are soliciting. A campaign aimed at the general population will involve a different approach than one targeting a population subgroup. Depending on the circumstances, the approach may include mass marketing, target marketing, or micromarketing.

Mass Marketing

Mass marketing involves the development of generic messages that are widely broadcast to the entire service area. There is no attempt to target specific audiences, identify likely best customers, or tailor the message to a particular subgroup. This approach involves the use of mass media (e.g., newspaper, radio, television) to blanket the market area. The message has to be general and typically touts the merits of the organization rather than any specific services.

Hospitals' use of mass marketing in the past reflected their desire to promote the organization overall (rather than specific services) and the belief that they could be all things to all people. No attempt was made to distinguish between different segments of the population, and only the crudest distinction based on geography was made between markets. This type of approach is effective at disseminating a small amount of information to a large number of people and can be useful when marketing a basic product that appeals to a homogenous audience.

Target Marketing

Target marketing refers to marketing initiatives that focus on a market segment to which an organization desires to offer goods and/or services. Target marketing is the opposite of mass marketing, which aims promotional efforts at the total market. Target markets in healthcare may be defined on the basis of geography, demographics, lifestyles, insurance coverage, usage rates, and/or other customer attributes. Thus, target marketing is likely to involve the use of customer segmentation systems.

Micromarketing

Micromarketing is a form of target marketing. Companies that use micromarketing tailor their marketing programs to the needs and wants of consumers narrowly defined in terms of geography, demographics, psychographics, or the benefits they desire. Customers and potential customers are identified at the household or individual level and marketed to directly using customized communication techniques. Micromarketing is most effective when marketers want to reach consumers with a narrow range of attributes.

Healthcare Products and Customers

The definition of marketing offered early in this chapter refers to the promotion of ideas, goods, or services. (The term *product*, used throughout the text, is often used interchangeably with healthcare *service*.) As mentioned in previous chapters, the product to be marketed in healthcare is often difficult to specify, unlike the products of other industries. Most of what healthcare organizations offer takes the form of services, and, unlike goods, they tend to be harder to precisely describe.

In addition, the nature of the product in healthcare has changed dramatically over the past couple of decades. Twenty years ago, one could define the product simply as a medical procedure, an orthotic device to correct a physical disability, or a consumer health product. In today's climate, healthcare products include not only these traditional products but also such products and services as prepaid health insurance plans offered by health maintenance organizations or a group purchasing contract offered by a provider network. (The nature of healthcare products is discussed further in Chapter 7.)

Many healthcare organizations offer a variety of products to their customers. Certainly, the hospital is an example of an organization that offers a wide range of services and goods. A major hospital offers hundreds, if not thousands, of different procedures. In addition, hospitals offer a variety of goods (in the form of drugs, supplies, and equipment) that are charged to the customer. One can describe an organization's product mix as it relates to the combination of services, goods, and even ideas it offers. These concepts are addressed in the sections that follow.

Ideas

Much of what healthcare organizations promote takes the form of *ideas*—intangible concepts that are intended to convey a perception to the consumer. The organization's image is an idea that is likely to be conveyed through marketing activities. The organization may want to promote the perception of quality care, professionalism, value, or some other subjective attribute. The development of a brand, for example, involves the marketing of an idea. The intent is to establish a mind-set that places the organization at the top of the consumer's mind on the assumption that familiarity will breed use.

When healthcare organizations first incorporated advertising, most of the attention was focused on promoting ideas. In particular, early marketers attempted to promote the organization's image and establish it as the preferred provider in its market. Although the trend has shifted away from image advertising and toward service advertising, many healthcare organizations continue to market ideas to their target audiences.

Goods

For the purposes of this text, products can refer to goods or services. A *good* is a tangible product that is typically purchased in an impersonal setting on a one-at-a-time basis. The purchase of a good tends to be a one-shot episode, while the purchase of services may be fulfilled through an ongoing process. Although healthcare is generally perceived in terms of a service, the sale of goods is ubiquitous in the industry. Consumer health products (e.g., adhesive bandages, condoms, toothpaste) are household products. Pharmaceuticals—whether prescription or over the counter—are purchased by nearly everyone at some point. Consumers are even gaining access to home testing kits and therapeutic equipment, and the sale/rental of durable medical equipment is a major industry. Even in a hospital setting, the bill for care is likely to include a number of goods among the itemized charges.

Services

Relative to goods, *services* are difficult to conceptualize. Services (e.g., physical examinations) are intangible in that they do not take the concrete form of goods (e.g., drugs). Services are more difficult to quantify, and consumers evaluate them differently from tangible products. Because services are often more personal (especially in the case of healthcare), they are likely to be assessed in subjective rather than objective terms. They are variable in that they cannot be subjected to the quality controls placed on goods but reflect the variations that characterize the human beings who provide the services. Services are inseparable from the producer in that they are dispensed on the spot without separation from the provider. Services are perishable in that they cannot be stored, and once provided, they have no residual value. Finally, services defy ownership rules in that, unlike goods, they do not involve transfer of tangible property from the seller to the buyer.

Consumers

Consumer, as the term is usually used in healthcare, refers to any individual or organization that is a potential purchaser of a healthcare product. (This definition differs from the more economics-based notion of a consumer as the entity that actually *consumes* the product.) Theoretically, everyone is a potential consumer of health services, and consumer research, for example, is generally aimed at the public at large. The consumer is often the end user of a good or service but may not necessarily be the purchaser. The term *consumer behavior* refers to the utilization patterns and purchasing practices of the population of a market area.

Customers

In healthcare, the *customer* is typically thought of as the actual purchaser of a good or service. Although a patient may be a customer for certain goods and services, the end user (e.g., the patient) is often not the customer. Someone else may make the purchase on behalf of the patient. Further, treatment decisions may be made by someone other than the patient. For this reason, hospitals and other complex healthcare organizations are likely to serve a range of customers, including patients, referral agents, admitting physicians, employers, and a variety of other parties who may purchase goods or services from the organization. For this reason, the customer identification process in healthcare is more complicated than it is in other industries.

Clients

A *client* is a type of customer that consumes services rather than goods. A client relationship implies personal (rather than impersonal) interaction and an ongoing relationship (rather than a single encounter). Professionals typically have clients, whereas retailers, for example, have customers or purchasers. The relationships between service providers and clients are likely to be more symmetrical than the relationships between service providers and patients, who are typically dependent and powerless relative to the service provider. Many also believe the term *client* implies more respect than the term *patient*.

Patients

Although the term *patient* is used loosely in informal discussion, a patient is someone who has been defined as sick by a physician. This definition almost always implies formal contact with a clinical facility (e.g., physician's office, hospital). Technically, a symptomatic individual does not become a patient until a physician officially designates the individual as such, even if the prospective patient has consumed over-the-counter drugs and taken other measures for self-care. Under this scenario, an individual remains a patient until discharged from medical care.

Nonphysician clinicians may treat patients, but because they do not provide medical services, they are discouraged from using the term. For example, behavioral health counselors are likely to refer to their patients as clients. Dependent practitioners, who work under the supervision of physicians (e.g., physical therapists), however, are likely to define their charges as patients.

Enrollees

Although health insurance plans have historically called their customers *enrollees*, use of this term has only recently become common among healthcare providers. However, with the ascendancy of managed care as a major force in healthcare, other healthcare organizations began to adopt this term. Thus, providers who contracted to provide services for members of a health plan began to think in terms of enrollees. This shift in nomenclature is significant because enrollees and patients have different attributes. Enrollees may also be referred to as *members, insureds,* or *covered lives.* Exhibit 3.3 discusses how different definitions of healthcare customers have implications for the operation of the system.

EXHIBIT 3.3
What's in a Name: Implications of Redefining the Patient

One of the developments in healthcare over the past couple of decades that has significant implications for marketing is the redefinition of health services users. The historical term *patient* is being replaced by *consumer, client,* and *customer.* Although the nomenclature changed in part to reflect the different parties that deal with the patient, this redefinition represents a paradigm shift in the system's orientation toward the health services user.

The term *patient* refers to a person who is formally under the care of a physician. Although other clinicians may also refer to their charges as patients, the term implies that a symptomatic person has been formally diagnosed as sick and now takes on a new set of attributes. Conceptually, a patient is more clearly differentiated from a nonpatient than, for example, a customer is from a noncustomer.

The patient role (also referred to as the "sick role"), like any social role, involves certain characteristics. Someone performing this role is considered to be "abnormal" and, thus, different in important ways from other people. The patient role implies a degree of helplessness and a state of dependence on clinicians and health facilities. It also implies a condition of relative powerlessness and an inability to take an active part in the therapeutic process. A patient is also typically characterized by a relative lack of knowledge concerning the situation in question. The patient remains in this role until officially discharged by a physician.

A client is similar to a patient in many ways. In the healthcare context, a client is a patient of a nonphysician. Outside of healthcare, a client is someone who uses the services of a professional, and certain health professionals, including mental health professionals, social workers, and other nonmedical personnel, may refer to their customers as clients.

The difference between patients and clients extends well beyond the different professionals involved. Being a client involves a more symmetrical power relationship with the service provider than that involved in the doctor–patient relationship. Clients are typically not thought of as being dependent to the extent that patients are, and clients can fire their providers much more readily than patients can fire their doctors. Thus, a client is theoretically less dependent, more involved in the decision-making process, and more knowledgeable about the issue at hand than a patient is. Ultimately, a client has more control over the situation than a patient does.

As healthcare became more marketing oriented, terms like *consumer* and *customer* were introduced. Although some purists may consider use of these terms a sacrilege, the fact is that, like it or not, patients are steadily taking on the characteristics of consumers and customers, not because of redefinition by marketers but because of the dramatic changes that have occurred in healthcare.

For our purposes, a consumer is anyone who has the potential to consume a healthcare good or service. In other industries, a consumer is often thought of as the end user of the product, but this is not necessarily a comfortable concept in healthcare. From a marketing perspective, anyone could be considered a consumer because nearly everyone is a potential user of health services. Whereas patients or clients are effectively under the direction, if not control, of health professionals, consumers are thought to independently determine the choices they make with regard to consuming health services. Thus, the consumer decision-making process is referred to more often than the patient decision-making process, which implies that the consumer is objectively evaluating options with regard to health services and making choices based on the variety of factors that affect decision making with regard to other goods and services.

A customer, for our purposes, is a consumer who is currently consuming a good or service. The customer has chosen, for whatever reason, to purchase a healthcare product or use a healthcare service. In many cases, this definition may be synonymous with the concept of patient, but from a marketing perspective, customers are thought of in different terms.

Unlike a patient (even if it is the same person), a customer is someone who is knowledgeable about the available options and has made a rational choice with regard to consuming particular goods

(continued)

EXHIBIT 3.3 (*continued*)

or services. A customer is considered to be more independent and assertive than a patient and is likely to have expectations that are different from those of patients. A patient might be concerned about humane treatment and effective outcomes, whereas a customer is also likely to expect fast, efficient service, convenient locations, respectful treatment by practitioners, value for the money, and a meaningful role in the process.

This new patient-customer is having a major impact on the healthcare system, and the baby boom generation now coming to dominate the patient pool epitomizes this new patient-customer. These persons want the outcomes of the healthcare system as patients and, at the same time, the benefits of being a customer. This development not only has implications for the delivery of care but also is important from a marketing perspective. Marketers solicit customers and patients in different ways. Customers and patients bring different traits to the examination room and use different criteria for measuring their satisfaction with services.

Healthcare marketers must be able to recognize the differences among the various users of health services and adapt marketing approaches accordingly. Clearly, the marketing approach taken, the message, the medium, and the means of evaluation will differ depending on whether the marketer is addressing patients, clients, consumers, or customers.

The Four Ps of Marketing

The marketing mix is the set of controllable variables that an organization involved in marketing uses to influence the target market. The mix includes product, price, place, and promotion. These four Ps have long been the basis for marketing strategy in other industries and are increasingly being considered by healthcare organizations. However, as will be seen, these aspects of the marketing mix do not necessarily have the same meaning for health professionals as they do for marketers in other industries.

Product

The first P, the *product* of healthcare, represents what healthcare providers are marketing. The product takes the form of goods, services, or ideas offered by a healthcare organization. The product is difficult to precisely define in healthcare, which creates a challenge for healthcare marketers. As noted above, products can refer to goods or services. A good is a tangible product that is typically purchased in an impersonal setting on a one-at-a-time basis. Services (e.g., physical examinations), on the other hand, are difficult to conceptualize and are intangible in that they do not take the concrete form of goods. For example, if a psychiatric problem is being treated with drugs, the product is easy to specify (e.g., so many pills of a certain dose per day). If the same condition is being treated through counseling, the description of the product is not as precise or standardized (e.g., an unpredictable number of counseling sessions).

In the past, healthcare providers seldom gave much thought to the product concept. A surgical procedure was considered just that and not something that had to be packaged. Today, however, the design of the product, its perceived attributes, and its packaging are all becoming more important concerns for healthcare providers and healthcare marketers.

Price

Price refers to the amount charged for a product, including the fees, charges, premium contributions, deductibles, copayments, and other out-of-pocket costs to consumers of health services. In economic terms, price is thought of in terms of an exchange. In other words, a healthcare provider offers a service in exchange for its customers' dollars. An employee paying an annual premium to a health plan, an insurance company reimbursing a physician's fee, or a consumer purchasing over-the-counter drugs are all exchanges involving a price. The price to the customer could also include the pain, discomfort, embarrassment, anxiety, frustration, and other emotional costs of dealing with providers, plans, and the disease or injury that prompted the experience. An obvious objective of marketing is to convince consumers that they will receive benefits for the price they pay.

Given the manner in which financing is structured in healthcare, price has not historically been a basis for competition. The issue of pricing for health services is a growing concern for marketers as the healthcare environment changes, and a number of factors are increasing the role of the pricing variable in developing a marketing strategy. For marketers, the challenge is understanding what a customer is willing to exchange for some want-satisfying good or service and developing a pricing approach compatible with the organization's goals and cost constraints.

Place

The third P, *place*, represents the manner in which goods or services are distributed for consumer use. Place relates to all factors of the transaction or relationship experience that make it easy rather than difficult for consumers to obtain an organization's products. Although the obvious factors of location and layout are included, so are hours, access, obstacles, waits for appointments, claims payment, and so on. In most cases, negative place aspects of an encounter impose such costs as lost time, frustration in finding the service site, parking fees, boredom, or other emotional burdens. Positive place aspects usually nullify such costs. For example, when a physician offers early morning or evening hours, patients can obtain care on the way to or from work and thus avoid having to take time off from their jobs.

In some cases, place factors may enhance perceptions of the product's quality, as when the physician's office or hospital is in a trendy location or on a campus that facilitates efficient treatment. Systems or health plans may speed up scheduling by allowing patients to make appointments over the Internet, for example. The online availability of medical records has added a different dimension to the concept of place. Allowing patients to sign up for health plans, check their status, and make benefit changes online at a work-site kiosk or home computer also adds place value.

Promotion

Promotion is the fourth P of the marketing mix. For many people, promotion has historically meant advertising, and advertising has meant marketing. Promotion represents any way of informing the marketplace that the organization has developed a response to meet its needs. Promotion involves a range of tactics involving publicity, advertising, and personal selling.

Promotion covers all forms of marketing communication and includes materials that deliver content in addition to those that foster transactions. For example, health plans can devise communications that help new members better understand their coverage, thereby enabling them to use their health plan more effectively. Providers can advise new patients on how to avoid place frustrations and costs, and address symptoms and concerns online before appointments to improve quality and patient satisfaction. The "promotional mix" describes the combination of techniques used by the marketer to achieve promotional goals.

Applying the Four Ps

Many observers find applying the traditional four Ps of the marketing mix to healthcare problematic. Some believe these dimensions of marketing are inappropriate for a service-oriented organization like healthcare. The uncomfortable fit between the four Ps of marketing and healthcare has even led some to pronounce the death of the four Ps and suggest their replacement with some other, more appropriate model in healthcare. Indeed, in today's competitive environment, some contend that additional Ps should be added to the list. Exhibit 3.4 presents an update of the four Ps for healthcare.

EXHIBIT 3.4
The 7 Ps of Marketing
By Brian Tracy

Once you've developed your marketing strategy, there is a "Seven P Formula" you should use to continually evaluate and reevaluate your business activities. These seven are: product, price, promotion, place, packaging, positioning and people. As products, markets, customers and needs change rapidly, you must continually revisit these seven Ps to make sure you're on track and achieving the maximum results possible for you in today's marketplace.

Product

To begin with, develop the habit of looking at your product as though you were an outside marketing consultant brought in to help your company decide whether or not it's in the right business at this time. Ask critical questions such as, "Is your current product or service, or mix of products and services, appropriate and suitable for the market and the customers of today?"

Whenever you're having difficulty selling as much of your products or services as you'd like, you need to develop the habit of assessing your business honestly and asking, "Are these the right products or services for our customers today?"

Is there any product or service you're offering today that, knowing what you now know, you would not bring out again today? Compared to your competitors, is your product or service superior in some significant way to anything else available? If so, what is it? If not, could you develop an area of superiority? Should you be offering this product or service at all in the current marketplace?

Price

The second P in the formula is price. Develop the habit of continually examining and reexamining the prices of the products and services you sell to make sure they're still appropriate to the realities of the current market. Sometimes you need to lower your prices. At other times, it may be appropriate to raise your prices. Many companies have found that the profitability of certain products or services doesn't justify the amount of effort and resources that go into producing them. By raising their prices, they may lose a percentage of their customers, but the remaining percentage generates a profit on every sale. Could this be appropriate for you?

(continued)

EXHIBIT 3.4 (*continued*)

Sometimes you need to change your terms and conditions of sale. Sometimes, by spreading your price over a series of months or years, you can sell far more than you are today, and the interest you can charge will more than make up for the delay in cash receipts. Sometimes you can combine products and services together with special offers and special promotions. Sometimes you can include free additional items that cost you very little to produce but make your prices appear far more attractive to your customers.

In business, as in nature, whenever you experience resistance or frustration in any part of your sales or marketing activities, be open to revisiting that area. Be open to the possibility that your current pricing structure is not ideal for the current market. Be open to the need to revise your prices, if necessary, to remain competitive, to survive and thrive in a fast-changing marketplace.

Promotion

The third habit in marketing and sales is to think in terms of promotion all the time. Promotion includes all the ways you tell your customers about your products or services and how you then market and sell to them. Small changes in the way you promote and sell your products can lead to dramatic changes in your results. Even small changes in your advertising can lead immediately to higher sales. Experienced copywriters can often increase the response rate from advertising by 500 percent by simply changing the headline on an advertisement.

Large and small companies in every industry continually experiment with different ways of advertising, promoting, and selling their products and services. And here is the rule: Whatever method of marketing and sales you're using today will, sooner or later, stop working. Sometimes it will stop working for reasons you know, and sometimes it will be for reasons you don't know. In either case, your methods of marketing and sales will eventually stop working, and you'll have to develop new sales, marketing and advertising approaches, offerings, and strategies.

Place

The fourth P in the marketing mix is the place where your product or service is actually sold. Develop the habit of reviewing and reflecting upon the exact location where the customer meets the salesperson. Sometimes a change in place can lead to a rapid increase in sales.

You can sell your product in many different places. Some companies use direct selling, sending their salespeople out to personally meet and talk with the prospect. Some sell by telemarketing. Some sell through catalogs or mail order. Some sell at trade shows or in retail establishments. Some sell in joint ventures with other similar products or services. Some companies use manufacturers' representatives or distributors. Many companies use a combination of one or more of these methods.

In each case, the entrepreneur must make the right choice about the very best location or place for the customer to receive essential buying information on the product or service needed to make a buying decision. What is yours? In what way should you change it? Where else could you offer your products or services?

Packaging

The fifth element in the marketing mix is the packaging. Develop the habit of standing back and looking at every visual element in the packaging of your product or service through the eyes of a critical prospect. Remember, people form their first impression about you within the first 30 seconds of seeing you or some element of your company. Small improvements in the packaging or external appearance of your product or service can often lead to completely different reactions from your customers.

Packaging refers to the way your product or service appears from the outside. Packaging also refers to your people and how they dress and groom. It refers to your offices, your waiting rooms, your brochures, your correspondence and every single visual element about your company. Everything counts. Everything helps or hurts. Everything affects your customer's confidence about dealing with you.

Positioning

The next P is positioning. You should develop the habit of thinking continually about how you are positioned in the hearts and minds of your customers. How do people think and talk about you when you're not present? How do people think and talk about your company? What positioning do you have in your market, in terms of the specific words people use when they describe you and your offerings to others?

In the famous book by Al Reis and Jack Trout, *Positioning*, the authors point out that how you are seen and thought about by your customers is the critical determinant of your success in a competitive

(continued)

EXHIBIT 3.4 (*continued*)

marketplace. Attribution theory says that most customers think of you in terms of a single attribute, either positive or negative. Sometimes it's "service." Sometimes it's "excellence." Sometimes it's "quality engineering," as with Mercedes Benz. Sometimes it's "the ultimate driving machine," as with BMW. In every case, how deeply entrenched that attribute is in the minds of your customers and prospective customers determines how readily they'll buy your product or service and how much they'll pay.

Develop the habit of thinking about how you could improve your positioning. Begin by determining the position you'd like to have. If you could create the ideal impression in the hearts and minds of your customers, what would it be? What would you have to do in every customer interaction to get your customers to think and talk about you in that specific way? What changes do you need to make in the way you interact with customers today in order to be seen as the very best choice for your customers of tomorrow?

People

The final P of the marketing mix is people. Develop the habit of thinking in terms of the people inside and outside of your business who are responsible for every element of your sales and marketing strategy and activities.

It's amazing how many entrepreneurs and businesspeople will work extremely hard to think through every element of the marketing strategy and the marketing mix, and then pay little attention to the fact that every single decision and policy has to be carried out by a specific person in a specific way. Your ability to select, recruit, hire and retain the proper people, with the skills and abilities to do the job you need to have done, is more important than everything else put together.

In his best-selling book, *Good to Great*, Jim Collins discovered the most important factor applied by the best companies was that they first of all "got the right people on the bus, and the wrong people off the bus." Once these companies had hired the right people, the second step was to "get the right people in the right seats on the bus."

To be successful in business, you must develop the habit of thinking in terms of exactly who is going to carry out each task and responsibility. In many cases, it's not possible to move forward until you can attract and put the right person into the right position. Many of the best business plans ever developed sit on shelves today because the people who created them could not find the key people who could execute those plans.

Source: Tracy (2008). Used with permission from Brian Tracy International: www.briantracy.com.

Other Marketing Processes

Following is an explanation of additional marketing concepts that will be useful to the reader. Each of the concepts will be addressed in greater detail later in the book.

Marketing Planning

Marketing planning may be defined as the development of a systematic process for promoting an organization, a service, or a product. This straightforward definition masks the wide variety of activities and potential complexity that characterize marketing planning. Marketing planning may be limited to a short-term promotional project or may be a component of a long-term strategic plan. It can focus alternatively on a product, a service, a program, or an organization. The marketing plan should summarize a company's marketing strategy and serve as a guide for all those involved in the company's marketing activities.

Of the various types of planning that could be carried out by a healthcare organization, marketing planning is most directly related to the customer. Marketing plans are, by definition, market driven, and they are single-minded in their focus on the customer. Whether the targeted customer is the patient, the referring physician, the employer, the health plan, or any number of other possibilities, the marketing plan is built around someone's needs. Although a consideration of internal factors is often pertinent (and internal marketing may be a component of many marketing plans), the marketing plan focuses on the characteristics of the external market with the objective of changing one or more of these characteristics.

Marketing Management

Marketing management refers to the analysis, planning, implementation, and control of programs designed to create, build, and maintain beneficial exchanges with target buyers for the purpose of achieving organizational objectives. The steps involved in the marketing management process include

(1) analyzing marketing opportunities, (2) selecting target markets, (3) developing the marketing mix, and (4) managing the marketing effort.

Although marketing management is a well-defined function in most industries, it is still in its infancy in healthcare. The fragmented approach to much of the marketing that has taken place and the immature status of marketing in healthcare are reflected in the slow development of marketing management skills.

Marketing Research

Marketing research is the function that links the consumer, customer, and public to the marketer through information used to identify and define marketing opportunities and problems; to generate, refine, and evaluate marketing actions; to monitor marketing performance; and to improve understanding of the marketing process. Often used interchangeably with the term *market research*, marketing research also encompasses product research, pricing research, promotional research, and distribution research. The marketing research process serves to identify the nature of the product or service, the characteristics of consumers, the size of the potential market, the nature of competitors, and any number of other essential pieces to the marketing puzzle.

Summary

As the healthcare industry has come to accept marketing as a legitimate function, health professionals have been exposed to a new vocabulary—the language of the marketer. Because health professionals hold various misconceptions about marketing, it is important that all be on the same page when it comes to marketing terminology. Many marketing terms could be adopted by healthcare organizations unchanged, whereas others require modification based on the unique characteristics of healthcare.

Health professionals have many misperceptions about what marketing is and what its functions are. Marketing cannot be pigeonholed as advertising, direct mail, or any specific activity; it involves a whole range of activities, from conducting marketing research to evaluating a completed promotional campaign. Further, the functions of marketing are numerous and range from big-picture functions, such as determining the strategic direction of the health system, to highly focused functions, such as increasing participation in a patient education class.

The healthcare industry presents a challenge in the application of marketing techniques. The concept of "market" does not exist in healthcare like it does it other industries, health professionals do not think in terms of products, and the nature of the customer is highly complex. A change of mind-set on the part of health professionals is required for marketing to be effectively used within the healthcare arena.

The traditional four Ps of marketing—product, price, place, and promotion—have been adapted to healthcare, although not without some limitations. All four are somewhat problematic when applied to healthcare because of the peculiar characteristics of the industry. As a result, attempts have been made to modify these components of the marketing mix or replace them with concepts that are more suitable to the healthcare environment.

Key Points

- The field of marketing has its own vocabulary with which health professionals must become familiar.
- The healthcare field can adopt many marketing concepts directly from other industries, but others must be modified to address the uniqueness of healthcare.
- Marketing should be viewed in the broadest possible light—not simply as a set of marketing tools, but as a contributor to organizational development.
- Marketing serves a number of functions in healthcare, and healthcare administrators should be sensitive to the implications marketing has for different levels of the organization.
- A wide range of marketing techniques are available to marketers, and their choice of technique depends on the circumstances.
- The traditional four Ps of the marketing mix—product, price, place, and promotion—can be applied to healthcare with modifications.
- The marketing function involves much more than promotions and must consider such processes as marketing research, marketing planning, and marketing management.

Discussion Questions

- Why is it difficult to directly apply the marketing approaches used in other industries to healthcare?
- Why do many health professionals have a misconception concerning the nature of marketing, and what are these misconceptions?
- What is the distinction between goods and services, and what are the implications of these differences for healthcare?

- What is the role of marketing as it relates to the various levels of the healthcare organization (e.g., senior managers versus product line managers)?
- Which components of healthcare marketing have health professionals been comfortable with historically, and which techniques are gaining more acceptance today?
- What factors have contributed to the conversion of the patient into a consumer, customer, or client, and what are the implications of this conversion on marketing?
- What characteristics of healthcare make it difficult to apply the four Ps of marketing directly to the healthcare organization?

Additional Resources

American Marketing Association website: www.marketingpower.com
MarketingProfs website: www.marketingprofs.com

MARKETING AND THE HEALTHCARE ORGANIZATION

Different types of healthcare organizations accepted marketing as a corporate function at different times and at different rates. At any point in time, different healthcare organizations are at different stages in the marketing progression. The role of marketing for various organizations is reviewed in this chapter, along with healthcare organizations' perspectives on marketing as a profession and as a component of the healthcare delivery system. This chapter also describes the evolving relationship between the marketing profession and the various types of healthcare organizations, and considers the challenge of integrating marketing with more traditional healthcare functions.

Factors Affecting the Adoption of Marketing

For-profit commercial businesses in consumer or industrial settings have historically led the way in terms of formal marketing activities. From the start of the marketing era, traditional businesses employed the full range of marketing techniques, including advertising. The same was true of traditional businesses in healthcare, such as consumer products companies and retail-oriented healthcare organizations. As early as the 1950s, numerous healthcare brands had become household names as a result of aggressive marketing.

Marketers of consumer health products typically used the same techniques as companies marketing other types of consumer products. However, some approaches unique to healthcare emerged. Insurance companies pioneered the concept of group sales, for example, and pharmaceutical companies developed physician-oriented sales approaches. In general, however, the primarily nonprofit nature of the industry mitigated against the widespread acceptance of marketing. Healthcare purists often equated marketing with advertising and considered it as incompatible with the principles of a charitable organization. These organizations were inherently conservative and generally thought that allocating resources for marketing purposes was in bad taste at best and unethical at worst.

Beginning in the 1970s, academic marketing experts asserted that marketing activities were common and acceptable among not-for-profit organizations (see, for example, Kotler 1975). Despite their assertion, health professionals as a group continued to resist the intrusion of formal marketing techniques. Further, as a practical matter, marketing was not a reimbursable expense for hospitals under the Medicare program. By the end of the 1970s, however, the mind-set of not-for-profit healthcare organizations was beginning to change, and a new attitude toward business practices began to emerge. Exhibit 4.1 reviews some of the changes that occurred in not-for-profit healthcare organizations.

EXHIBIT 4.1
Putting the Profit in the Not-for-Profit Organization

Many healthcare entities are chartered as not-for-profit organizations (NFPs). Not-for-profit organizations are typically conservative, particularly with regard to the expenditure of funds. They tend to restrict their spending to activities that directly relate to their mission. Historically, marketing activities have not been considered by NFPs as worthy uses of scarce organizational resources. Further, NFPs tended to view their goals as altruistic, setting them apart from their more avaricious for-profit kin. This stance fostered the perception that NFPs have nobler intentions than for-profit healthcare organizations.

NFPs have historically eschewed the pursuit of profit as an activity beneath them, largely as a result of their lack of exposure to basic business practices. NFPs that have been exposed to standard business practices have resisted applying them, arguing that they are not in business but in a higher calling. During the 1980s, however, many NFPs in healthcare—particularly provider organizations—found that their world was changing and that they needed to rethink their stance on profit. The adage "no margin, no mission" was increasingly expressed during this period as NFPs began to realize the importance of profit for organizational survival. Although healthcare professionals are still loath to use the "p word," the pursuit of profit or net revenue under some other moniker came to be accepted. As a result of this new attitude, NFPs began to adopt many of the business practices of other industries and of the for-profit organizations that were prominent in healthcare at the time.

> Marketing was one of the business practices that healthcare organizations came to accept. The margin necessary to support ongoing operations and continued development of the organization had to be nurtured, and the role of marketing in this process came to be recognized. If revenue was to flow to the bottom line, the organization had to increase customer traffic, sales volumes, market share, and all of the other indicators normally used in industry. Marketing was recognized as critical to the processes that would ultimately contribute to the bottom line. NFPs came to recognize the need to turn a profit and the importance of profitability to their continued viability, and ultimately came to appreciate the contribution that marketing made in this regard.

The scope and nature of healthcare marketing had broadened considerably by the mid-1980s, and, like every industry, healthcare continuously modified its marketing approach to fit its particular needs. Few of the marketing techniques from other industries could be adopted unchanged, but many techniques could be adapted for healthcare. At the same time, novel approaches were required to address the unique attributes of the healthcare industry.

Attributes that complicate marketing in healthcare include, for example, the fact that most healthcare organizations serve multiple markets and/or consumer groups. A traditional business can focus on prospective customers in the general population, but healthcare organizations may have to consider physicians, nurses, patients, employee assistance personnel, managed care plans, and regulators. An organization offering a mental health or substance abuse program for adolescents might have to accommodate the needs of judges, probation officers, and social workers. Organizations marketing a sports medicine program would have to consider employers, schools, and health plans among their potential customers, in addition to individual consumers.

Early on, major employers were not considered to be an important market for healthcare organizations, although companies typically bore their employees' healthcare costs. Today, however, major employers often attempt to control rising healthcare costs by dealing directly with providers to meet their employees' healthcare needs. As a result, healthcare organizations have an opportunity to compete for employers' business.

The situation for healthcare providers is also unique in that the health insurance plans in which consumers are enrolled are likely to influence their choice of medical facility. Although there may be allowances for using out-of-network practitioners and/or the option of paying more out of pocket for the privilege, most health plans specify which facilities and practitioners the insured can use. Healthcare organizations of all sizes spend an inordinate amount of time and effort negotiating contracts with health plans, and the more aggressive healthcare organizations see this situation as a marketing opportunity.

Healthcare Organizations and Marketing

The variety of organizations is endless, so generalizations cannot be made about healthcare organizations with regard to marketing. The following discussion addresses the marketing experiences of a range of healthcare organizations, including healthcare providers, suppliers, consumer products companies, pharmaceutical companies, insurance companies, and vendors of support services.

Healthcare Providers

When people think about healthcare marketing, most think of the campaigns initiated by healthcare providers. The term *provider* originated in the insurance arena to refer to practitioners or organizations that provide health services to health plan members. Hospitals are the most visible provider organizations, and their marketing activities are likely to be significant. Marketing by general hospitals can be traced back to the late 1970s, when a few hospitals hired marketers or established basic marketing departments. The real surge in marketing occurred in the early to mid-1980s, when many hospitals became enamored with advertising. Ads for hospitals and their services flooded the print and electronic media, and some hospitals used billboards to reach the public. Although the ultimate benefit of these expenditures was hard to determine, increased competition among providers during this period fueled the use of advertising. See Exhibit 4.2 for an example of hospital advertising.

By 1990, hospital administrators were rethinking the advertisement-focused marketing strategy they typically used. Advertising budgets and, in some cases, marketing departments and personnel were cut back. A much more balanced approach to marketing, which integrated advertising with public relations and communications activities and added direct sales capabilities, came to replace the former strategy. Hospitals adopted more contemporary forms of marketing by establishing marketing databases and call centers. Customer relationship marketing, direct-to-consumer marketing, and Internet marketing—the ultimate contemporary approach—were also adopted in the 1990s. These trends demonstrated a shift from a sales approach to more of a relationship management approach to marketing.

EXHIBIT 4.2
Sample Print Advertisement

many times the first
sign of heart disease is
sudden death

Heart disease can be scary. That's no excuse for ignoring it. Take charge of your heart health with your free online HeartAware assessment. We'll assess your risk and guide you to better health.

heartaware

Take the free 5 minute test that could save your life.

▶ edward.org/heartaware

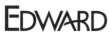   **For people who don't like hospitals**

Source: Edward Hospital, Naperville, IL. Used with permission.

Media advertising was the approach of choice for cultivating the general public, and specialty hospitals in particular attempted to maintain high visibility in their communities. National healthcare chains often conducted nationwide advertising campaigns supplemented by customized advertising in the local communities they served. Many of these chains employed sales forces that called on potential referrers of psychiatric or substance abuse patients. Public relations approaches, including holding open houses and disseminating feature stories, also were commonly used. A compelling Internet site has become customary for specialty hospitals, just as it is for other health facilities.

The target market for nursing home services is much more limited than that for general hospital services, and marketing in this area is typically less visible and more subdued. Nursing homes do not need the volume of patients other facilities require because of their patients' long stays. Further, someone other than the patient may be involved in the admission decision, so nursing homes must consider both prospective patients and their caregivers. They tend to emphasize advertising as a means of remaining top of mind and, where appropriate, solidifying relationships with referral agencies. Word of mouth is an important means of promoting nursing homes. Exhibit 4.3 describes research on the factors that contribute to positive nursing home recommendations.

EXHIBIT 4.3
Nursing Home Marketing: What Are Customers Looking For?

As baby boomers age, the demand for nursing services is expected to increase. In preparation, healthcare marketers must develop a better understanding of the factors that influence choice of nursing home. Customers for nursing home services include not only residents but also third-party payers, employees, doctors, hospitals, and caregivers. In this era of the graying of America, with an enormous potential market for senior services of all sorts, keeping current customers satisfied is vital for positive word of mouth. It also is vital for nursing homes to recognize family and friends as customers who may generate positive word-of-mouth publicity. Both the resident and these proxies may be considered customers for nursing home services, so it is important to understand the needs of both groups. Meeting the needs of the resident is the organization's mission, but meeting the needs of the proxies may ensure that they continue to generate referrals to the business.

Data obtained from 2,709 residents living in 26 different nursing homes across the nation provide some insight into marketing issues. Of the residents surveyed, 71 percent were women. The average age of residents was 75 for males and 80 for females. Many of the residents were relatively new to their facility: 43 percent of the men had lived in the facility for less than one month, compared to 30 percent of the women. In addition, 21 percent of the female residents had been in the facility for more than three years, whereas only 12 percent of the male residents had been there that long. The reported health status of the residents (as measured on a 5-point scale, where 1 indicated "very poor" and 5 indicated "very good") did not vary by gender. Fifty-six percent of the residents were identified as having less than good health (fair, poor, or very poor ratings).

Survey administrators found that only 31 percent of the questionnaires were completed by residents. The others were completed by a family member other than a spouse (40 percent), a spouse (12 percent), some other person (10 percent), a legal guardian (4 percent), or a friend (3 percent). Completion of the questionnaire by a proxy was strongly associated with the resident's health.

The questions covered 39 service issues related to the nursing home experience. The questionnaire also contained a question to assess "positive word of mouth," which was defined as the "likelihood you would recommend the (facility) to others." Respondents reported that the nursing homes did well in the areas of courtesy and friendliness but not as well with noise, food, and responsiveness. The service variables with the lowest scores were noise level in and around the room, followed by variety of food selections and quality of the food. The highest marks were given to courtesy of the admitting staff, friendliness of nurses, and courtesy of the housekeeping staff. The issues found to require the greatest attention were those dealing with services provided by the aides (e.g., information from aides, assistance with meals, and response to the call button).

Interestingly, the satisfaction ratings differed depending on who was doing the rating. For example, residents were more positive about the aides and the facility than were family and friends. In fact, when the overall satisfaction scores were compared for each type of respondent, the residents gave the highest scores. Friends, family, and guardians gave lower scores than residents, although the difference between the scores the residents and other respondents gave was significant only where the other respondents were friends. Nevertheless, the likelihood of recommending the nursing home was higher among

(continued)

EXHIBIT 4.3 (*continued*)

family members than among residents, and was significantly higher among family members than among friends.

Fortunately for the facilities, the items with the lowest scores were not among those with the highest correlation to likelihood to recommend. Items that had the highest correlation to likelihood to recommend included respectful, dignified treatment and nurses' technical skill, ability to explain care, and friendliness—domains in which nursing facilities tend to score relatively well. Among the eight service domains, nursing was most strongly related to likelihood to recommend the facility. Experiences with dining and aides were also important predictors of likelihood to recommend. Admission issues, not surprisingly, influenced the families' and residents' likelihood to recommend, but not the other respondents' likelihood to recommend. Similarly, finance issues were strongly related to likelihood to recommend only for the residents and their legal guardians. When taken together, the service domains explained about 60 percent of the variation in likelihood to recommend.

Residents tended to give higher ratings than their proxies. This difference may indicate that residents are reluctant to criticize staff or service delivery processes on which they depend. In contrast, family members' responses were particularly critical of the aides and of housekeeping.

On the other hand, some of the score differences may stem from anxiety or guilt associated with placing a loved one in a nursing home. Family members want to be certain that the quality of care meets an appropriate standard. Clearly, there are many components to quality of care, and patient and family assessments are just one element. Nevertheless, these ratings can help organizations identify perceived strengths and weaknesses in service delivery and take corrective action to meet customer needs and manage word of mouth in the community.

The difficulty in identifying the customers for nursing home services creates special challenges in determining and meeting customer requirements. Should the facility operate with an eye to resident ratings or family ratings? Or should it attempt to meet the expectations of the respondents who gave the lowest scores, assuming that meeting the requirements of that group will exceed the requirements of the other groups? Nursing homes would be wise to collect data from all identified customers—patients and proxies—and make efforts to satisfy both. The net result would not only be more data from "other" consumers, but potentially more data from the healthy residents whose voices previously have been lost to the proxy.

Irrespective of customer segment, the data suggest that nursing homes can maintain positive word of mouth by ensuring that nursing, aide services, and dining needs are met. Because the scores for nursing are already relatively high, the greatest opportunity appears to be in improving scores for aides and food quality.

Source: Adapted from Becker and Kaldenberg (2000).

Assisted living facilities are more like nursing homes than hospitals in their approach to the market. They do not require a large volume of patients but a small number of qualified prospects. As with nursing homes, someone other than the resident may be involved in the decision to enter an assisted living facility, so marketing must be geared not only to potential residents but also to their caregivers. Although fewer nursing homes are being built, assisted living facilities continue to spring up around the country. Print and electronic advertising is important for ongoing positive publicity. As with nursing homes, word-of-mouth endorsement is important for assisted living facilities.

Residential treatment centers have historically operated in a manner similar to that of specialty hospitals in terms of marketing. They tend to focus on ads for the general public and relationship building with potential referral agents. They often employ sales forces and may aggressively seek prospective customers.

Taken as a group, inpatient facilities have historically used public relations, advertising, and community outreach as their primary marketing tools. Many have also used direct sales. More contemporary approaches, such as customer relationship management, database marketing, and Internet marketing, are becoming common. The trend among healthcare facilities, especially hospitals, has been toward relationship development and more sophisticated and/or information technology-oriented approaches. They have also turned toward more low-cost/high-exposure types of marketing. See Case Study 4.1 for a discussion of some of these approaches.

Marketing by healthcare providers is also influenced by characteristics peculiar to the healthcare industry. For example, hospitals do not generally attract patients directly but must depend on their medical staffs to refer patients for admission. Similarly, many medical specialists do not accept patients directly but rely on referrals from primary care physicians and other specialists.

CASE STUDY 4.1
Low-Intensity Marketing

Like many healthcare organizations, Yale-New Haven Hospital (YNHH) was being asked to do more with less when it comes to marketing. Given its moderate advertising budget and the area's high media costs, YNHH had focused its advertising in the past on billboards, newspapers, and the Yellow Pages. Advertising via radio, television, and magazines was considered too expensive. From 1995 to 1999, the bulk of its advertising dollars went into three-quarter-page display ads in daily newspapers across Connecticut. These ads, developed through a lengthy review process with a traditional advertising agency, were ineffective in increasing consumer awareness because the limited budget prevented consistent exposure to the public.

To find a more effective yet inexpensive means of advertising, YNHH considered banner ads in newspapers. These ads are small strips that are 2 to 3 inches tall and range from 5 to 12 inches long. Usually one topic is covered per ad, and they may or may not include artwork. Banner ads are designed to pop out by using color and regular placement in the same place in the newspaper. They generally run on a daily basis and are placed at the top and bottom of the front page. The cost of the banner ad depends on its size and location. Most banner ads include a "call to action," giving the reader an opportunity to respond to the pitch.

As an experiment in early 1999, YNHH placed a half-inch by 12-inch strip ad at the bottom of the front page of the local newspaper twice a week. After monitoring the impact of the strips for a few months, there was no noticeable increase in calls to YNHH's call center for information or referral to a physician. A meeting was held with the local paper's sales executives to share the unfavorable results. The hospital informed the newspaper that it would cease running the banner ads if the newspaper did not develop a better approach. The paper came back with a new design that required discussions with and approval of the editorial side of the newspaper and major redesign of the paper's front page to develop space for a bigger ad at no additional cost.

YNHH expanded its banner ad initiative in the fall of 2000, and since then, more than 350 newspaper ads have been developed. Most of these ads promoted clinical programs such as heart, cancer, maternity, and diabetes, as well as ongoing clinical trials. Other ads were specific to the call center and promoted the physician referral program, the health information library, the nurse advice line, and the women's heart line. A third group of ads promoted consumer-oriented services, such as Web-based services, press conferences to announce newborn babies, and support groups. The final category of ads promoted general awareness of YNHH programs and announced special events, such as Nurses' Day.

Follow-up research indicated that the banner ad campaign was highly successful. Between the fall of 2000 and 2002, consumer awareness of YNHH in the southern Connecticut market increased from 29 percent to 49 percent. The proportion of consumers associating YNHH with state-of-the-art care increased from 22 percent to 40 percent. Because the hospital's marketing budget had declined 30 percent between 2000 and 2002, and there had been no increases in other marketing activity, the bulk of the change in consumers' attitudes and behaviors was attributed to the banner ads. In addition, 49 percent of the calls routed to the call center were generated by the banner ads during this period, and a large portion of follow-up calls for other services was stimulated by the banner ads. Evidence also suggested that callers who had found YNHH through the Yellow Pages often had been encouraged to seek them out after seeing the banner ads.

Although banner ads are not a panacea for marketing challenges, they have been generally beneficial to YNHH. They have generated considerable inquiries and have allowed the organization to spread its marketing budget much further than traditional advertising would have allowed. The volume of consumer interaction with the hospital has grown dramatically, and most of the increase in admissions during this period was attributed to the campaign. Furthermore, the banner ad campaign contributed substantially to the development of the YNHH customer database: As of 2003, 40,000 additional names had been added since the ads began running. These positive results were obtained at a time of declining newspaper readership. YNHH marketers found that their best customers were among the most loyal newspaper subscribers; with their inevitable health problems, older people were the last loyal customer group for this medium.

There is little downside to the use of banner ads as the focal point of a marketing campaign. Organizations must ensure, however, that they have the capability to respond to demand and must maintain a wide range of publications and other resource materials as references when responding to inquiries.

Source: Adapted from Gombeski et al. (2003).

(continued)

CASE STUDY 4.1 *(continued)*

Discussion Questions
- What prompted YNHH to rethink its use of banner ads in newspapers?
- What changes were implemented to make the banner ads more effective?
- What types of services appear to lend themselves to this type of advertising?
- What was the impact of the new banner ads in terms of "traffic" generated for YNHH?
- How would the declining importance of newspapers affect YNHH's reliance on this marketing technique?
- What are the implications of the demographics of loyal newspaper subscribers for the use of this medium to reach healthcare consumers?
- Are there more contemporary forms of media in which banner ads might be more effective?

Given that most patients are not going to walk off the street into a specialist's office but are going to be referred, advertising to the end user has limited value for many medical practices. These types of referral relationships typically do not exist in any other industry, and their presence complicates the marketing approach for providers.

Marketing activities among healthcare providers are also constrained by ethical and regulatory considerations. For the most part, it is inappropriate for healthcare providers to offer the incentives typical of other industries to potential sources of business. For example, it is considered unethical and even illegal for hospitals to offer physicians incentives to admit patients.

Clinicians have, for the most part, lagged behind hospitals and other healthcare organizations in their marketing efforts. Until recently, many physicians did not face the same competitive situations that hospitals began facing in the 1980s. In addition, ethical constraints limited the amount of advertising considered acceptable by the medical profession. Individual physicians and professional medical associations were long hostile to the notion of formal marketing, although most engaged in various forms of marketing to promote their practices.

Today, in contrast, increasing numbers of physicians and physician practices are using advertising to gain visibility and increase volume. These practices are often specialty groups that are trying to distinguish themselves from other specialists in their field. Physicians who offer elective procedures are involved even more heavily in advertising. Thus, ophthalmic surgeons performing laser eye surgery and cosmetic surgeons, for example, are more likely than specialists offering more traditional services to advertise their services directly to consumers. Because insurance usually does not cover these services, these practitioners depend less on referrals from colleagues and more on direct solicitation of potential customers.

Physicians have historically emphasized networking and relationship development for marketing purposes. More recently, some have ventured into advertising, although much of the more hard-sell advertising has been initiated by physicians involved in retail or elective aspects of healthcare. Physicians may use direct mail to reach selected audiences or to announce changes in the practices. Physicians are increasingly using the Internet as a means of promoting their practices and maintaining contact with their patients. In some markets, larger groups are using managed care and health plan contracting as a means of market development.

The level of marketing and the approach that clinicians use vary by profession and market. Independent practitioners such as dentists, podiatrists, and chiropractors may use low-key advertising to attract patients and maintain their visibility. Some may also rely on referral relationships. Direct mail may be occasionally used to contact prospects directly, but Internet marketing has not become widespread among these providers.

Various types of alternative therapists use a wide range of marketing techniques. Many advertise their services, often targeting select populations that are thought to be better prospects. An outreach approach is often important for alternative therapists in that they may have to educate the public about their forms of therapy. Internet marketing has gained more traction among providers of unconventional health services than perhaps any other group.

Certain types of health programs face unique challenges when it comes to marketing their services. For example, behavioral health programs designed for psychiatric and/or substance abuse patients have to be sensitive to their audience. Advertising for such programs tends to be more subtle than for other programs, and particular care has to be taken in formulating the message to be conveyed. Much of the marketing related to these types of programs, especially for private-pay patients, is carried out via behind-the-scenes relationship building.

The marketing approach for services such as human immunodeficiency virus (HIV)/acquired immunodeficiency syndrome (AIDS) programs is particularly problematic, and challenges are faced on a number of fronts. For various reasons, affected individuals may be difficult to identify and contact. There may be resistance to receiving unwanted information and concerns about confidentiality related to such a controversial condition. Marketing for

HIV/AIDS service agencies needs to attract the attention of those in need of services without attracting undue attention to the agency. Such organizations may adopt vague names (e.g., Adult Special Services) or minimal signage to limit the potential for stigmatization of their clients.

Most public health activities do not directly involve healthcare consumers. For example, activities aimed at maintaining clean air and water and ensuring a safe food supply typically involve activities unrelated to the delivery of care. On the other hand, public health agencies deal with a range of issues that do involve interface with the public. Some activities, such as child immunizations and nutritional counseling, may be noncontroversial and promoted through traditional information-and-referral channels and word of mouth. More controversial programs, such as those dealing with family planning, teen pregnancy, sexually transmitted diseases, and HIV/AIDS, require more aggressive yet more sensitive approaches. Many public health agencies also provide some medical treatments, and these programs need to be promoted as well.

Public health agencies have relied on information-and-referral approaches and standard public relations approaches in the past to publicize their services. They have also made use of community outreach programs to promote their services in the community. However, given the increasing significance of certain problems considered to be in the public health domain, such agencies have become much more aggressive in terms of marketing and have added various forms of health communication to their stable of marketing approaches. A variety of social marketing initiatives have been launched, many coordinated by the Centers for Disease Control and Prevention or some other federal agency. Initiatives aimed at sexually transmitted diseases, HIV/AIDS, and tuberculosis, as well as nonclinical programs such as nutritional counseling and family planning, have also begun to use social marketing approaches.

Healthcare Suppliers

In healthcare, suppliers include a wide range of organizations that supply the goods and equipment that support the operation of the system. Healthcare organizations use an extensive range of supplies, from office supplies (e.g., computer forms) to cloth products (e.g., uniforms, linens) to disposables (e.g., gloves, syringes). A large physician practice may have a vendor list of dozens of suppliers, and a hospital may have a list of hundreds.

Healthcare organizations also use a wide range of equipment and deal with a variety of vendors for these products. In addition to standard office machines, they use equipment related to clinical activities, including sterilizers, blood pressure cups, stethoscopes, x-ray machines and other imaging equipment, monitors of various types, and laboratory equipment. They also use a considerable amount of durable medical equipment, such as examination tables, hospital beds, wheelchairs, and other items designed for extended use. (Information technology will be addressed later.)

Supplies and equipment may be obtained directly from producers, but more often they are obtained from distributors who handle a range of products. In either case, supply and equipment vendors are likely to use trade advertising geared toward business customers in publications aimed at hospitals, physicians, or other types of facility or personnel. They also rely on sales representatives who use direct sales approaches with healthcare facilities and healthcare professionals. Supply and equipment vendors also use sales promotion in the form of appearances at professional meetings and exhibitions that representatives of healthcare facilities and healthcare professionals are likely to attend.

Unlike the patient care side of healthcare, organizations marketing medical supplies, biomedical equipment, and durable medical equipment can operate in much the same manner as their corollary organizations in other industries. The primary difference is the logistics involved in connecting with a physician or the right person at a hospital to make a presentation. The decision makers in other industries are often much more available and easier to identify. The types of marketing healthcare suppliers generally use include direct sales, business-to-business marketing, advertising, and sales promotion. They are also increasingly using the Internet for online marketing and promotion.

Consumer Products Companies

Although marketing on the part of healthcare providers is still evolving, the marketing of consumer goods in healthcare is a well-established phenomenon. Consumer health products have long been marketed to the American public, and, arguably, some of the best-known early consumer brands were associated with health-related products. Brand names like Bayer, Johnson & Johnson, and Ex-Lax were household terms long before the modern healthcare system emerged in the United States.

Today, pharmacy shelves are filled with consumer health products. Households are typically well supplied with headache remedies, cold medicine, adhesive bandages, heating pads, and a variety of other products used for personal health needs. Feminine hygiene products and goods for baby care are common household items, too. Household inventories may also include products for foot care, dental care, and eye care. Recent advances in home diagnosis and treatment have added new lines of products and equipment to the options available to the household. (Over-the-counter drugs will be discussed later in the chapter.)

Traditional over-the-counter medical remedies and personal health products have been supplemented by a wide range of nutritional products and a plethora of "cosmeceuticals" and "nutraceuticals." There has been an explosion of products that bridge the gap between cosmetics and drugs and promise such results as younger skin or hair regrowth. Products that combine nutritional benefits with medicinal benefits are now common, too.

The emergence of alternative therapies has also contributed to the rapid growth of personal health products. A variety of natural products have entered the market as alternatives for or supplements to more conventional health products or treatments. Growing interest on the part of the American consumer in alternative medicine and holistic health has made alternative therapy a major industry.

The market for consumer health products continues to grow dramatically as the U.S. population becomes more health conscious, new products are developed, and a do-it-yourself attitude becomes more pervasive among healthcare consumers. The variety of products and the level of competition make the continuous use of high-level marketing essential to the business strategy of producers of consumer health products.

Consumer health products tend to be marketed in a manner similar to that used to promote other types of consumer products. Producers of personal health products rely heavily on media advertising (both print and electronic), along with advertising inserts in popular publications. They also use such sales promotion techniques as discount coupons, rebates, and contests. Marketers of personal health products also emphasize in-store advertising and secure highly visible shelf space.

Perhaps the most important development in marketing consumer health products has been the emergence of the Internet as a new marketplace for a wide range of products. Although mainstream brands typically rely on traditional retail marketing approaches, marginal products and newcomers to the market have latched on to the Internet as their primary promotional channel. To a certain extent, many of these new products are shut out of the mainstream market (e.g., because of lack of access to retail shelf space); at the same time, however, these products often cater to a market that is receptive to innovation and prefers to use the Internet to access goods and services.

Pharmaceutical Companies

Pharmaceutical manufacturing is an enormous and highly profitable industry in the United States. Sales of prescription drugs in 2008 were approximately $291 billion, accounting for 10 percent of annual healthcare expenditures in the United States (IMS 2009). Profits on pharmaceutical sales average 15 percent or three times the average for all industries. Despite its huge profit potential, the drug industry is highly risky and competitive. After receiving approval from the Food and Drug Administration, a new drug often faces stiff competition from other drugs already on the market and is granted patent protection for only a limited length of time.

Prescription drug use has grown dramatically since the research break-throughs of the post–World War II period. The increased availability of more effective pharmaceuticals has shifted the therapeutic emphasis away from invasive procedures toward drug therapy. Patients today spend less time in the hospital and more time at the prescription counter. As a result, U.S. health-care expenditures, including expenditures on prescription drugs, are rising. Between 2002 and 2008, drug expenditures increased nearly 80 percent (IMS 2009).

Because of the competitive nature of the industry and the pressure to recoup investments in research and development, the drug industry has developed sophisticated, aggressive, and expensive marketing strategies. Approximately $57.5 billion was spent on pharmaceutical marketing in 2007, accounting for approximately 3 percent of all healthcare expenditures in the United States (Gagnon and Lechin 2008). Marketing expenditures accounted for 30 percent or more of revenue; pharmaceutical companies spent $3.7 billion advertising to consumers in 2008 through television, radio, magazines, newspapers, and outdoor billboards. They spent an additional $6.7 billion marketing to physicians through sales representatives and journal advertisements (Kaiser Family Foundation 2008).

Pharmaceutical companies promote themselves through professional literature in at least three ways: medical journals, industry-oriented news-letters/newspapers, and research compendia. They are heavy advertisers in medical journals (although many journals will not accept advertising). They also sponsor research that they hope (if favorable) will be published in medical journals. (Unfortunately, some pharmaceutical companies have been found guilty of paying medical scientists to write favorable reports on their drugs even when the research didn't support positive outcomes.)

Drug companies also send unsolicited "throwaway journals" to doctors' mailboxes. These newsletters/newspapers contain summaries of research published in other journals that doctors do not have time to review. They also may take the form of trade journals in which pharmaceutical companies advertise, or to which they (or medical professionals in their employ) submit articles. Often, a pharmaceutical company will produce its own newspaper in an attempt to promote its products through a "journalistic" format.

As the volume of published medical information has mushroomed, drug companies have provided doctors with alternatives to tedious forays into the medical literature. By acting as intermediaries in providing information to doctors, drug companies save doctors' time and expense while maintaining some control over what they see and hear. These services have historically taken print form but are increasingly being broadcast on television or disseminated via the Internet.

Continuing medical education (CME) is one area of medical communication that is massively subsidized by the drug industry. Since the 1970s, physicians and other clinicians have been required to complete a minimum amount of accredited training each year to maintain their hospital privileges and professional certification. As a result, thousands of CME conferences are held each year. Drug companies may participate as passive financial sponsors of CME conferences or actively plan and implement them. Thus, most CME conferences now have pharmaceutical industry support, and although some limitations have been enacted in recent years on drug companies' influence, CME is still largely sponsored by them.

Field representatives (or detailers) are a crucial link in the information chain between drug companies and clinicians. More than 30,000 pharmaceutical company representatives—one for every 15 American doctors—make tens of millions of office visits to doctors. Drug representatives dispense promotional brochures and medical literature and speak with physicians about their products, as well as offer them free samples. Physicians obtain much of their information on drugs from pharmaceutical detailers, making this activity, at least from the drug company's perspective, a successful marketing technique.

Gifts to physicians were a cornerstone of pharmaceutical marketing for many years. The most abundant category of gifts includes reminder items, such as pens or notepads, which prominently display the name of a drug. Gifts are often offered to physicians in exchange for their attention to promotional material or presentations. "Drug lunches" in large hospitals and clinics are one such example. A pharmaceutical company provides lunch for an audience, usually medical students and junior physicians, and a representative from that company gives a presentation while they eat. Pharmaceutical companies also sponsor dinner meetings during which speakers promote the company's products. Physicians in attendance are typically paid an honorarium for their time. Exorbitant gifts and cash payments of any amount were banned by the American Medical Association in 1990 and have been replaced in many cases with gifts of medical textbooks or medical instruments. The length to which pharmaceutical companies should be allowed to go in marketing to doctors continues to be a source of controversy, however.

Current trends in the healthcare system are changing the way prescription drugs are chosen, and marketing techniques have rapidly adapted to this new environment. The growth of managed care in the United States has had a profound effect on drug prescribing, with managed care organizations accounting for an increasing share of drug sales. The managers of both private and public health plans are in a position to control billions of dollars of drug purchases each year. As a result, pharmaceutical marketers are turning more attention toward "wholesale" purchasers, and physicians and consumers have become less important targets.

During the late 1970s and the 1980s, the relatively small industry of mail-order pharmacy houses grew dramatically, fueled by the greater pharmaceutical needs of an aging population and the cost advantages these wholesale businesses offered. Because they provide drugs at lower costs than many retail pharmacies, these companies have obtained exclusive contracts to supply prescriptions to many managed care organizations. They also influence which drugs millions of people use, so they have become targets for acquisition by drug companies. By controlling the mail-order pharmacies, a pharmaceutical company can influence prescribing patterns.

The major development of the 1990s was the emergence of direct-to-consumer (DTC) marketing on behalf of the pharmaceutical industry. Pharmaceutical companies that once marketed almost exclusively to physicians now market directly to consumers. DTC advertising often prompts patients to seek treatment for previously untreated conditions and pressures physicians to consider prescribing drugs their patients have been exposed to through DTC advertising. A significant portion of the nearly $4 billion the pharmaceutical industry spends on consumer marketing involves DTC advertising, and various surveys have found that DTC ads encourage patients to ask their doctors about drug therapy and, much less frequently, about a specific drug.

The introduction of generic drugs was another development that affected pharmaceutical marketing. These unbranded drugs are comparable to the highly advertised brands (although not identical) and sell for a much lower price. Pharmacies can reduce prescription drug costs substantially through the substitution of generics. Pharmacists who counsel and educate patients at the point of care are primarily responsible for this phenomenon. Not surprisingly, pharmaceutical companies have sought to limit the presence of generic drugs that might substitute for their name-brand drugs. Because of the access and cost barriers some U.S. patients face in obtaining drugs, companies in other countries (most notably Canada and Mexico) have begun to market both brand-name and generic drugs to U.S. consumers.

Many pharmaceuticals that do not require a prescription are sold over the counter (OTC). OTC drugs are marketed in a manner similar to that used to promote other consumer health products, but they often have the power of pharmaceutical marketing behind them. Growth in the sales of OTC drugs has been boosted by the introduction of a wide range of alternative therapies and natural products that may not face the same advertising restrictions to which more traditional pharmaceuticals are subject.

The most significant trend over the past few years has been the growth of drug marketing via the Internet. Online drug sales are carried out by mainstream pharmaceutical companies, mail-order drug houses, and, increasingly, entrepreneurs hoping to capture the ever-growing demand for drugs on the part of American consumers. Most online drug sellers are legitimate and adhere to ethical and professional guidelines, but some online drug distributors may sell prescription drugs without a doctor's order, while others, mostly overseas, are outright scams. The growth in sales of drugs online has significant implications for marketing, as Internet access to this information reduces the importance of traditional marketing techniques.

Health Insurance Companies

Health insurance companies were among the earliest healthcare organizations to develop marketing techniques in the period after World War II. In the early days of health insurance, policies were generally sold to individuals or families, and health insurance plans were marketed in the same manner as other types of insurance. Health plans advertised their programs using a variety of techniques and carried them out through a network of agents. Because health insurance was a relatively novel phenomenon until the 1960s, the marketing approach often involved educating the prospect.

By the 1960s, health insurance was predominantly sold in wholesale fashion through employers who purchased group plans on behalf of their employees. Group plans came to be the norm, and individual policies became increasingly uncommon. The spread and entrenchment of employer-based insurance was abetted by a substantially unionized workforce for which health benefits became an almost inalienable right. Although insurance companies advertised group plans (e.g., through print and electronic media or billboards), they were primarily sold to large employers through sales forces representing a particular insurance company or brokers representing several health plans.

The major development in health insurance during the last quarter of the twentieth century was alternative forms of financing for healthcare coverage, created for purposes of competing with traditional indemnity insurance. During the 1970s, health maintenance organizations (HMOs) emerged as a form of prepaid insurance that minimized the fee-for-service aspect of reimbursement. HMOs and other alternatives to indemnity insurance came to be generically referred to as "managed care."

Although there had always been a certain level of competition among health plans, the competition for enrollees was typically low key. The emergence of managed care incited much more intense competition with existing indemnity plans (and with each other). The marketing of managed care plans involved the same approaches used for group plans and individual plans. Legislation was passed that required employers to offer their employees a managed care plan, which meant employees were likely to have a choice of two or more plans. Thus, a managed care marketer's first task was to convince employers to offer his organization's plan to their employees. Subsequently, he had to encourage employees to choose his organization's plan over any others offered. Managed care plans began to offer special benefits to encourage enrollment and to retain employees once they were enrolled.

During the late 1990s, managed care enrollment leveled off, with at least half of all insured enrolled in some type of managed care plan. The defined contribution approach to health insurance benefits also emerged during this decade. Traditional insurance and managed care plans alike offered defined benefits, which meant the provisions of the plan were established up front and all enrollees received the same benefits regardless of their circumstances or preferences. Employees were given credit for a certain amount of insurance resources and could disburse these funds in the manner they saw fit by choosing options from a menu of benefits. The introduction of defined contribution plans made modification of existing marketing approaches necessary, as plans could now be customized for individual enrollees. The standardized approach to benefits that had become common gave way to a tailored approach. This development was propelled by health plans' use of the Internet to offer enrollees access to information on their benefits.

By the end of the 1990s, the conventional approach to group insurance had lost ground for various reasons. A growing number of employers were no longer offering insurance as a benefit, were cutting back their coverage, or were becoming "self-insured." In addition, a growing number of Americans were going without health insurance. This population came to include not only marginal participants in the economy but an increasing number of working-class and middle-class individuals who did not have access to group insurance. This state of affairs led to a revival of the individual insurance policy, a development that has been driven by Internet marketing and distribution. Insurers are offering health plans via the Internet and advertising them through print and electronic media. Because they are national plans, they can enroll millions of individuals and thereby create a large enough pool of plan members to spread the risk.

One other important aspect of health insurance marketing involves government-sponsored insurance programs. Medicare and Medicaid are entitlement programs with criteria for enrollment. Historically, there has been no competition for Medicare enrollees because seniors are automatically enrolled in Medicare when they reach the specified age. Although alternatives to simple Medicare enrollment have been around since the 1970s, the federally approved (and subsidized) Medicare Advantage program was reorganized in 2003. Medicare Advantage plans are offered by private insurers on a fee basis to Medicare enrollees who seek additional advantages over straight Medicare benefits. The federal government does not have to market the Medicare program to seniors because they are automatically enrolled, but

Medicare Advantage plans employ various techniques to convince seniors that they are a more favorable option than traditional Medicare or competing Medicare Advantage plans. More recently, the introduction of Medicare drug benefits (Part D) required a social marketing effort on the part of the Medicare program to encourage Medicare beneficiaries to participate.

Medicaid enrollees have traditionally been signed up by their respective states on the basis of federally approved eligibility criteria. However, states have increasingly contracted out management of their Medicaid programs to private healthcare networks. Government agencies responsible for Medicaid programs have historically employed social marketing techniques to ensure that eligible individuals knew about these programs and the services they offer. In particular, new supplemental insurance programs, such as those for children, need to be promoted to those who can benefit from them.

Support Services

Much of the growth in the healthcare workforce has occurred among organizations providing support services to healthcare organizations. Although hospitals and other facilities may provide many types of support services in-house, there have always been services that internal resources could not easily provide. Since the 1980s, healthcare organizations have been outsourcing an increasing number of services to specialized service providers.

Among the support services hospitals require are transcription services, billing and collections services, utilization review, recruitment and staffing services, hazardous waste disposal, laboratory services, and information technology. Information technology services have become particularly important as healthcare's dependence on technology increases. In many cases, hospitals and other healthcare organizations have benefited from outsourcing these services.

Vendors that provide these services typically market via direct sales and often sponsor community events. They may also advertise in print or electronic media or use direct mail to maintain visibility. The Internet, too, has increasingly gained popularity as a vehicle for marketing a wide range of support services.

Marketing's Intent

The variety of marketing techniques described in the preceding sections can be examined in terms of the intent of the marketing effort. Early on, the intent of marketing for provider organizations was to disseminate general information on the organization, report new developments, maintain visibility among the general public, and make people aware of the organization and its services. This blanket approach to marketing was general and low key. As marketing became more aggressive, its intent was to induce referrals to the organization's services and to solicit customers from the general population. This process was much more specific in terms of its approach, message, and targets. However, this more aggressive approach still involved one-way communication and provided no opportunities for formal feedback.

The development of customer databases, call centers, and websites in the 1990s ushered in a new phase of healthcare marketing. These marketing tools offered opportunities for customer interaction and input. With the two-way communication they afforded, relationships with existing or prospective customers could be developed. Websites in particular became a draw for patients and other consumers seeking general information or dealing with a particular health condition. The ability to schedule appointments, check on laboratory results, and interact with providers via the Internet created a bond not afforded by other forms of marketing.

As healthcare marketing became more sophisticated, its intent shifted to relationship management. As healthcare providers become more numerous and competition increased, it became important for providers to hold on to their existing customers. Progressive healthcare organizations began to shift their emphasis from techniques useful in attracting new customers to techniques useful in retaining existing customers.

Marketing's Role

As healthcare marketing matured, marketing's role in the industry shifted. In the early stages, some activities directed toward marketing ends were not considered as marketing per se. Many provider organizations even avoided using the term. As the need to market more aggressively developed, a more formal marketing function emerged. Organizations expanded and formalized their publicity and communication efforts. Realizing the need to advertise, providers often contracted consultants with marketing know-how and engaged outside agencies to develop creative materials and purchase advertising space.

As marketing became more important, many providers established marketing departments. These efforts often began with a single person and developed over time to include a strong marketing staff. Initially, marketing was often subsumed under public relations, planning, business development, or some other department. Eventually, it was carved out as a stand-alone function. It was accorded its own budget and more prominence on the corporate organizational chart.

As provider organizations came to appreciate the importance of marketing, their marketing departments took on an increasingly important role. Many organizations established a vice president of marketing or otherwise elevated their marketing staff. Once a function external to the organization and something considered as a necessary evil, marketing became an important internal function and was redefined as a major contributor to the organization's success. Marketing dollars, once viewed as an unnecessary expense, came to be seen as an investment essential to maintaining a healthy bottom line. Marketing personnel were moved closer to the center of the organizational structure. Instead of entering the picture after decisions had been made by others, marketers emerged as major contributors to corporate decision making.

Summary

The acceptance of marketing as a corporate function in healthcare occurred at different times for different organizations. Even today, different healthcare organizations are at different stages of marketing maturity. For-profit commercial healthcare businesses have historically led the way in terms of formal marketing activities, while more ubiquitous not-for-profit organizations have been much slower to accept marketing as a corporate function.

Although the scope of healthcare marketing had broadened considerably by the mid-1980s, few marketing techniques could be applied from other industries unchanged. Most healthcare organizations had multiple markets or customer types to target. Whereas a traditional business is able to target one type of customer, a complex healthcare facility may have to consider a wide variety of customers. Marketers were faced with having to develop novel approaches that took into consideration the unique attributes of the healthcare industry.

Generalizations about healthcare organizations with regard to marketing cannot be made. Hospitals are the most visible of healthcare organizations, and their marketing activities are likely to be significant in scope. Specialty hospitals have been particularly active in marketing, and nursing homes, assisted living facilities, and other residential facilities face their own marketing challenges. Most physicians have long engaged in informal types of marketing, although most were loath to advertise. Today, however, increasing numbers of physician practices are using advertising as a means of gaining visibility and attracting patients.

Public health agencies promote activities such as child immunizations and nutritional counseling through traditional information and referral channels and through word of mouth. Controversial programs, such as those dealing with family planning, teen pregnancy, sexually transmitted diseases, and HIV/AIDS, require aggressive yet sensitive approaches.

Organizations marketing medical supplies, biomedical equipment, and durable medical equipment typically operate in much the same manner as similar organizations in other industries, and consumer health products are aggressively marketed. Pharmaceutical companies have developed sophisti-cated, aggressive, and expensive marketing strategies, allocating more of their budget to marketing than any other category of healthcare organization does.

Health insurance companies were among the earliest healthcare or-ganizations to employ marketing techniques. In the early days of health in-surance, policies were generally sold to individuals or families, and health insurance plans were marketed in the same manner as other types of insur-ance. By the 1960s, health insurance was predominantly sold in wholesale fashion to employers on behalf of their employees. By the end of the 1990s, individual policies experienced a resurgence prompted in part by the ability to purchase insurance via the Internet.

The role of marketing in healthcare organizations has evolved through a number of stages, moving from more traditional public relations and com-munication approaches, to advertising and direct sales, to more contempo-rary technology-based techniques, such as database marketing and Internet sales. As the field has matured, the role of the marketer has shifted from that of an outside resource to a full participant in the organization's decision-mak-ing process.

Key Points

- Healthcare organizations were much slower than other industries to adopt marketing practices.
- For-profit entities like pharmaceutical companies, medical supply companies, and insurance companies adopted marketing practices much faster than did organizations providing patient care.
- The nature of healthcare—and particularly the dominance of not-for-profit organizations—contributed to the slow adoption of marketing practices.
- Although organizations in other industries typically have one target audience, the constituents for healthcare services are multiple and varied.
- Healthcare organizations have adopted marketing practices at varying rates of speed, and the type of technique chosen varies with the type of organization and its maturity with regard to marketing.
- Historically, pharmaceutical companies' approach to marketing was unique in that they did not market directly to the end user but to an intermediary— the physician—who then prescribed the products to the patient.
- As healthcare marketing has matured, the role of marketing and the marketer has evolved.

Discussion Questions

- What are some factors that account for the different rates at which healthcare organizations have adopted marketing techniques?
- What types of organizations were the fastest (and slowest) to adopt marketing? Why was marketing adopted at different rates?
- What lessons did healthcare learn about marketing from industries such as hospitality and financial services?
- How does the marketing of cardiology services by a hospital differ from the marketing of cosmetic surgery by a plastic surgeon?
- In what ways are the approaches used by pharmaceutical companies to market prescription drugs unique to the healthcare industry?
- In what ways would the marketing of individual health plans by insurance companies differ from the marketing of group insurance plans?
- What marketing techniques were so routinely used by healthcare organizations that they were not recognized as marketing?
- What role has technology played in the evolution of marketing in healthcare?
- How has the healthcare industry progressed from an emphasis on sales to an emphasis on developing long-term customer relationships?

Additional Resources

Andreasen, A. R., and P. Kotler. 2007. *Strategic Marketing for Non-Profit Organizations*, 7th edition. Upper Saddle River, NJ: Prentice Hall.

Peterson, M. 2008. *Our Daily Meds: How the Pharmaceutical Companies Transformed Themselves into Slick Marketing Machines and Hooked the Nation on Prescription Drugs*. New York: Sarah Crichton.

Thomas, R. K. 2008. "Marketing Your Healthcare Practice." Self-Study Course. Chicago: Health Administration Press.

———. 2007. *Health Services Marketing: A Guide for Practitioners*. New York: Springer.

Thomas, R. K., and M. Calhoun. 2007. *Marketing Matters: A Guide for Healthcare Executives*. Chicago: Health Administration Press.

II

UNDERSTANDING HEALTHCARE MARKETS

All marketing efforts begin with an assessment of the market to be served. This assessment typically involves identifying potential customers and determining their characteristics. In healthcare, this task is a challenge because the market for health services is different from the markets for any other industry. Marketers must define their customers, products, and marketing targets, understand consumer decision making, and be knowledgeable about the sources of information consumers use. In healthcare, there is a bewildering variety of customers, providers, and payers with which marketers must contend.

Chapter 5 describes the context in which healthcare marketing takes place. Marketing activities do not take place in a vacuum; the form they take is influenced by sociocultural factors. Effective marketing depends on an understanding of the societal framework in which healthcare operates.

Chapter 6 introduces the reader to the healthcare consumer and the factors that influence consumer behavior in the healthcare arena. The decision-making process involved in the consumption of health services is different from that in other industries, and marketers must develop an appreciation for the unique aspects of consumer behavior in healthcare.

Chapter 7 describes healthcare products—the ideas, goods, and services marketers promote. Health professionals are not accustomed to thinking in terms of products, and marketers often have difficulty conceptualizing healthcare products.

Chapter 8 addresses the factors that contribute to the demand for health services and healthcare products and describes how demand is converted into sales. It also proposes methods marketers can use to measure demand and introduces readers to indicators of health services utilization. The factors that determine the demand for and ultimate consumption of health services are numerous and their interplay complex.

THE NATURE OF
HEALTHCARE MARKETS

Marketing professionals in any industry must demonstrate an understanding of the market in which they operate. This issue is particularly important in healthcare because of the unique nature and variety of healthcare markets. This chapter discusses these unique characteristics, describes markets relevant to healthcare organizations, and reviews the various methods of defining markets and delineating market areas.

Introduction

Marketing activities do not take place in a vacuum but are products of the sociocultural environment in which they occur. To understand the intersection between healthcare and marketing, it is necessary to understand the societal framework in which both enterprises exist. For effective marketing to occur, marketers must first fully understand the nature of the existing system in which they function. For healthcare organizations to be successful in today's environment, they must develop an appreciation for the markets their organizations serve and the salient characteristics of those markets. To do so requires an in-depth understanding of the social, political, and economic characteristics of the target population, along with their lifestyles, attitudes, and other prominent traits. (These factors are discussed in more detail in Chapter 6.)

Although it is not possible to describe all of the social and health systems dimensions that are important in developing marketing initiatives, the key issues are addressed in the sections that follow. Previous chapters have addressed the characteristics of American society and their implications for healthcare marketing. This chapter focuses on the types of markets for healthcare goods and services that have emerged and their implications for healthcare organizations.

Although physicians and most not-for-profit healthcare organizations have resisted in the past the use of the term *marketing* in regard to any of their activities, they have nevertheless been concerned with markets on a daily basis. Physicians must consider the characteristics of the population they serve, and specialists must be cognizant of the physician-referrers who constitute their markets. Hospitals must appreciate the market represented by their medical staff, and health plans must develop an understanding of the individual or corporate entities that constitute the market for health insurance. Some of these target audiences may not represent markets in the traditional sense of, say, retailers, but they are *real* markets for the health professionals who deal with them.

As noted in Chapter 3, the establishment of a marketing function implies the existence of a market, with *market* referring to both a marketplace and potential customers in that market, both individuals and organizations. Although a strict definition of marketing would refer to the set of actual and potential buyers of a product, this notion of a market has been expanded in healthcare. Increasingly, for healthcare marketers, a market is defined as a group of consumers who share some characteristic that affects their needs or wants and makes them potential buyers of a healthcare product.

Defining Markets

A market for healthcare goods or services can be delineated in a number of different ways. The definition used depends on the purpose of the analysis, the product involved, the competitive environment, and the type of organization cultivating the market. Further, the nature of the market depends on the orientation of the organization involved in marketing. For example, the market for cardiac care may be identified as a five-county referral area regardless of which providers offer cardiac care. In other words, everyone in that geographic area who potentially needs cardiac care is identified as the market. On the other hand, *market* may refer to the geographic area served by a particular healthcare organization—that is, Hospital X controls a five-county market area (regardless of the services it offers).

The term *market area* as used here is comparable to the term *service area* for all practical purposes. Historically, *service area* has been used to identify the geographic area served by not-for-profit organizations or areas that are officially defined as the territory of a particular organization. For example, a health clinic that has been assigned a service area by a regulatory authority or a territory delimited on the basis of a health plan contract can be thought to have an identified service area. For-profit healthcare organizations, pharmaceutical companies, and distributors of consumer health products, on the other hand, are more likely to think in terms of market areas. As the health-care industry has become more competitive and has come to accept market-ing as a healthcare function, an increasing number of healthcare organizations have begun thinking in terms of market areas.

Geography

The most common method of defining a market is based on geography. A *geographically based market* is delineated in terms of specified geographic units. Most market research, in fact, focuses on a census tract, zip code, or county (or a group of any of these units) as the basis for analysis. This type of market area is typically delineated in terms of the "official" boundaries of the geographic units chosen for analysis. Geographically based markets are popular because analysts and decision makers are familiar with established geographic boundaries; the de facto operating spheres of many organizations often correspond with specified geographic boundaries; and market data are typically collected and reported for established geographic units. Exhibit 5.1 describes the most common geographic units used by marketers.

EXHIBIT 5.1
Units of Geography in Healthcare Marketing

Nearly all healthcare marketing activities are linked to some geographic area. Public health agencies and community-based organizations typ-ically have specific geographic areas over which they have authority or that they are designated to serve. Private-sector healthcare orga-nizations typically plan for markets that are delineated on the basis of geography. For purposes of this discussion, the geographic units that healthcare marketers use can be divided into three major categories: political/administrative units, statistical units, and a third category of miscellaneous types of units.

Political/Administrative Units
Political or administrative divisions are the most commonly used geo-graphic units in marketing. Many healthcare organizations have market areas that coincide with the political boundaries of cities, counties, or states. Not only is it convenient for private-sector organizations to use standard political or administrative units to establish their boundaries; the use of political units also facilitates data collection, as most statis-tics are compiled using these boundaries. Political units are also useful in spatial analysis because many statistics are compiled on the basis of

(continued)

EXHIBIT 5.1 (*continued*)

political boundaries. The following political and administrative units are frequently used in marketing.

Nation

The nation (in this case, the United States) is defined by national boundaries. Although some national chains or consumer health products companies may be interested in data at the national level, few healthcare organizations operate in a national market. Nevertheless, statistics for the nation (e.g., mortality rates) are often important as a standard to which other levels of geography are compared.

States

The major sub-national political unit is the state. Data are typically available for 50 states, the District of Columbia, and several U.S. territories. Because individual states are responsible for a broad range of administrative functions, states tend to be useful sources of social, demographic, economic, and environmental data. State agencies are also an important source of health-related data.

Counties

The county (or, in some states, boroughs, townships, or parishes) is the primary unit of local government. The nation is divided into more than 3,100 county units (including some cities that are politically designated as counties). The county is a critical unit for marketing, as many healthcare organizations view their home county as their primary service area. States typically report most of their statistics at the county level, and the county health department is likely to be a major source of health data.

Cities

Cities are officially incorporated urban areas delineated by boundaries that may or may not coincide with other political boundaries. Although cities are typically contained within a particular county, many city boundaries extend across county lines. Because cities are incorporated according to the laws of the state in which they are located, there is little standardization with regard to boundary delineation. For this reason, cities are not useful units for market analyses. In many cases, however, certain city government agencies are involved in data collection activities that may be useful to marketers.

Congressional Districts

Congressional districts are established locally and approved by the federal government. They are typically delineated by means of political compromise and do not correspond well with any other geographic unit. Although the Census Bureau reports data for congressional districts, limited data are collected at the congressional district level. In addition, the boundaries tend to change over time, making these units not particularly suitable for marketing purposes.

State Legislative Districts

State legislative districts have characteristics similar to those of congressional districts. They are drawn up by states primarily on the basis of political compromise. Although the Census Bureau reports data for state legislative districts, few data are collected on them. Further, their boundaries are subject to periodic change. For these reasons, they are not useful as units for purposes of healthcare marketing.

School Districts

School districts are established for the administration of the local educational system. Although such districts theoretically reflect the distribution of school-aged children in the population, such factors as the migration of students into and out of a district may play a role in determining the configuration of school districts in a community. Although school districts may be useful sources of data in developing population projections, few statistics are generated for this unit of geography, thereby limiting the usefulness of this source for marketing.

Statistical Units

Statistical areas are established to allow government agencies to collect and report data in an efficient and consistent manner. The guidelines for establishing most statistical units are promulgated by the federal government. The following are the most important statistical units in marketing.

Regions

The federal government establishes regions for statistical purposes by combining states into logical groupings. The Census Bureau has grouped the 50 states into four regions—Northeast, South, Midwest, and West—on the basis of geographic proximity and economic and social homogeneity. Although this unit is seldom used for marketing

(continued)

EXHIBIT 5.1 (*continued*)

purposes, some federal health agencies report statistics at the regional level. (The term *regional* is also alternatively used to refer to a group of counties or states delineated for some other purpose than data compilation, as in the "Delta Regional Authority.")

Divisions

For statistical purposes, the federal government divides the nation's four regions into nine divisions. Each division includes several states, providing a finer breakdown of the nation's geography. Divisions are seldom used as a basis for health services marketing. The following list breaks down the nine census divisions by region.

Census Regions and Divisions

Northeast Region
New England Division: Maine, New Hampshire, Vermont, Rhode Island, Connecticut, Massachusetts
Middle Atlantic Division: New York, New Jersey, Pennsylvania

Midwest Region
East North Central Division: Ohio, Indiana, Illinois, Michigan, Wisconsin
West North Central Division: Minnesota, Iowa, Missouri, North Dakota, South Dakota, Nebraska, Kansas

South Region
South Atlantic Division: Delaware, Georgia, Florida, Maryland, District of Columbia, Virginia, West Virginia, North Carolina, South Carolina
East South Central Division: Kentucky, Tennessee, Alabama, Mississippi
West South Central Division: Arkansas, Louisiana, Oklahoma, Texas

West Region
Mountain Division: Montana, Idaho, Wyoming, Colorado, New Mexico, Arizona, Utah, Nevada
Pacific Division: Washington, Oregon, California, Alaska, Hawaii

Metropolitan Statistical Areas

The federal government delineates metropolitan statistical areas (MSAs) as a means of standardizing the boundaries of cities and urbanized areas. Because states have differing criteria for incorporating cities, the MSA concept provides a mechanism for creating comparable statistical areas. An MSA includes a central city, a central county, and any contiguous counties that are logically included in the urbanized area. Data available on MSAs are increasing, and this unit is often used to define market areas.

Census Tracts

Census tracts are small statistical subdivisions of a county established by the Census Bureau for data collection purposes. In theory, census tracts contain relatively homogeneous populations ranging in size from 1,500 to 8,000. For many purposes, the census tract is the ideal unit for compiling market data. It is large enough to be a meaningful geographic unit and small enough to contribute to a fine-grained view of larger areas. The Census Bureau collects extensive data at the census-tract level, although this information is available only every ten years from the decennial census. In general, limited health data are available at the census-tract level, although some government agencies do collect and report data for this unit of geography.

Census Block Groups

Census tracts are subdivided into census block groups that include approximately 1,000 residents. A tract is composed of a number of block groups, each containing several blocks. The block group provides an even finer picture of a community than at the tract level, although fewer data elements are likely to be compiled at the block group level. Few health data are available at the level of the census block group.

Census Blocks

Census block groups are subdivided into census blocks, the smallest unit of census geography. The term *block* comes from the four-sided shape formed from the perpendicular intersection of four streets, although some other visible feature (e.g., railroad track, stream) or invisible feature (e.g., city limits) sometimes serves as a boundary. Census blocks tend to be the most homogeneous of any unit of census geography, and the average block houses approximately 30 persons. Virtually no health data and only limited demographic data are available for census blocks.

Zip Code Tabulation Areas

Zip code tabulation areas (ZCTAs) were developed by the Census Bureau for tabulating summary statistics from the 2000 census. ZCTAs are generalized representations of U.S. Postal Service zip code service

(continued)

EXHIBIT 5.1 (*continued*)

areas. They are created by aggregating the Census 2000 blocks (whose addresses use a given zip code) into a ZCTA, and then that zip code is assigned that ZCTA's code. These units represent the predominant U.S. Postal Service five-digit zip codes found in a given area. The Census Bureau's intent was to create zip code–like areas that would remain more stable from census to census.

Other Geographic Units

Healthcare marketers also use other geographic units that are often more suited to business development activities than are political or statistical units.

Zip Codes

Unlike the geographic units previously discussed, zip codes are not formal government entities. Their boundaries are set by the U.S. Postal Service and are subject to change as population shifts occur or the needs of the postal service dictate. This lack of stability means zip codes have limited value for historical analyses or for tracking phenomena over a long period. Further, zip codes seldom coincide with census tracts or other political or statistical boundaries, making the synthesis of data for various geographies extremely difficult. Zip codes tend to be much larger than census tracts, sometimes including tens of thousands of residents.

Nevertheless, the zip code is a useful unit for defining the market areas of smaller physician practices, smaller hospitals, and even specialty niches for larger health systems. Commercial vendors compile a great deal of information at the zip code level. More important, healthcare organizations typically maintain zip codes for nearly every consumer they come in contact with, making this unit an accessible geographic identifier linked to every customer record.

Areas of Dominant Influence

Taken from media advertising, the *area of dominant influence*, or ADI, refers to the geographic territory (typically a group of counties) over which a form of media (e.g., television, newspaper) maintains predominance. This concept is useful when healthcare marketers are interested in media promotions and want to determine the reach of a particular marketing campaign.

In actuality, few markets (for healthcare or anything else) neatly follow political, statistical, or administrative boundaries. In fact, markets nearly always change faster than their formal boundaries, and there will inevitably be some slippage between a geographically defined market area and the actual market area. Furthermore, market areas are often gerrymandered to conform to geographic boundaries that represent a reasonable approximation of the service area under study, primarily because the available data are usually organized on the basis of these geographic units. In addition, a market is difficult to visualize unless it is considered in terms of concrete, recognized boundaries.

Population Segments

A market may be defined in terms of a population segment or some component of the population. Marketers often report that the "market for product x" is this or that market segment. In these cases, they are typically not referring to a geographically defined market area but to a more nebulous market defined in terms of demographics, psychographics, or some other population characteristic. Examples of markets defined in this manner include active seniors, women of childbearing age, and psychographically defined segments such as "Generation Y."

Markets conceptualized in terms of population segments can be broad or narrow. For example, a market defined as "seniors" cuts a broad swath through the U.S. population. On the other hand, a market defined as "seniors who require nursing home care" is a much narrower segment of the population. Similarly, the nature of the market could depend on whether one is speaking in terms of a broad range of services (e.g., comprehensive inpatient services) or a narrowly defined individual service (e.g., outpatient eating disorder treatment).

Consumer Demand

A third way of delineating a market is from the perspective of the service itself—that is, the market is defined by consumer demand. For example, healthcare organizations may seek to identify geographic areas in which there are large concentrations of potential patients for a particular service. Geographically defined and demographically defined markets start with the general characteristics of the population and work down to its specific healthcare needs, whereas demand-based markets start with a particular need or service and work backward to identify the relevant population of consumers. In this instance, markets are defined in terms of their healthcare needs rather than broad geographic or demographic categories. Examples of markets defined in this manner are populations in need of geriatric services or behavioral health services. A hospital may consider nearly the entire population in its defined service area as part of the market for hospital services, whereas a home health agency may envision a narrowly defined sub-segment of the population as its potential market. Although markets defined in terms of consumer demand may coincide with established boundaries, they are just as likely to cut across geographic boundaries.

Opportunities

A fourth way of looking at markets is in terms of the healthcare opportunities that exist in a given area. A geographic area might be viewed with interest because there is a shortage of providers or lack of facilities in that area. An area characterized by a lack of competition is obviously attractive to an opportunistic organization. In other cases, the number of providers may be adequate, but their fragmentation may offer an opportunity for an organization that can appropriately package its services.

Areas (or populations) characterized by a high level of unmet healthcare needs may present additional opportunities. In other words, an area (or a population) may appear to need a certain level or type of service, but, for whatever reason, the service is not available. For example, a specified population, according to a demand model, should record a certain number of mammograms per year based on its size and composition. If the number of mammograms performed annually is significantly lower, this population may have an unmet need. Note that many unmet needs exist in populations with limited ability to pay for services. Depending on the type of organization performing the research, these populations may or may not be appropriate target candidates.

Similarly, opportunities may exist in areas where a gap analysis indicates a service shortfall or a mismatch between needs and services. The number of physicians or hospital beds that a given population can support is usually determined using various computer models. If the number of physicians and/or hospital beds located in the area falls below the expected number, there may be opportunities in that market.

Markets Without Walls

There is a fifth way to define a market, although in this case, the phrase "a market without walls" might be appropriate. Increasingly, certain markets are no longer defined in terms of geographic units or population segments. For example, the markets for contact lenses, health food supplements, and certain home testing products have become less dependent on location. These products may be purchased by mail order, through television shopping services, or via the Internet. In addition, the advent of telemedicine allows a specialist in one location to receive electronically transmitted test results for a patient in a different location, and patients and their doctors can interact via the Internet, thereby diminishing the importance of geographically defined markets.

Delineating Geographic Market Areas

The first step in developing an understanding of the market to be served is delineating the current market area for the healthcare organization. A number of methods can be used to specify the market area, and the method will vary with the type of organization and service involved.

Existing Patient Distribution

One method for delineating a geographic market area uses the internal data the organization maintains on its patients. The point of origin of existing customers can be determined (e.g., in terms of county, zip code, or even address) and their residences plotted on a map to determine their spatial distribution. A growing number of healthcare providers are mechanizing this process, either by purchasing mapping software or accessing online marketing systems that facilitate strategic marketing activities. The geographic area (e.g., zip code, county) from which a pre-specified percentage of admissions are drawn may be designated as the provider's market area. As a rule of thumb, the area from which 75 to 80 percent of the patients are drawn represents the core market area. (Although it may be worthwhile in some cases to target the area covered by 100 percent of organization's patients, from a marketing perspective it may make more sense to focus one's efforts.)

Market areas can also exist at different levels—for example, primary, secondary, and even tertiary market areas might be identified. The area that accounts for 60 percent of patients could be considered the primary market area, and the area that accounts for the next 25 percent of patients might constitute the secondary service area. The area accounting for the remaining 15 percent of patients would be considered the tertiary market area. By taking this approach, the healthcare organization is able to develop a more refined view of its overall market area. This information helps the marketer craft campaigns that address the respective needs of those in the primary, secondary, and tertiary markets.

Multiple market areas may exist for organizations that provide multiple services. The market area for the hospital's obstetrics services may differ significantly in size and configuration from its market area for trauma care or orthopedic surgery. Typically, the market area for general hospital services is likely to be different than that for more specialized offerings. For example, urgent care centers may be more dependent on drive-by traffic of residents from other communities than on the residents proximate to the facility.

The delineation of market areas in this manner assumes that patients are originating at their residences when they seek care. Although this assumption is the case more often than not, the analysis should also account for patients who do not come from their residences but from other facilities (e.g., nursing homes) or from industrial or commercial sites (Pol and Thomas 2001).

Ideal Markets

In some situations, the existing market area may not match the organization's objectives. The composition of the identified market area may be changing. The characteristics of resident consumers may have changed, or the organization's clientele may have moved away from the facility, as in the case of an inner-city hospital whose patients have moved to the suburbs but continue to patronize the facility. The question to ask becomes: Is this market area appropriate to use as a framework for marketing?

Further, in establishing the market area for a new service or new location, data on the patient origin for existing patients will not be available. One approach to delineating the market area might be to determine the maximum distance or driving time consumers are willing to travel for a given health service. Computer software is available to perform this task, although in rapidly changing areas, driving times can become significantly different over a relatively short time.

Prospective Markets

A third method focuses on establishing market area boundaries for a service not yet offered. Delineating these boundaries is much more difficult and usually requires the use of multiple techniques. One approach may be to determine the residential distribution of patients using similar services. If another organization is offering the same or similar services, its market area boundaries might be used as a guide. Distance and/or driving time data may be evaluated as well. However, a more subjective approach may be required because the service in question is new to the area. Data on the same service in a different market area may be available through professional networks. These data could help establish time/distance parameters. Surveys of potential consumers of these services (e.g., physicians and patients) may also provide valuable time/distance information.

Once delineated, market area boundaries must be continuously monitored for change. Traffic patterns and driving times change, and the entrance or exit of competition may significantly alter market area boundaries over a short time. Changes of taste and preference regarding physician services (e.g., increased interest in home infusion therapy) or changes in patient type (e.g., increased demand for outpatient services) must also be monitored to determine their effect on market area boundaries.

Nongeographic Boundaries

The identification of non–geographically based markets involves a potentially more complicated process. Typically, these markets are defined in terms of size and composition, and the geographic area provides only the context. Thus, a national market would consider only the geographic boundaries of the United States as a framework in which to identify submarkets. An example would be the population of women who gave birth in the previous six months. With respect to a given service (e.g., mental health services for postpartum depression), the size of the effective market can be estimated at the national level.

When identifying market area boundaries on the basis of the location of non–geographically defined markets, the situation becomes more complicated. In an ideal world, the mere presence or absence of a target population (e.g., active seniors, women of childbearing age, Latinos, or baby boomers) would be adequate. However, situations are seldom this clear-cut, and a non–geographically defined market is likely to be interspersed with populations that have other characteristics. In other words, marketers seldom find an either/or situation but find that market concentrations are more a matter of degree. Thus, measures of the concentration of the target population in a geographic area need to be developed.

Often the emphasis in data analysis is placed on identifying areas with high or low concentrations of persons susceptible to certain illnesses or areas with shortages or surpluses of healthcare providers. For example, if a healthcare provider is interested in geographic areas with high concentrations of older persons, several procedures can be used. Suppose the larger market is a particular state, and the sub-state markets of interest are counties in that state. The goal is to identify the counties with the highest concentrations of persons aged 65 or older. The percentage of the population aged 65 to 74 and 75 or older is used as the basis for index construction. The indicator chosen will depend on a number of factors, including the nature of the population, the type of service, and/or the marketing methodology being used. Ultimately, use of a methodology that combines both the number and percentage of seniors may be appropriate.

When viewing markets from a nongeographic perspective, a different identification strategy is used. The point of reference is a larger population, such as the United States or a region within the boundaries of the United States. The purpose of the exercise is to find concentrations of persons with certain characteristics in subgroups of the population. For example, if health insurance plans want to identify the segments of the population that had the highest rates of uninsureds, they might examine the composition of the nation's uninsured population.

An additional way of defining non–geographically based markets is in terms of consumer propensity to obtain a particular good or service. Market analysts in other industries have long identified population segments on the basis of their willingness, ability, and/or interest in a particular product. Although healthcare services cannot be viewed in exactly the same manner as these other products, there is increasing interest in identifying potential markets in terms of their propensity to be affected by a particular condition or to use/need a particular service. This approach is often based on demographic or psychographic profiling. If, for example, a propensity score of 100 indicates average use of a particular service, a score of 200 for a specific population segment suggests a propensity to use this service that is twice the average for the total population. On the other hand, a propensity score of 50 indicates a use rate that is half the average.

Proxy Data

Because propensity data are unlikely to exist for the residents of a particular geographic area, inferences have to be made on the basis of knowledge gained from the analyses of other populations. For example, if the likelihood of the presence of human immunodeficiency virus (HIV) infection among Latinos is a function of Puerto Rican ancestry, a specified level of education and income, and residence in a highly mobile urban area, it should be possible to develop a propensity score for the presence of HIV in various Latino populations. Thus, the propensity score for Latinos in parts of New York City might be 250, while that for Latinos in Miami might be only 45. In another example, the propensity for undergoing laser eye surgery might be related to certain psychographic or lifestyle segments. Thus, five lifestyle segments might be found to have a propensity score for laser eye surgery of 300 or more (or three times the average), in contrast to ten other lifestyle segments who almost never undergo laser eye surgery. To the extent that the distribution of lifestyles can be specified for a target area, it becomes possible to determine the potential market by using such an approach. The variation in health services utilization from market to market cannot be overemphasized. Exhibit 5.2 presents evidence that supports the existing disparities in the use of health services.

EXHIBIT 5.2
Geographic Variations in Health Services Utilization

Healthcare analysts realized long ago that significant variation exists in the utilization of health services from community to community in the United States. As early as the 1970s, research revealed that the rate of procedures performed from community to community, even in adjacent states, varied to a degree not explained by population differences. The procedure rate could range from 10 percent of the patient population in some markets to 50 percent in others. These studies suggested that the volume of health services delivered was less a function of disease prevalence than it was a reflection of the characteristics of the medical community and the practice patterns of local physicians.

Typical of the findings on this issue are the results of a study that compared the cities of Boston, Massachusetts, and New Haven, Connecticut, in terms of their health services utilization patterns (Wennberg, Freeman, and Culp 1987). Although the two cities are similar in terms of the factors that *should* determine the use of health services, they differ dramatically on almost every indicator of health services utilization. The hospital admission rate, for example, was nearly twice as high in Boston as it was in New Haven. Further, residents of Boston were much more likely to be hospitalized for various acute and chronic conditions than were residents of New Haven. The average annual per capita expenditure on healthcare in Boston was twice that of New Haven. However, the comparative utilization patterns were not always consistent. The rates of performance for certain procedures were much higher in Boston, but for others, they were much higher in New Haven.

A number of factors account for these seemingly inexplicable differences. A major factor is the variation in physician practice patterns from community to community. In some communities, it is standard practice to treat a problem with surgery; in other communities, the standard calls for less invasive treatment. In some communities, conventional medical wisdom calls for hospitalization for certain diagnostic tests and procedures, whereas in others, it is customary to handle such cases on an outpatient basis.

Other factors contributing to different utilization rates include the relative supply of facilities and services. There is pressure, for example, to fill hospital beds if they are available and to use medical technology in which the organization has invested. In contrast to other industries, competition in healthcare often drives up both utilization levels and costs, thereby accounting for an additional degree of variation. Even the presence of a medical school may influence the level of utilization and the types of procedures performed. Increasingly, the level of managed care penetration is a significant factor influencing utilization rates.

Given these variations, how does an analyst determine the appropriate level of utilization? Is the reported level of utilization high or low? What should be realistically expected? Of course, one way to address this question is to use a standard rate of utilization, such as the health services utilization rates developed by the National Center for Health Statistics from national surveys (see www.cdc.gov/nchs/

(continued)

EXHIBIT 5.2 (*continued*)

products/series.htm#sr13). These rates provide useful benchmarks, but because most analyses focus on local markets, how appropriate are they for the market in question? There is no easy answer to this dilemma. The analyst must be able to gain enough knowledge about the local healthcare environment to make reasonable assessments about the appropriate level of utilization.

Profiling Healthcare Markets

Once geographic boundaries have been established for a market or the parameters for a non–geographically defined market have been established, key attributes of the population within those boundaries can be specified. The development of a market profile involves collecting and analyzing detailed information about the market area(s) in question. Any and all characteristics relevant to service provision must be obtained from whatever primary and secondary data sources are available.

Market Size

Markets can be distinguished by several different dimensions. The first dimension is market size. *Size* here refers to the absolute number of potential consumers in a specific market area. The marketer typically begins by determining the total population within the market area. This figure indicates the universe of potential customers that exists and must be refined to reflect the portion of the population relevant for the analysis. This refined assessment of the market would include only segments that represent prospective customers for the organization or its specific services.

Market Composition

The second aspect addressed in a profile is market *composition*, or the makeup of the identified population. Composition is usually framed in terms of the number of persons in a particular area who have certain characteristics (i.e., demographic, socioeconomic, and psychographic data). This profile is also likely to include characteristics such as marital status, household structure, education level, and income characteristics. More detailed data on economic characteristics (e.g., labor force characteristics, housing values) may also be considered.

The demographic analysis is often accompanied by an assessment of the psychographic characteristics of the market area population. Information on the lifestyle categories of the target audience can be used to determine the likely health priorities and behavior of a population subgroup. Consumer attitudes are also likely to be considered as a component of psychological segmentation. The attitudes of consumers in a market area are likely to have considerable influence on the demand for almost all types of health services.

During the profiling process, the situation with regard to insurance coverage is typically assessed. The emphasis on insurance coverage will vary depending on the nature of the organization. The payer mix of a market area (and of the organization that is the focus of the marketing plan) is clearly significant for healthcare providers whose financial viability depends on it.

Although many providers attempt to limit the number of self-pay patients they serve, there is a multibillion-dollar market for elective services that are not typically covered by insurance plans. The entire vanity market, including face-lifts, tummy tucks, and other cosmetic procedures, is strictly driven by patients who do not have insurance that covers these procedures. Another example is the alternative therapy industry that has emerged to challenge mainstream medicine and depends almost entirely on out-of-pocket expenditures by its customers.

Community type is also a consideration when collecting baseline data on the market. The dominant community type within the market area, whether urban, suburban, or rural, will have important implications for health status and health behavior. Consumer attitudes are also likely to be different among the various community types, and the existence of submarkets within the market area may be a complicating factor when developing a marketing plan.

Health Status

The health status of the market area population is the third dimension considered in a market profile. The level of morbidity in a population is a major concern for health services planners. Incidence and prevalence rates are likely to be important in a marketing analysis. This category includes measures of morbidity in terms of disease prevalence along with disability indicators. To the extent possible, planners need to project future rates of incidence and prevalence to plan for anticipated developments in the medical arena.

The health status of the market area population defines the range of health service needs that is likely to exist. The services healthcare organizations provide are ideally designed to address the health problems that characterize the population of the market area. These health conditions should indicate the segments of the market to be targeted as well as the needs of the population the organization hopes to meet.

Health Services Demand

The fourth dimension involves translating health conditions into demand for health services. The types of diseases and other health problems identified in the market area population should indicate the types of services needed. A market's need for childhood immunizations, for example, can be translated into demand for a specific number of health department clinics and clinic personnel. The wants of a market in terms of face-lifts and laser eye surgery can be translated into demand for plastic surgeons and ophthalmic surgeons.

In many cases, actual data on the market may not be available, and estimates of need must be calculated. Fortunately, a number of models have been developed for estimating and projecting the demand for a service using data on population characteristics and known utilization rates. These modeling techniques require an understanding of the service area and the manner in which these models operate. Modeled data are never as good as actual data, but the estimates generated by methodologically sound models are adequate for most purposes. In any case, modeled data must be used if the level of need is being projected for some future period. See, for example, the prospective risk assessment developed by Health and Performance Resources for use in determining health services demand (Reuters 2008).

Typically, the level of need will be expressed in terms of a percentage of the population or a rate of some type. For example, calculations may reveal that 20 percent of the adult population is affected by a clinically identifiable emotional condition or that the crude birthrate is 15 births per 1,000 population. The most common measures of need would be the prevalence and incidence rates epidemiologists and public health officials use. These measures of the level of morbidity provide the baseline data on which the rest of the analysis depends.

Once the level of need has been determined for the defined market area, the number of potential cases in that area can be estimated. A high prevalence rate by itself does not ensure a meaningful market. Healthcare is a numbers game, and a critical mass is needed to support any service.

The extent to which the identified needs are being met is indicated, at least partially, by the health behavior of the market area population. Health behavior includes both formal utilization of health services and informal actions designed to prevent health problems and to maintain, enhance, or promote health. In terms of formal activities, potential indicators include hospital admissions, patient days, average length of stay, use of nonhospital facilities, physician office visits, visits to nonphysician practitioners, and drug use. In recent years, the use of freestanding medical facilities and alternative therapies has also become an important indicator.

Availability of Resources

The fifth dimension considers the availability of healthcare resources. Resources include existing healthcare personnel, facilities, and programs. The types of resources identified will depend on the nature of the organization.

A general hospital, for example, would want to determine the availability of resources comparable to its own, whether they are offered by a competing hospital or another healthcare organization. A medical specialty group, on the other hand, would be interested in the much narrower range of available resources in its specialty area.

Of the resources available to the community, healthcare organizations should hone in on those that are considered competition. In the past, hospitals knew other hospitals were their competition, cardiologists knew other cardiologists were their competition, and so forth. The environment has changed, and today, competition can take a number of forms. Many types of nonhospital organizations now compete with hospitals. These competitors are not always external to the hospital; in some cases, members of the hospital's own medical staff may set up rival services. The boundaries of specialty practice have become blurred as aggressive specialists seek to expand the range of services they offer. Purveyors of alternative therapies have also emerged to challenge mainstream physicians on many fronts.

In profiling the market area, the temporal dimension is another important consideration. Whether determining the needs of the target market or identifying competing services, marketers must take the three time horizons—past, present, and future—into account. Although the current characteristics of the market area are a good starting point, it is important to develop a sense of its historical trends. Is the population growing or declining? Are the characteristics of the population different today than they were five years ago? Is the number of competitors increasing? The most important time frame, however, is the future, whether two, five, or ten years down the road. The market area profile should project the future characteristics of the population, the future health services needs of that population, and likely future developments with regard to competing organizations.

From Mass Market to Micromarket

When the healthcare industry first began to recognize the importance of marketing, the total population was considered the market for most services. Hospitals, for example, believed they provided all services to all people. They did not attempt to distinguish segments of the population and made only crude, geography-based distinctions between markets.

Healthcare organizations operating in this mode typically take a mass marketing approach. *Mass marketing* involves developing generic messages and broadcasting them in a wide, untargeted manner to the entire service area. There is no attempt to target specific audiences, identify likely best customers, or tailor the message to a particular subgroup. This approach involves the use of mass media (e.g., newspaper, radio, television) to blanket the market area. The message has to be general, and it typically touts the merits of the organization rather than specific services.

As healthcare entered the marketing era, healthcare marketers adopted target marketing techniques. Target marketing involves the identification and subsequent cultivation of segments of the market area population that have certain attributes. These segments of the population may reside in a geographic area that is being emphasized, may be demographic or psychographic sub-segments of the population, or may be individuals otherwise classified as prospective customers.

The intent of target marketing is to deliver a particular message to a particular audience to attract members of this segment of the population as customers. Target marketing is an efficient and cost-effective means of communicating a message to the targeted audience. By eliminating segments of the population, marketing effort and expense are minimized. Target marketing, thus, offers the marketer more "bang for the buck." Although target marketing typically involves the use of traditional media, communication channels can be tailored to reach the target audience. Thus, wide-circulation newspapers and network television would be eschewed in favor of special-interest publications, radio stations appealing to specific audiences, and cable channels with certain viewer demographics.

In targeting audiences for specific goods and services, certain established rules should be applied. Targeted markets must be amenable to rating in terms of their potential, the markets must be realistic in size, the targeted customers must be reachable, and the targeted customers must have some minimum level of response potential. Assuming that the market is of adequate size, another consideration besides the potential number of cases is the geographic distribution of prospective customers within the market area. The importance of customer distribution varies with the type of service and the characteristics of the population. Some services are supported by a local population and others by a more far-flung population. On the other hand, some populations are much more mobile than others or are otherwise more or less sensitive to travel times and/or distances.

In recent years, many healthcare organizations have gone a step further and adopted a micromarketing approach. *Micromarketing* involves identifying and soliciting specific individuals or households. Identification of prospective customers at this level is usually not necessary to support healthcare marketing campaigns. However, there may be situations in which it is more efficient and cost-effective to identify the individuals or households that are the best prospects for a particular service. For example, if an ophthalmic surgeon has determined that individuals with certain demographic and psychographic traits are better candidates for laser eye surgery than those with other traits, the most effective approach may be to contact people with those attributes directly through direct mail or telemarketing rather than use a more broad-based approach. Similarly, a hospital implementing a major donor drive may target only households that have the resources and propensity to make a substantial contribution.

The Effective Market

In healthcare, the potential market for a service may not correspond to the population that actually uses that service. Because the target population's level of need for a particular health service may (or may not) reflect its level of interest in that service, it is important to determine the extent to which members of the target population really want the service. Although it may be possible to conduct a preliminary analysis of the market area population and develop an estimate of the level of interest in a particular service, many situations require primary research. Ideally, no new program or service should be introduced without a consumer survey, and the newer the service or less familiar the market, the greater the need for such a survey. Many new programs have failed because the target population's actual level of interest was much lower in reality than it was on paper.

Ascertaining the level of interest may be relatively straightforward. Market surveys often query consumers about their interest in the availability of a service and whether they would use it if it were available. Marketers in healthcare found early on, though, that these responses have to be carefully qualified. Typically, respondents express an interest in any new service that appears to benefit them specifically or even the community in general. However, when their likelihood of using the service is qualified by introducing location or price considerations, the level of interest may change. For example, one survey found that a large portion of consumers in a target area were interested in a hospital-sponsored fitness program. When the likely location was disclosed, interest waned somewhat. It waned even further when the proposed fee schedule was introduced. Obviously, the more elective the service under consideration, the more important these qualifiers become.

Payer Mix

A factor that has become increasingly important in developing a market profile is the consumer's ability to pay for health services. The analyst must determine the potential payer mix of the target population and estimate the expected level of reimbursement for a particular service. Given that different payers (e.g., commercial insurers, Medicare) offer different levels of reimbursement, the effective payer mix will ultimately determine the actual level of payment.

The two bases for determining a target population's ability to pay are household income and type of health insurance coverage. For major health problems (i.e., problems requiring hospitalization and/or intensive services), the level of insurance coverage is the more important consideration. Employer-sponsored commercial insurance generally affords the highest level of reimbursement. Other forms of private insurance (e.g., Blue Cross) are also desirable. Although payments under Medicare and Medicaid are essentially guaranteed, reimbursement rates under these government insurance programs have historically been lower than those of commercial insurance plans. For elective services, the level of income is usually more important than the type of insurance coverage.

In some areas, underinsurance is an issue, especially during an economic downturn. On the other hand, certain segments of the population may have insurance coverage, but copayment provisions, restrictions on benefits, and/or limitations on reimbursement may reduce its value.

The emergence of managed care as a force in the market has obviously changed the playing field. Unfortunately, information available on managed care at the market level is limited, and primary research is often needed to gain an understanding of managed care penetration and the market shares of managed health plans.

Competition

The market potential for health services must also be adjusted to take existing competitors into account. Except in rare cases where a market is not served at all, competitors in various guises will inevitably exist. Indeed, the proliferation of competitors has been a major development in U.S. healthcare. Some of these competitors may already be entrenched within the target area or population. Others may be entering the market to challenge those that are already active.

Regardless of the nature of the competition, the available market must be adjusted to account for it. A family practitioner opening an office in a community may face competition from other family practitioners, other primary care providers, public health clinics, urgent care centers, government-sponsored clinics, and even alternative therapists. A realistic assessment of the potential market must consider all of these factors.

A related activity involves measuring market share for the organization and, if possible, for its competitors. The numerator in these calculations would be the number of cases recorded for the organization (or its competitors), and the denominator would be the total instances of that phenomenon for the market area. Internal records on procedures, discharges, and/or diagnoses may serve as the numerators for market share calculations. Denominators may be derived from data made available in response to data reporting requirements. For example, hospital discharge data are often collected by state

EXHIBIT 5.3
Calculating Hospital Market Shares for Obstetrical Admissions

Hospital	2005 OB Admissions	Market Share
Hospital X	200	14%
Hospital Y	400	29%
Hospital Z	600	43%
All Other	200	14%
Total	1,400	100%

health departments and aggregated at geographic levels, such as the county level. A simple calculation divides the number of discharges from Hospital X in County Y by the total number of discharges in County Y. See Exhibit 5.3 for an example of a market share calculation.

In the absence of a clearinghouse for utilization data, another way to gather data for rate denominators is to generate estimates of the number of procedures and discharges using population and incidence information. For example, the number of diabetes cases in a market area can be estimated by multiplying national or regional incidence rates by population data specific to age or other enumerated factors known to differentiate the probability of being diagnosed with diabetes. Estimates can be used as proxies for the actual data when there is no market-specific count of procedures, discharges, or diagnoses that can serve as the market share denominator. Case Study 5.1 describes the steps involved in determining the effective market for a particular service.

CASE STUDY 5.1
Determining the Effective Market

Southern Health Systems (SHS), a fictional organization, established a satellite hospital in a growing suburban area ten years ago. Since then, the hospital has become relatively successful. It has attracted adequate medical staff and gradually increased its occupancy rate. At the time it opened, SHS was not authorized to offer labor-and-delivery services. Now, however, there appears to be a significant market for maternity services, as the population has reached a critical mass and many young families have moved into the community.

(continued)

CASE STUDY 5.1 *(continued)*

In 2007, the SHS marketing staff was instructed to assess the situation and determine the potential for maternity services within this market area then and in the future. This assessment was needed if SHS was to make a rational decision with regard to expansion. Because the state requires a certificate of need to add any new service, the data were needed to make a case for adding obstetrics beds. The SHS market analysts were cognizant of the need to not only identify the apparent potential for maternity services but also specify the effective demand.

As in any market research project, the analysts began by delineating the service area likely to be served by the proposed obstetrics program. Once satisfied that a defensible service area had been specified, the analysts profiled the population within that service area. They determined the size and characteristics of the current population and developed projections for the future that reflected anticipated changes in its demographic characteristics.

According to the data available at the time (three-year-old census data), the population of the service area in 2004 was approximately 42,000 residents. Estimates for the service area purchased from a demographic data vendor projected a 2014 population of 50,000. The SHS analysts thought this figure represented the maximum population capacity of the area because virtually all available residential land would be built up by 2014. The demographic characteristics of the population in 2004 also were determined and projected forward to 2014. The analysts focused on data on the age structure of the population (especially the number in their childbearing years), the marital status of the population (unmarried suburban residents typically don't have children), and the racial and ethnic composition of the population. This latter attribute was considered important given the disparities in birthrates among the various racial and ethnic groups. The psychographic (or lifestyle) characteristics of the service area population were also analyzed on the grounds that people in different lifestyle clusters exhibit different attitudes toward childbearing.

The analysts also researched the situation with regard to insurance coverage. Because this information was not readily available, they had to conduct primary research. A sample survey of the area's households revealed that 75 percent of the service area population was covered by some form of commercial insurance. Small proportions were covered by Medicare, Medicaid, or some form of military insurance. A negligible number of residents were uninsured. The high level of insurance coverage was a positive finding.

Satisfied that the number of women of childbearing age was adequate (23 percent of the population compared to 19 percent countywide) and that a significant proportion of the households were married couples with or without children (55 percent compared to 35 percent for the county), the market analysts calculated current and anticipated levels of fertility for the market area population. Because detailed data were not available on fertility patterns of the market area population, known figures from a similar population were applied.

The analysts calculated a proxy estimate of the birthrate for this population (15 births/1,000 people), which turned out to be well above the county rate of 10/1,000. This estimate was not surprising, given that this population is skewed toward women of childbearing age. The general fertility rate also was calculated to determine the fertility rate for women of childbearing age (i.e., those aged 15–44), which turned out to be lower than that for the county overall (58/1,000 women aged 15–44 compared to 65/1,000). This calculation provided a more realistic view of the likely level of fertility for this population than the crude birthrate because it adjusted for the size of the childbearing age population.

On the basis of these figures, the analysts estimated that the population would yield almost 700 births annually by 2014, with a 2007 estimate of 570 births. Thus, 700 births became the base figure for calculating the effective market for obstetrical services. This figure had to be adjusted for various factors that were likely to affect its conversion into demand for the hospital's proposed maternity services. One of the demographic factors that needed to be considered was the projected growth in the proportion of the service area population that was African American. Given the higher fertility rate for the African-American population, the anticipated number of 2014 births was adjusted to 750. However, psychographic data gathered on the service area population indicated that the career orientation of many of the area's women was likely to lower the potential number of births. Thus, the anticipated number of births was adjusted back down to 725.

A major consideration was the drag on potential demand represented by competition from other providers of obstetrics services. After all, this service would be new, and with the exception of existing patients of SHS facilities who might transfer their business to the satellite facility, SHS would have to cultivate a new set of obstetrics customers. Realistically, many, if not most, of the women of childbearing age in

(continued)

CASE STUDY 5.1 *(continued)*

the community were likely to have existing relationships with obstetricians/gynecologists (OB/GYNs). These potential patients would have to be convinced to change to an OB/GYN affiliated with the new facility, or SHS would have to convince its existing OB/GYNs to join the staff of the new facility. Further, many potential customers would be constrained in their use of facilities by the health plans that cover their obstetrical care. Last, some of these potential maternity customers had already delivered children at another facility (or had otherwise positive experiences with a competing hospital) and would not be inclined to change hospitals without a good reason.

On the basis of their experiences elsewhere, SHS analysts believed the combined effect of these three factors (i.e., existing provider relationships, insurance steering, and previous experience) would reduce the potential market share to approximately 50 percent of the total in the short run, and SHS would grow this share to 60 percent by 2014. In the best of all worlds, the analysts believed a market share of 75–80 percent was the most they could ultimately hope for, so a 60 percent share in 2014 was considered a reasonable estimate.

On the basis of adjustments necessitated by these facts, the analysts estimated that SHS would capture approximately 285 births during its first year of operation and approximately 420 births annually by 2014. Given that a minimum of 200 annual births were required to justify the cost of establishing the facility, the SHS analysts concluded that the effective demand was adequate to support the proposed maternity service.

Discussion Questions

- Why did SHS market analysts have to assess the size of the market before going forward with the development of a new obstetrics service?
- Why couldn't the analysts simply use the total population as the basis for determining the demand for obstetrics services?
- To what extent might the lifestyle orientation of women in the market area influence their attitudes toward childbearing?
- How important are the presence of other obstetrics service providers and the existing relationships between market area women and obstetricians in determining the effective demand for obstetrics services?
- What challenges do marketers face in introducing a new service to a market area, particularly a service as personal as obstetrics care?

The Changing Nature of Healthcare Markets

The healthcare arena has historically been characterized by relative stability and predictability. However, this situation has given way to an environment that is increasingly unstable and unpredictable. This dynamic must be considered when markets are being analyzed because it has implications for identifying, profiling, and evaluating healthcare markets, making an understanding of the changes occurring in the healthcare market necessary for effective decision making on the part of marketers.

Several factors have contributed to the changing nature of healthcare markets. Many of these factors are inherent in the market areas themselves and are not directly health related. Market areas are constantly undergoing changes in terms of demographic characteristics; changes in population size, composition, and distribution are everyday occurrences. Lifestyle changes have also become common in U.S. society.

The demand for services in a particular market or population segment may be influenced by a variety of factors, ranging from changing consumer preferences to newly introduced technology. National or regional trends with respect to service usage, especially in the consumption of elective services (e.g., liposuction), also contribute. Technological advances that make new procedures possible—and old procedures better—reshape the constellation of services offered and the way services are delivered (e.g., inpatient versus outpatient). Changing insurance arrangements could easily affect the level of demand for services in a specific market.

Another factor that contributes to changing markets is the fluid competitive situation. Existing competitors are constantly changing locations, services, or marketing strategies. New competitors are continually entering the market, and other competitors are dropping out. This situation has been complicated by the emergence of national chains that may enter a market and, almost overnight, upset the competitive balance. National and state legislation that facilitates the creation of the new partnerships (e.g., health alliances) or alters regulatory powers or procedures (e.g., for health maintenance organizations) reshapes and, in some instances, creates markets for services.

The ubiquity of change is one more reason to establish market research as an ongoing process rather than an ad hoc activity. Identifying, profiling, and evaluating markets are not onetime activities to be returned to three, five, or ten years later. These three tasks should be an ongoing *process* used to continually search for market opportunities and to provide continuous evaluation of current strategy. Making these procedures routine, investing in the requisite hardware and software, and training personnel to perform these functions are essential tasks for nearly all health services providers. Case Study 5.2 describes the steps involved in identifying true market potential.

CASE STUDY 5.2
Is There Really a Market for It?

The primary objective in analyzing any market is to determine the potential demand for some good or service being offered to that market. The market analysis process typically determines the size and composition of the target market and profiles the identified area in terms of its demographic and socioeconomic characteristics. The market is also typically profiled in terms of such health-related characteristics as disease incidence, utilization rates, and referral patterns.

The initial market analysis attempts to estimate the market potential. The analyst will typically determine, for example, the age distribution, racial characteristics, and marital status of the target population, along with such socioeconomic characteristics as income levels, workforce characteristics, and educational levels. Through this process, the analyst compiles all of the information necessary to determine the potential market for the goods or services being offered.

Years of experience with market analysis suggest that such characteristics need to be verified from as many perspectives as possible and interpreted on the basis of any information on the community that may have a bearing on the issue. An analyst must be able to read between the lines and capture the essence of the market, which may not be obvious from the raw data.

In some cases, especially when entering a new market, the analyst may have only secondary data. The analyst should verify this information through ground-level research using whatever means available, even primary research. In fact, the analyst may not be able to determine the effective level of demand in a market without surveying the residents.

A case in point involved a growing suburban area outside a medium-size southern city. The community had all the earmarks of an up-and-coming suburb. Its population was growing rapidly, and an increasing number of upscale housing units were being constructed. Income levels were rising, and the socioeconomic status of the resident population was steadily increasing. An examination of the available data suggested a highly attractive market in terms of its demographics.

Analysis of the secondary data revealed that the market was composed of an upwardly mobile population with a moderately high level of ambulatory care needs. The population appeared to be ripe for innovative programs (e.g., freestanding birthing centers), progressive services (e.g., behavioral healthcare), and even trendy venues (e.g., fitness centers). In short, the community appeared to be a dream for marketers offering new services. Even better, virtually no competition had emerged in the community.

The analyst conducted a survey of community residents to confirm the conclusions drawn with regard to the services this population would likely demand. The first clue that things were not as they seemed surfaced early in the interviewing process, when interviewers encountered high refusal rates and a generally hostile respondent population. Analysis of the survey data revealed that, contrary to the initial analysis, the population was anything but progressive. The residents of this suburb were traditional in their approach to healthcare and resistant to new or innovative services. They had little interest in such programs as women's services, fitness centers, and behavioral health programs, despite large numbers of residents who fit the profile for these services.

The high proportion of military personnel and retirees in the area also influenced the respondents' attitudes. These residents' situations were much different than those of typical suburban residents in that their military affiliation and retirement health plans influenced their health service utilization patterns.

Ultimately, the community was offered a basic package of primary care services. The gap between the residents' lifestyles and their socioeconomic status and the presence of a large military and retired population precluded the development of the types of services typically offered to a growing, upscale suburban population. Luckily for the hospital planning the services, its market analyst obtained the information necessary to prevent a serious strategic miscalculation based on the paper profile of the market area.

Discussion Questions

- What characteristics of this fast-growing suburban population made hospital administrators envision a potential market?
- When the suburb's population was initially examined, what types of services did analysts think would appeal to the community?
- What type of research was carried out to verify the conclusions based on secondary data for this population?
- How did the findings from the consumer survey conflict with what was deduced from the secondary data?
- What did the market analyst discover about this population that discouraged the development of innovative health services?
- Rather than cutting-edge services, what types of programs might the market analysts conclude are more appropriate for this population?

Summary

An understanding of the market to be served is a critical requirement for marketing professionals in any industry. To appreciate the interface between healthcare and marketing, they must understand the societal framework in which both enterprises exist. Marketing professionals also must have thorough knowledge of the social, political, and economic characteristics of the target population, along with the lifestyles, attitudes, and other traits of the market area population.

The market for healthcare goods and services can be delineated in a number of ways. Markets can be conceptualized on the basis of geographic scope, population characteristics, level of demand, and market potential. With the emergence of the Internet, markets without walls have also become common. The market area for an organization can also be delineated in various ways, and the approach used depends on the circumstances. The geographic division used to define the market (e.g., zip code, county) depends on the characteristics of the organization and the type of services provided. Over time, healthcare marketers have moved away from a mass marketing approach to a target marketing or micromarketing approach in an effort to increase marketing precision.

Once defined, a market must be profiled in terms of its salient characteristics, including demographic and socioeconomic traits, psychographic or lifestyle attributes, health status, and patterns of health behavior. The population's ability to pay for care is an increasingly important consideration. Market characteristics are constantly changing, and market areas must be assessed in terms of past, present, and future traits.

A number of factors must be considered in determining the effective market for a healthcare organization. The total demand must be adjusted for such factors as ability to pay, consumer preferences, existing relationships, and presence of competitors. A distinction must also be made between consumer needs and wants when evaluating a potential market.

Key Points

- The decision to implement marketing implies that a market exists, but the word *market* has a different meaning in healthcare than it does in other industries.
- A healthcare market can be defined in a number of different ways.
- A number of geographic units may be used to delineate a healthcare market.
- Large healthcare organizations are likely to have a number of different markets to consider.

- Healthcare markets can be profiled in terms of their size, population composition, health status, and level of health services demand.
- Healthcare is unique in that not all people with a particular health status will necessarily be considered potential customers.
- Healthcare marketers must determine what portion of the total market represents the effective market for the organization's goods or services.
- Healthcare markets are often more dynamic than markets in other industries, as they must respond to developments in health conditions, treatment modalities, and reimbursement patterns.

Discussion Questions

- What are some of the ways marketers define healthcare markets, and what determines how market delineation differs for various types of healthcare organizations?
- What are some of the bases on which markets can be delineated, and what determines which approach is used?
- How can a start-up organization delineate a market in which it has no history?
- What determines the geographic division (e.g., county, zip code, census tract) at which a market area should be delineated?
- Why is it sometimes difficult to delineate a market area using standard political boundaries?
- How can marketers identify unmet healthcare needs that may indicate an untapped market?
- To what extent has the Internet changed the way markets are organized?
- What are the most salient demographic characteristics considered in profiling a population, and how may these traits differ according to the type of healthcare organization?
- What arguments can be made for the use of psychographic analysis in healthcare marketing today?
- Why is the ability to pay for healthcare an important factor to consider in a target market assessment?
- What factors have prompted the transition from a mass marketing orientation to a target marketing orientation in healthcare?

Additional Resources

Pol, L. G., and R. K. Thomas. 1997. *Demography for Business Decision Making*. New York: Quorum.

U.S. Census Bureau. 2008. *Statistical Abstract of the United States.* Washington, DC: U.S. Government Printing Office.

HEALTHCARE CONSUMERS AND CONSUMER BEHAVIOR

In any industry, the goods and products offered reflect the needs, desires, and preferences of that industry's consumers. Although this generalization is true in healthcare to some extent, the industry defies this basic tenet in many ways. In healthcare, a distinction is made between healthcare patients, clients, consumers, and customers—although all of these terms are used at different times to define the purchasers and/or end users of healthcare services and products. In this chapter, the different categories of customers are described, and their attributes' implications for marketing are discussed. The unusual nature of consumer behavior in healthcare is also described, along with the steps involved in the consumer decision-making process.

The Healthcare Consumer

Consumer, as the term is typically used in healthcare, refers to a person with the potential to consume a good or service. As noted in Chapter 1, anyone who has a want or need for (and presumably the ability to pay for) a product can be considered a potential customer. According to this definition, the entire U.S. population is a market for some type of healthcare good or service.

Healthcare organizations have not historically viewed consumers in this manner. Individuals were not considered consumers of health services until they became sick. Until recently, the general assumption was that none of the 305 million U.S. citizens was a prospect for health services *until* one sought care. Thus, healthcare providers made no attempt to develop relationships with non-patients. Marketers in the consumer goods industries pursue potential customers much more aggressively than do marketers in healthcare, assuming that nearly everyone has a need (or at least a want) that can be met.

How Healthcare Consumers Are Different from Other Consumers

Healthcare consumers differ from the consumers of other goods and services in a variety of ways. For one, healthcare purchases are largely nondiscretionary in that serious consequences could result if no action is taken. A health professional typically orders services for the good of the patient. In virtually no other industry are goods or services prescribed for the consumer and then pressure placed on the consumer to comply with the prescription.

In addition, healthcare consumers often do not know the price of the services they consume, which reflects the unusual financing arrangements characterizing healthcare and the patient's lack of access to pricing information. Unlike that of consumers in other industries, the behavior of healthcare consumers is seldom affected by cost factors.

Further, healthcare consumers have little knowledge about the operation of the healthcare system and may have little or no direct experience with it. They have no basis in reality for evaluating the quality of the services they receive and must make judgments about their treatment on the basis of subjective criteria.

Most healthcare episodes have an emotional component not present in other consumer transactions. Medical care involves a certain level of anxiety for both the patient and those close to the patient. As noted in Chapter 1, emotions like fear, pride, and vanity influence the behavior and decisions of patients and their families. Exhibit 6.1 presents differences between healthcare consumers and other types of consumers.

How Healthcare Consumers Are Similar to Other Consumers

Although much has been made of the unique characteristics of healthcare consumers, they are more similar to consumers in other industries than the previous discussion suggests. Some healthcare episodes do involve emergency or life-threatening conditions, but most do not. Thus, most healthcare episodes involve some discretion on the part of the end user or those involved in the decision-making process. Further, the consumption of many types of services is considered elective. Much like other consumers, healthcare consumers are likely to distinguish between needs and wants when consuming services. Clearly, most healthcare consumers would view angioplasty to correct a heart condition as a need but laser eye surgery to improve vision as a want. The latter would typically be considered a discretionary "purchase," whereas the former would be regarded as nondiscretionary.

EXHIBIT 6.1
Healthcare Consumers Versus Other Consumers

Consumers of Health Services	Consumers of Other Services
Seldom determine their own need for services	Usually determine their own need for services
Seldom are the ultimate decision maker	Usually are the ultimate decision maker
Often make decisions subjectively	Usually make decisions objectively
Seldom have knowledge of the price	Always have knowledge of the price
Seldom make decisions based on price	Usually make decisions based on price
Are reimbursed by third party for most costs	Are rarely reimbursed by third party for costs
Usually make nondiscretionary purchases	Usually make discretionary purchases
Usually require a professional referral	Rarely require a professional referral
Have limited choices	Have unlimited choices
Have limited knowledge of service attributes	Have significant knowledge of service attributes
Have limited ability to judge quality of service	Are usually able to judge quality of service
Have limited ability to evaluate outcome	Are usually able to evaluate outcome
Have little recourse for unfavorable outcome	Have ample recourse for unfavorable outcome
Seldom are the ultimate targets for marketing	Always are the ultimate targets for marketing
Are not susceptible to standard marketing techniques	Are susceptible to standard marketing techniques

Healthcare consumers are like other consumers in that the level of demand for goods and services is elastic. Years ago, the conventional wisdom was that the demand for health services was essentially inelastic. It was assumed that those who were sick consumed services and those who were well did not. Not only does this assumption reflect a dated notion of health and illness; it also does not account for the vast number of discretionary transactions that occur in healthcare.

Today the demand for health services is seen as extremely elastic. The level of healthcare utilization is influenced by a wide range of factors independent of health status, including availability of services, access to health insurance, and physician practice patterns. Furthermore, the demand for health services can be manipulated—for example, by physicians who order greater or lesser amounts of a particular service, or by marketing campaigns that make consumers aware of a service they did not know existed. Pharmaceutical advertising, for example, has convinced many consumers that they suffer from a condition they had never heard of before.

One final similarity relates to the ability to pay for services. Most patients pay for healthcare through some form of insurance. Those without insurance must pay out of pocket or resort to a healthcare "safety net," such as a public health clinic or charity hospital. Historically, healthcare was thought to be such a necessity that people would find a way to pay for required services even if they had to go into debt to do so. Many argued that community safety nets would ensure that all health problems were addressed in one way or another.

Clearly, the ability to pay for care is a major consideration affecting the demand for healthcare goods and services. Admittedly, for elective procedures and other products not considered medically necessary, consumers may be unwilling to pay out of pocket and thus reduce the demand for services. During periods of economic prosperity, the volume of cosmetic surgery, laser eye surgery, and other vanity services increases; conversely, during periods of economic downturn, the volume of such discretionary expenditures may decrease. Even medically necessary treatment may be cut back; as a result of the recession that began in 2008, the number of visits patients made to physicians' offices decreased (AAFP 2009).

Since the emergence of modern medicine in the United States, the ability to pay for care has had implications for health services utilization. There are endless accounts of patients who have been unable to obtain care because they did not have the resources to pay for it. Today, physicians and hospitals are likely to expect payment on the front end from people who lack insurance. As result, people without health insurance or personal financial resources may be reluctant to seek treatment and are less likely to obtain care, even care considered medically necessary. The inability to pay for healthcare is even more pronounced when prescription drugs are involved. A deathly ill patient can eventually be admitted to an emergency department, but necessary drugs cannot be obtained from a pharmacy without payment. Ultimately, healthcare consumers must weigh the economic implications of consuming goods and services just as consumers in any other industry must.

The Variety of Healthcare Customers

One of the more important attributes of healthcare customers is their variety. Not only are there individual consumers of healthcare goods and services; health professionals and facilities are also major consumers of goods and services. Although organizations' needs may be different than individuals' needs, many of the same marketing issues pertain.

Healthcare consumers are classified in a variety of different categories, each with specific needs. In the eyes of the general public, the typical patient is someone requiring life-saving services. Life-threatening situations, however, are rare occurrences, but when they do occur, they require dedicated personnel, equipment, and facilities for their management. Most healthcare encounters involve a different category of consumer: people requiring routine health services, who present themselves for treatment at a doctor's office, clinic, or therapy center. A third category includes consumers who desire elective health services (i.e., products and services that are not considered medically necessary).

Another major category of consumer comprises those involved in self-care. Research has indicated that the prevalence of self-care among consumers is much greater than previously thought and that many people access the formal healthcare system only after they have exhausted other options. Thus, symptomatic individuals are likely to first self-diagnose and self-medicate using the wide range of do-it-yourself remedies available. Pharmacy shelves are stocked with products and devices for home testing and treatment, and the Internet has expanded the availability of such products.

For these and other reasons, a number of different terms are applied today to the purchasers and end users of healthcare goods and services. Today, the term *patient* is giving way to other terms that more clearly reflect the contemporary healthcare environment. Major terms were described in depth in Chapter 3. Exhibit 6.2 summarizes those terms for reference. Note that these categories of customers are not mutually exclusive and that the term of choice depends on the context. Someone who has become a psychiatric patient could just as easily be categorized as a *client*. At the same time, this patient/client is the *end user* of a service (i.e., psychotherapy) and an *enrollee* in a health plan that pays for the treatment. Further, the patient is considered a *customer* for this service.

Professional and Institutional Customers

While patients are the first group that comes to mind when thinking about customers in healthcare, there are numerous other groups of customers to

EXHIBIT 6.2
A Typology of Healthcare Customer Terms

Term	Meaning	Determinant	Application
Patient	Person under the care of a health care provider	Formal diagnosis by a medical practitioner	Traditional term for a person receiving medical care
Client	Person who has a formal relationship with a healthcare provider	Entry into a therapeutic relationship with a provider (with or without a formal diagnosis)	Most often applied to relationships with nonphysician providers (e.g., mental health professionals)
End user	Person who receives a service or consumes a good	Receiver of the product, regardless of who orders it or pays for it	Used to distinguish between the person receiving the care and other parties (e.g., the party that pays the bill)
Enrollee	Person who is enrolled in a health plan or other group arrangement that finances healthcare	Formal membership by qualifying and paying a premium	Enrollment status determines covered services, copayments, and deductibles
Consumer	Anyone in the population who might use a health service	Inclusion in the population under consideration	Universe of potential customers to be targeted by marketers
Customer	Person who uses a service or purchases a good	Receiver of a good or service in exchange for something of value	Consumer who has been converted into a buyer of goods or services

consider. Two major groups are health professionals and healthcare organizations, both of which consume a wide range of goods and services.

Physicians

Although physicians are thought of as providers of services rather than as consumers, physician practices are major customers for many goods and services. Hospitals solicit physicians to join their medical staffs. Provider networks and health plans solicit the participation of physicians and other clinicians. Nursing homes, home health agencies, and hospices may depend on physicians for referrals. Many physicians depend on referrals from other physicians.

Physicians are customers of a variety of organizations providing support services, including billing and collection services, utilization review companies, medical supply distributors, biomedical equipment companies, and biohazard management companies. Physicians are customers of information technology vendors who sell or service practice management systems, imaging systems, and electronic patient record systems. Physicians have also traditionally been pharmaceutical companies' primary customers.

Other Clinicians

Other clinicians are customers for many of the same goods and services as physicians. Dentists, optometrists, podiatrists, chiropractors, mental health counselors, and other independent practitioners have many of the same needs physicians have and are cultivated by similar marketing entities. These providers require supplies, equipment, billing and collections services, information technology, and other services, just as physicians do.

Hospitals and Other Institutions

Hospitals and other institutional settings are customers for a wide range of healthcare-specific goods and services in addition to the normal products any large organization consumes. These organizations require many types of medical supplies and biomedical equipment, and some may require durable medical equipment, such as wheelchairs and hospital beds. They are customers for a variety of support services, including billing and collections, physician recruitment, and marketing. By providing food service, gift shops, and parking services, hospitals are customers for a spectrum of non-health-related goods and services. They are routine consumers of such goods as office supplies and janitorial supplies. Hospitals and other healthcare facilities are heavy consumers of information technology and are major customers of information technology vendors and consultants.

Employers

Major employers are customers of health plans, managed care plans, providers, and provider networks. Most health plans are employer based, and competing health plans seek to contract with employers for the management of their employees' health. Individual providers may seek to contract with employers that are self-insured or otherwise open to negotiated services. Employers are also customers for a variety of direct provider services, including occupational health services, employee assistance programs, fitness center programs, and other services that providers may market directly to employers.

Other Customers

Like organizations in other industries, healthcare organizations have internal customers. Chief among these internal customers are their employees. Every organization should view the members of its workforce as customers. In this regard, healthcare has generally lagged other industries. The mission, goals, and objectives of the organization should be continuously marketed to internal customers, and their input should be regularly solicited.

Another customer in this category is the organization's board of directors. In most organizations, the board of directors is charged with setting the organization's direction and monitoring its progress. This body typically plays a critical role in the operation of the organization and should be considered an important internal customer.

Other secondary customers should be considered as well. One example of a secondary customer is the general public. Most provider organizations and many other types of healthcare organizations must maintain a positive public image. Not only is it important to create and sustain corporate goodwill; at some point, the organization may need to demonstrate that it is a good community citizen and, in the case of not-for-profit organizations, that it deserves to retain its tax-exempt status.

The media is yet another customer of healthcare organizations. The media must be cultivated to ensure that the organization's story is told—and told in the right manner. Long before hospitals and other healthcare organizations had formal marketing functions, they had public relations departments to deal with the media.

Many healthcare organizations have one or more branches of government as customers. Health facilities and health professions are regulated by government agencies and often maintain separate government relations offices to interface with them. If the organization has not-for-profit status, its continued exemption from taxes depends on good relationships with the appropriate government agencies. The same goes for organizations located in areas where certificate-of-need requirements exist.

Segmenting the Market for Healthcare Products

Market segmentation, long a practice in other industries, is used to single out and call marketers' attention to certain segments of the population. Not every subgroup in a population qualifies as a target market, and certain rules of thumb help marketers identify a meaningful market segment. To be useful to a marketer, a segment should be *measurable* in that accurate and complete information on the segment's characteristics can be acquired in a cost-effective manner. The segment should be *accessible* in that marketers are able to communicate effectively with its members using standard marketing methods. It should be *substantial* enough to be considered for dedicated marketing activity. And it should be *meaningful* in that it includes consumers who have attributes relevant to the aims of the marketer.

A viable market segment should also evidence a desire for the healthcare product in question and be able to pay for it. Further, the growing emphasis on consumer engagement has raised sensitivity to the issue of healthcare consumers' readiness for change. Some of the more common forms of market segmentation are described in the sections that follow.

Demographic Segmentation

Commonly used in consumer goods industries, market segmentation based on demographics is the best-known approach to identifying target markets. This type of segmentation defines demographically distinct subgroups on the basis of their need for various goods and services. The links between demographic characteristics and health status, health-related attitudes, and health behavior have been well established. For this reason, demographic segmentation is always an early task in any marketing planning process.

Marketers will typically segment the healthcare market in terms of age, sex, and race or ethnicity. Depending on the service to be offered, the market may be further segmented according to income level, educational level, or even marital status. The population may then be even further classified according to region of the country or type of community (e.g., rural, suburban, urban). Research has indicated, for example, that the demographic segment most likely to sign up for fitness programs includes affluent women between 35 and 40 years old living in suburban communities in the Midwest. (Chapter 8 provides additional detail on the demographic characteristics of populations.)

Geographic Segmentation

An understanding of the spatial distribution of the target market has become increasingly important as a result of healthcare's reorientation toward the consumer. One of the implications of this trend has been an increased emphasis on the appropriate location of health facilities. A market-driven approach to health services requires healthcare organizations to take their services to consumers wherever they are, and major purchasers of health services are insisting on convenient locations for their enrollees. Knowledge of the manner in which the population is distributed within the service area and an understanding of the links between geographic segmentation and other forms of segmentation are critical to the development of a marketing plan. (Geographic units used for geographic segmentation were described in Chapter 5.)

Marketers can segment the population in terms of geography in a number of ways. They can identify the geographic areas that constitute the market area for an organization (e.g., the zip codes from which a physician draws patients), or they can segment the population by type of community, considering, for example, the area's rural, suburban, and urban residential components as separate markets. Or, they can relate other variables (e.g., demographic characteristics, lifestyle traits) to particular geographic areas. For example, marketers commonly segment the market area geographically in terms of income by identifying areas with low, medium, or high income levels. Exhibit 6.3 illustrates the geographic distribution of a demographic variable (income).

EXHIBIT 6.3
Income Distribution for Washington, DC (by census tract)

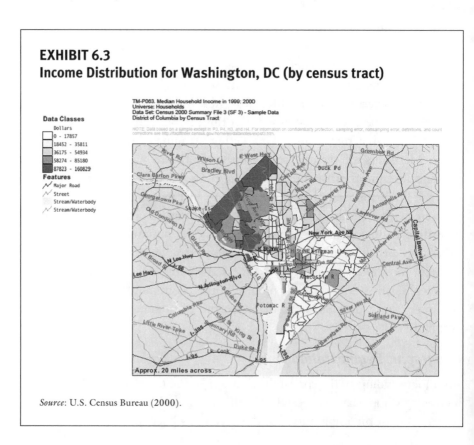

Source: U.S. Census Bureau (2000).

Psychographic Segmentation

For many types of goods and services, an understanding of the psychographic or lifestyle characteristics of the target population is essential. Lifestyle clusters in a population often transcend (or at least complement) its demographic characteristics. Most important, psychographic traits can be linked to the attitudes, perceptions, and expectations of the target population, as well as to its propensity to purchase certain services and products. Although use of psychographic analysis in healthcare has lagged other industries, health professionals are finding an increasing number of applications for this approach, and more healthcare data are being incorporated into psychographic segmentation systems.

Marketers can choose from a handful of different psychographic segmentation systems for use in partitioning the market area in terms of lifestyle. For example, the MOSAIC system developed by Experian assigns one of 60 lifestyle clusters to most households in the United States. (See www .demographicsnow.com/Templates/Static/Understanding%20MOSAIC .pdf for an explanation.) Knowing the cluster of a household opens the door to a variety of other information useful to marketers, in addition to lifestyle information. Exhibit 6.4 graphically presents the psychographic breakdown of a market area by major lifestyle grouping.

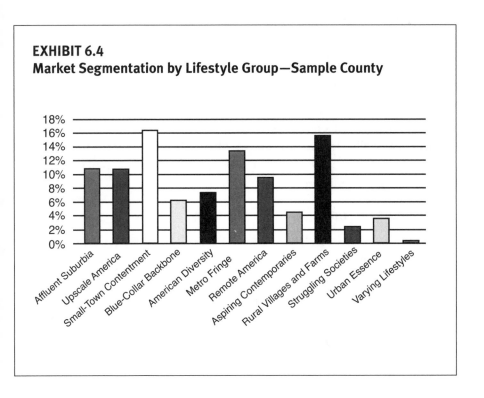

EXHIBIT 6.4
Market Segmentation by Lifestyle Group—Sample County

Health Risk Segmentation

An approach to market segmentation unique to healthcare involves partitioning the population in terms of its level of health risk. This approach is particularly important in determining the types of health services appropriate for a particular population and in crafting the marketing message for those services. Health risks may be measured in terms of a specific health condition (e.g., the risk level for diabetes) or in terms of a variety of health risks in combination. In either case, the level of risk is quantified and presented numerically or, more commonly, ranked as low, moderate, or high.

From a marketing perspective, the level of risk affects the type of marketing message used and the timing of its delivery. Consumers with low levels of risk need to receive information on prevention and health enhancement, along with information on the warning signs of health problems. Consumers at moderate risk need to be encouraged to take appropriate action. Consumers at high risk need to be made aware of the need for urgent action, informed of the types of health services available, and encouraged to comply with their prescribed treatment.

Usage Segmentation

Usage segmentation, a common approach in other industries, is now being applied to healthcare. The market area population can be divided into categories based on the extent of use of a particular service. In examining the use of urgent care clinics, for example, the population can be divided into heavy users, moderate users, occasional users, and nonusers. This approach can be applied to many services but may be most useful when elective goods and services are under consideration. This information provides a basis for subsequent marketing planning that can be tailored, for example, to existing loyal customers versus noncustomers. Consumers' willingness to use certain services, especially elective procedures, often reflects the extent to which they are open to change in general. See Exhibit 6.5 for a discussion of the adoption process for new healthcare services.

Payer Segmentation

A form of market segmentation unique to healthcare involves targeting population groups on the basis of their payer categories. The payer mix of the market area population has come to be one of the first considerations in profiling a target population. The existence of insurance coverage and the type of coverage available are major considerations in marketing most health services. Further, health plans cover some services and not others—an important consideration in marketing. For elective services paid for out of pocket, a targeted marketing approach is typically most effective.

EXHIBIT 6.5
Who Adopts Innovative Services?

Despite their emphasis on research and innovation, healthcare organizations are relatively conservative. They adopt new techniques or treatment modalities only after extensive testing, and even then, practitioners may be reluctant to forsake tried-and-true procedures. Similarly, most healthcare consumers tend to be conservative in their approach to care, preferring to stick with proven treatments rather than opt for more experimental approaches.

This perception of healthcare consumers, however, masks the wide range of approaches to the adoption of health services. The baby boom generation, for example, has been particularly open to innovative approaches. As a result, many novel health services have been introduced, from urgent care to alternative therapies. Clearly, some segments of society have a greater predilection for innovation than others.

Marketers have studied the process through which individuals come to adopt a new procedure or therapeutic modality by tracking the process from the point at which an individual first hears about an innovation to its final adoption by the consumer. In many ways, this process is similar to the consumer decision-making process discussed later in the chapter. Various studies have found that the population can be subdivided into the categories of innovators, early adopters, early majority, late majority, and laggards (Rogers 2003).

Innovators represent, on average, the first 2.5 percent of all those who adopt. They are eager to try new ideas and products; it's almost an obsession for them. They have higher incomes, are better educated, and are more active outside their community than non-innovators. They are less reliant on group norms, are more self-confident, and are more likely to obtain their information from scientific sources and experts.

Early adopters represent, on average, the next 13.5 percent to adopt a product. They try the product early in its life cycle and, compared to innovators (who have a more cosmopolitan outlook), are much more reliant on group norms and values and more oriented to the local community. Early adopters are more likely to be opinion leaders because of their closer affiliation with groups. Because of their personal influence on others, they are regarded as the most important segment in determining whether a new product will be successful.

(continued)

EXHIBIT 6.5 (*continued*)

The *early majority* are the next 34 percent to adopt. They deliberate more carefully before adopting a new product; they collect more information and evaluate more options than early adopters do. Although slower to adopt, they are an important link in the diffusion process because they are positioned between the earlier and later adopters.

The *late majority* are the next 34 percent to adopt. They are described as skeptics who eventually adopt an innovation because most of their friends have already done so. Subject to group norms, they adopt under the pressure to conform. They tend to be older, have below-average income and education, and rely primarily on word-of-mouth communication rather than the mass media.

Laggards are the final 16 percent to adopt. They are similar to innovators in their inattention to group norms. They are independent because they are bound to tradition, and they make decisions in terms of the past. By the time they adopt an innovation, it has probably been superseded by something else. Laggards have the lowest socioeconomic status.

Healthcare marketers can improve their effectiveness by determining how innovative their product is and using this information to target the components of the consumer population who are most likely to adopt the product. Efforts directed toward those who are unlikely to adopt new goods or services will be wasted.

Source: Adapted from Assael (1992) and Rogers (2003).

Market analysts typically categorize payers as commercial insurers (sometimes carving out managed care plans as a subcategory), Medicare, Medicaid, and other government programs (e.g., military). Those who are not covered by insurance and pay for health services out of pocket form a residual category that may be referred to as the *uninsured*. Exhibit 6.6 illustrates the payer mix of a target market area.

Benefit Segmentation

Different people buy the same or similar products for different reasons. Benefit segmentation is based on the idea that consumers can be grouped according to the principal benefit sought. The benefits consumers consider when making a purchase decision include such product/service attributes as quality, convenience, value, and ease of access. As healthcare has become more con-

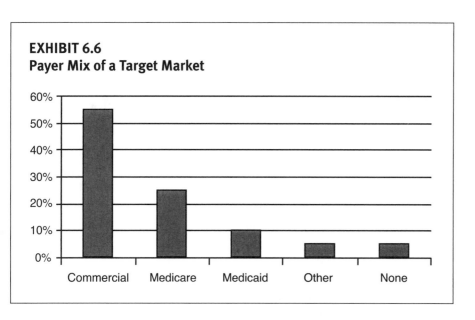

EXHIBIT 6.6
Payer Mix of a Target Market

sumer driven, market researchers have sought to determine which buttons to push to make a product or service resonate with potential customers. The same service can be positioned in different ways depending on the benefits sought by the target audience. Thus, the marketer might promote free, close-to-the-door parking to one segment, the quality of the staff to another segment, and competitive pricing to yet another segment. Exhibit 6.7 illustrates the results of a survey on benefits sought in a family practice clinic, and Exhibit 6.8 summarizes the different approaches to segmentation.

EXHIBIT 6.7
Attributes Sought in a Family Practice Center,
Ranked in Order of Importance

Attribute	Percentage of Respondents Seeking That Attribute
Convenient location	93%
Extended hours	85%
Same-day appointments	64%
Free, nearby parking	63%
Personal care manager	50%
Online consultation	42%
Low prices	31%

Source: Thomas (2005).

EXHIBIT 6.8
Approaches to Healthcare Market Segmentation

Basis for Segmentation	Focus	Example	Use
Demographics	Specific demographic groups	Women of childbearing age	Conducting product development, target marketing
Geography	Geographically concentrated consumer groups	A fast-growing new suburb	Selecting a site
Psychographics	Consumer groups exhibiting a particular lifestyle	Psychographic cluster of Generation X career women	Tailoring services or marketing messages to the lifestyle
Health risk	Segments identified in terms of their level of health risk	Segments with a high level of obesity	Targeting for prevention messages and social marketing initiatives
Usage level	Consumer groups reflecting various levels of product usage	Customers loyal to a particular brand	Tailoring marketing messages to level of usage
Payer category	Consumer groups with varying ability to pay for health services	Medicare enrollees	Assessing the financial potential of a market segment
Benefits sought	Product attributes desired by consumers	Busy consumers demanding speed and convenience	Determining the "hot buttons" of a targeted consumer group

Consumer Behavior

Consumer behavior refers to the patterns of consumption of goods and services that characterize healthcare consumers, along with the factors that contribute to this behavior and the processes that lead to a purchase decision. Because marketing is driven by consumer needs, an appreciation of the behavioral dimension of any target population is essential. Ultimately, this behavior is what a marketing campaign seeks to influence. While the behavior of professionals and organizations is important, this discussion focuses on individual consumers.

Despite the differences between healthcare consumers and other consumers, healthcare consumers' decision criteria can be classified in the same manner as those of consumers in other industries. The categories of factors that influence purchase decisions include technical, economic, social, and personal criteria. Technical criteria include quality of care, clinical outcomes, the environment, and the amenities associated with health services. Economic factors, perhaps the least relevant in healthcare, include the price of goods and services, the payment mechanism (e.g., insurance), and the perceived value of the service rendered. Social criteria include such factors as the status associated with the professional, the facility, or the procedure performed and the influence of the consumer's social group. Personal criteria include factors related to the emotional aspects of the service, self-image issues, and even moral and ethical considerations.

It is traditional to think in terms of a hierarchy of needs in setting the context for analyzing consumer decision making. Most refer to Maslow's theory of motivation. Maslow (1970) contended that the first order of need for human beings involves physiological needs for food, water, air, shelter, and so on. Once these basic needs are met, individuals can begin to think in terms of their safety and security needs, including freedom from threats and the establishment of security, order, and predictability in their lives. At this stage, health begins to emerge as a value in its own right.

With this foundation, individuals can begin to think in terms of the next level in the hierarchy—social or companionship needs. These needs include friendship, affection, and a sense of belonging. To these needs, esteem or ego needs are eventually added, including the need for self-respect, self-confidence, competence, achievement, independence, and prestige. Finally, at the top of the needs hierarchy, individuals feel the need for self-actualization, which includes the fulfillment of personal potential through education, career development, and other goals. Only a few societies in the history of the world have achieved this top level of fulfillment.

The level of the hierarchy at which an individual or a population functions says a lot about the healthcare needs it faces (and the approach a marketer should take). At the lower levels of the model, survival needs dominate the healthcare arena. Society members face threats from pathological agents and a hostile environment. At the higher levels of the model, the threats common at the lowest levels have been moderated and, rather than attempting to preserve life and limb, society members can focus on health maintenance and enhancement. Their needs shift from life-saving procedures and public health considerations to self-actualization needs, such as weight control, fitness programs, and cosmetic surgery.

From a marketing perspective, individuals who are at the survival level are likely to respond only to a marketing initiative that addresses their immediate needs. They are not going to respond to promotions for services that enhance their quality of life or require out-of-pocket expenditures (which explains the difficulty involved in convincing financially precarious people that they ought to invest in healthy lifestyles). As individuals progress up the hierarchy, they are more open to discretionary services and appreciate the importance of maintaining and enhancing their health status. At the self-actualization level, services like plastic surgery, breast implants, and teeth whitening become a means of raising status and enhancing self-esteem.

Ultimately, the types of healthcare goods and services a person responds to, the communication method used to reach that person, and the message that resonates with that person reflect his or her position in this model. Marketers are faced with the challenge of matching the product, medium, and message to the status of the target audience in relation to the needs hierarchy. Case Study 6.1 illustrates a marketing approach to a consumer behavior challenge.

CASE STUDY 6.1
Using Consumer Engagement to Encourage Wellness Behavior

A growing number of companies are developing employee health management programs in an effort to control their healthcare costs and maintain a healthier, more productive workforce. Employers are encouraging employees to identify their health risks and, when appropriate, take necessary actions to address those risks. Employee health programs facilitate participation in health risk assessments and typically offer incentives to encourage employees to sign up for wellness classes, weight management programs, chronic disease management programs, and so forth. The benefits of participating in such programs are well documented, not only for the health of the employee but also for the company's bottom line.

Despite the known benefits of these programs, employers face a number of challenges in effectively implementing them. Employees often resist participating in health risk assessments. Employers can't mandate participation, and even when incentives are offered, presentation rates for health risk assessments are low. This resistance creates a problem because a health risk assessment is typically required for placement in a wellness program. Even more significantly, after health risks have been identified, it is a challenge to get employees to commit to a wellness program. In the same way that incentives have little influence on participation in health risk assessments, they have a limited effect on participation in fitness programs, chronic disease management, and other wellness options.

Many observers contend that the inability to generate the desired level of employee participation in such programs is a marketing problem. Many, if not most, people would be willing to undergo a health risk assessment if approached in an effective manner. Similarly, most people who realize they are at risk for a health problem would be willing to change their behavior under the right circumstances. Ultimately, the question is how to engage employees in a manner that elicits the desired results.

In one company, the marketing department was asked to develop an approach to consumer engagement that allowed the employer to target different groups of employees with a message that resonated with their particular situation. They believed the right message at the right time would go a long way toward engaging the employees in the company's health improvement effort.

To this end, the marketing department developed a questionnaire, which all employees completed. Unlike the health risk assessment, the survey did not delve into the employees' detailed health conditions but asked a only few questions about their knowledge of health risk, their attitudes toward improving their health status, and actions they were taking or would be willing to take to improve their health. As a result of the survey, the marketers were able to divide the workforce into categories of workers who (1) had limited knowledge about health issues and their own health status, (2) knew they had health risks but were reluctant to take appropriate action, (3) were willing to take appropriate action but were not sure how to do it, and (4) were already involved in some type of wellness program.

(continued)

CASE STUDY 6.1 (*continued*)

Armed with this information, the marketers developed a consumer engagement initiative that targeted the needs of each group but emphasized for all groups a core theme of living well. For the first group, the initiative focused on information dissemination to raise these employees' level of knowledge. The material created for the second group aimed to change these employees' attitudes and encouraged them to develop an appreciation of proactive measures. In the third group, the marketers had to cultivate an awareness of available options and otherwise facilitate participation. The marketing message for the fourth group was designed to reinforce existing desirable behavior. The overall intent was to move employees from one group to the next group using well-timed and stage-appropriate marketing messages.

After the consumer engagement initiative had operated for a year, a follow-up survey indicated that (1) the level of awareness of health risks had increased, (2) an increased number of health risk assessments had been performed, (3) a higher proportion of employees had signed up for company-sponsored wellness programs, and (4) the dropout rate for existing programs had decreased. Although the employer is still refining this program, management concluded that a targeted consumer engagement approach influenced positive changes in knowledge, attitudes, and behavior among the employee groups. Although minor changes were made to make the program more attractive, the primary factor in its success was the implementation of an effective marketing initiative.

Discussion Questions

- Why do employers think it is beneficial to assess their employees' health status and offer them wellness program options?
- What factors prevent employees from reducing their health risks and taking steps to improve their health status?
- What factors led management to conclude that the ineffectiveness of the employee health program was a marketing issue?
- Along what dimension(s) did the marketers segment the employee population?
- In what ways is this consumer engagement initiative an example of target marketing?
- How was the effectiveness of this consumer engagement initiative evaluated?

Consumer Decision Making

In nearly every other industry, the end user is responsible for the purchase decision, and the decision maker actually consumes the good or service. In healthcare, the end user of the service (e.g., the patient) typically does not make the decision to purchase the service. Instead, a physician is likely to determine what, where, when, and how much of the service is provided. Alternatively, the decision maker may be a health plan representative, an employer, or a family member. The marketer is faced with the challenge of determining where to place the promotional emphasis under these circumstances.

As a result, the end user of a service may not be the ultimate target of a marketing initiative. Healthcare marketers have therefore identified a number of other categories of target audiences that may be more important than the end user. For example, various categories of *influencers* have been identified, who could be family members, counselors, or other health professionals who encourage consumers to use a particular good or service. The role of *gatekeepers* might also be considered, including primary care physicians, insurance plan personnel, discharge planners, and others responsible for channeling consumers into appropriate services.

Another category comprises the *decision makers* who make choices for the consumer, who could be family members, primary care physicians, or caregivers who act on behalf of consumers. *Buyers* of healthcare services compose the final category and include employers, business coalitions, and other groups that might indirectly control the behavior of consumers by determining which services they can and cannot use.

One of the most important findings relates to the role of women in the healthcare decision-making process. Data on health services utilization indicate that women use a disproportionate share of healthcare resources (NCHS 2009). Further, women generally make most of the decisions for their children and often for their husbands. They are also likely to be involved as healthcare decision makers for their parents or other dependent family members. Although women consume at least half of the personal health services in the United States, they account for more than 80 percent of the decisions to purchase healthcare goods or use healthcare services (HCPro 2007).

Steps in Consumer Decision Making

A basic understanding of the decision-making process consumers go through when purchasing goods and services is important for marketing planning purposes. The steps involved in the consumer purchase model are described in the following list. These steps are an amalgam of approaches adapted for the healthcare environment and should be taken into consideration when developing a marketing plan (Berkowitz and Hillestad 2004). The approach marketers take depends on the consumer's stage in the decision process.

- *Problem recognition.* The first step in the purchase decision process is consumer recognition of a problem or need. The marketer's task is to identify the circumstances or stimuli that triggered the need and to use this knowledge to develop marketing strategies that spark consumer interest.
- *Information search.* At this stage of the decision process, the consumer is interested enough to search for more information. The consumer may exhibit heightened attention to the condition recognized in the first step or initiate an information search. The similarities and differences between the approaches healthcare consumers and other types of consumers take to information gathering are discussed in Exhibit 6.9.
- *Initial awareness.* Awareness refers to the target population's initial exposure to the good or service being marketed. Thus, during the information search, the healthcare consumer becomes exposed to the various options that exist for addressing the problem.
- *Knowledge emergence.* Knowledge concerning the options crystallizes as the healthcare consumer begins to understand the nature of the good or service and to appreciate its potential for addressing the problem.
- *Alternative evaluation.* At this stage, the consumer uses the information he or she has accumulated to evaluate available options and make a rational purchase decision. The consumer may decide to rule out some options at this point.
- *Contract assessment.* This step is unique to healthcare in that many goods and services will not be considered for purchase if the provisions of the consumer's insurance plan do not cover them or the available provider does not accept the type of insurance carried by the consumer.
- *Preference assignment.* Preferences develop at the point the consumer expresses a tendency for one good or service (e.g., a podiatrist rather than an orthopedic surgeon) or decides between different providers of the same service (e.g., podiatrist A rather than podiatrist B).
- *Purchase decision.* The healthcare consumer makes a decision at this point (or someone else makes it) with regard to the good to be purchased or the service to be used. Healthcare is different from other consumer contexts in that a variety of players may be involved in the purchase decision.
- *Product usage.* At this point, the healthcare consumer buys the product or uses the service. This step could be as simple as buying adhesive

bandages at the neighborhood pharmacy or as complex as undergoing a heart transplant.

- *Post-purchase behavior.* In this last stage, the consumer assesses whether the outcome of the purchase is satisfactory. Family members or other parties also may express their opinions about the purchase. If satisfied, the consumer becomes an advocate for the product or service (or a detractor if dissatisfied).

EXHIBIT 6.9
Information Search by Healthcare Consumers

The information search process healthcare consumers follow tends to differ considerably from the process followed by consumers in other industries. The healthcare industry is unique in many ways and does not offer the sources of information typically available to other consumers. The availability of information, of course, differs according to the goods or services in question. Personal health *products*, such as adhesive bandages, over-the-counter pharmaceuticals, and nutraceuticals, are marketed in much the same manner as other consumer products. Healthcare *services*, however, are marketed differently than other consumer services.

The structure of the healthcare delivery system is complicated; even seasoned health professionals find it difficult to fully understand. Thus, when a healthcare consumer is faced with having to choose a practitioner, facility, or program, adequate information may not be available. There is a dearth of accurate and detailed information on the clinicians and organizations that provide health services. Furthermore, issues of quality, value, and outcomes as they relate to physicians, hospitals, and other providers cannot be communicated by promotional material as is the case with other services.

Faced with this lack of information, where does the healthcare consumer turn? Traditionally, healthcare consumers have access to two primary sources of information on healthcare—one informal and one formal. The primary sources of informal health information have historically been friends, relatives, neighbors, and work associates. These associates can offer insights based on their own experiences and information they have gathered. The formal sources—physicians and other health personnel—may be consulted less frequently but are more authoritative. Because of their position in the system and the knowledge

(continued)

EXHIBIT 6.9 (*continued*)

they are presumed to have, doctors in particular are a major source of information on healthcare.

These two sources have been supplemented by information gleaned from the media. Historically, print media (e.g., magazines and newspapers) and electronic media (e.g., radio and television) have been the primary sources. Newsletters geared to the needs of healthcare consumers also have become common, as have self-help books, of which the number and variety seem to have no end.

These sources of information continue to be important to healthcare consumers today, but they now share space with other sources. With the introduction of Medicare and Medicaid in the 1960s and the emergence of managed care in the 1980s, healthcare consumers turned to their health plans for information on healthcare providers, mostly in response to the restrictions health plans impose on the use of practitioners, facilities, and programs. This shift also indicated the growing importance of health plans as a valuable source of information on the healthcare system. Managed care plans have been particularly aggressive in establishing call centers and encouraging their enrollees to seek information before making health-related decisions.

Another source of healthcare information that came to the fore in the 1990s was the World Wide Web. The Internet has become a major source of health-related information; there are purportedly more sites in cyberspace related to healthcare than any other topic. Most wired healthcare consumers have at some point accessed the Internet for information on a health issue they or someone else faced. Consumers are increasingly armed with Internet-generated information when they present themselves at the doctor's office. Although the quality of the data available on the Internet and the implications of better-informed patients for medical practice merit discussion, the Internet is clearly replacing traditional information sources as the first resort in healthcare consumers' information search.

In addition to the purchase decision process, consumers progress through different stages of purchasing behaviors. As in the decision process, the point at which the target market is located in the consumer behavior progression will determine the focus of the marketing plan. Exhibit 6.10 describes a stages-of-change approach to modifying consumer behavior.

EXHIBIT 6.10
A Stages-of-Change Approach to Market Assessment

Marketers in any field spend much of their time trying to get potential customers to change their behavior. In healthcare, these efforts may involve increasing their level of knowledge about the service in question, changing attitudes toward a particular health service provider, encouraging people to switch from one service to another, or encouraging people to change their lifestyles to improve their health. For this reason, marketers have spent a considerable amount of time trying to understand the factors that cause individuals to modify their level of knowledge, their attitudes, and their behavior patterns.

One classic approach to understanding change was developed by Prochaska, Norcross, and DiClemente (1995). Through their study of initiatives aimed at changing behaviors that are detrimental to health (e.g., smoking), they developed a model that marketers could easily apply to other health behaviors. They found that an individual goes through five stages when dealing with change:

- *Pre-contemplation.* At this stage, the individual has not yet thought about taking action. For example, this individual could have a healthcare condition but is unaware of it (e.g., high cholesterol).
- *Contemplation.* At this stage, the individual becomes aware of the problem and is considering doing something about it. For example, the individual with high cholesterol found out about this condition at a health fair.
- *Preparation.* The individual has decided some action needs to be taken and starts taking steps toward addressing the problem in this stage. For example, he or she has become convinced that some action is required to address the cholesterol problem and begins to examine available options.
- *Action.* The individual proactively takes on the problem with whatever resources are available in the action stage. For the person with high cholesterol, "action" may mean visiting a primary care physician or a nutritional counselor.
- *Maintenance.* By this stage, the individual has taken action and now must be encouraged to continue the course of treatment

(continued)

EXHIBIT 6.10 (*continued*)

that has been prescribed. The person with high cholesterol, for example, needs to maintain a healthy diet and regularly take the drugs prescribed by the doctor in the action stage.

As in the purchase decision process, the marketer will target groups of people in the population who presumably are at a similar stage in the model, and the stage at which the target population resides determines the marketing approach he or she will take. Individuals in the pre-contemplation stage clearly need information. These people are not aware that a problem exists. Those in the contemplation stage have the requisite knowledge but have yet to take action; here is where the marketer needs to catalyze attitude change. Individuals in the preparation stage are planning to take action; here, the marketer must make sure that they are aware of the services available to them. Those who have reached the action stage need encouragement and support, which the marketer can provide by ensuring that the service is high quality and that customers are served in a friendly and efficient manner. Finally, at the maintenance stage, the individual must be encouraged to maintain the regimen that has been prescribed and should be supported by ongoing communication. From a marketing perspective, an ongoing relationship should be in place at this point to ensure the continued involvement of these customers with the provider.

Summary

Although the consumer is the primary concern of almost every industry, only in recent years has healthcare come to think in terms of consumers rather than patients. Most healthcare providers in the past gave no thought to consumers until they entered the system as patients. The pre-patient and post-patient phases were neglected, and healthy people were not considered candidates for health services.

As healthcare became more market driven, the importance of the consumer was increasingly recognized. Healthcare organizations redefined patients as customers and came to appreciate the variety of customers they serve. Today, healthcare constituents take the form of consumers, customers, clients, patients, and enrollees, all of which have unique characteristics. Other customers to be cultivated by healthcare organizations may include employers, board members, government agencies, the press, and the general public.

Because of the unique characteristics of the healthcare industry, healthcare consumers are different than consumers in other industries. At the same time, however, they share some of the characteristics of other consumer types. To reach the massive healthcare market efficiently, marketers segment the population on the basis of demographic characteristics, geographic distribution, psychographic attributes, service usage, payer category, and desired benefits.

Along with healthcare's increased emphasis on the consumer came increased attention to consumer behavior. Healthcare consumers generally follow the same steps as other consumers when making purchase decisions; they begin by recognizing a need and end with an assessment of their purchase. However, healthcare consumers' purchasing behaviors are influenced by aspects particular to healthcare that do not concern consumers of other products.

Key Points

- Healthcare providers are not used to thinking in terms of consumers as people in other industries do, and only in recent years has healthcare become consumer oriented.
- Marketers should be sensitive to the ways healthcare consumers differ from consumers of other products.
- At the same time, healthcare consumers share many of the attributes of consumers of other products.
- Although the patient is typically thought of as the primary consumer of health services, large healthcare organizations often have a wide variety of customers to satisfy.
- Redefining the patient as a consumer has encouraged wider use of marketing in healthcare.
- Users of health services are described in different ways depending on the context (e.g., patient, client, customer, enrollee, end user).
- Healthcare organizations themselves (e.g., hospitals, physician practices) are customers for a wide range of goods and services.
- The healthcare market can be segmented in a number of ways—in terms of demographic and socioeconomic characteristics, psychographic traits, usage level, and so on.
- Healthcare is unique in that customers are segmented in terms of their payer category (i.e., type of insurance coverage).
- The consumer decision-making process in healthcare is similar in most ways to the process for other consumer goods.
- Healthcare consumers seek information from a variety of sources, and the Internet is becoming an increasingly important resource.

- The consumer decision-making process is influenced by healthcare consumers' readiness to change and their willingness to innovate.
- The consumer decision-making process in healthcare is different in that someone other than the end user may make the decision and/or pay for the services.

Discussion Questions

- How is everyone in society arguably a potential consumer of health services?
- Why until recently has the healthcare industry not thought of its customers as consumers in the sense that other industries have?
- In what ways are healthcare consumers different from consumers of other goods and services?
- In what ways are healthcare consumers similar to consumers of other goods and services?
- How can one distinguish between the different varieties of healthcare consumers (e.g., patients, clients, end users, enrollees)?
- What are some examples of institutional customers for healthcare goods and services?
- Why do healthcare organizations often have a much wider range of customers than organizations in other industries have?
- What are some of the dimensions along which the healthcare market can be segmented?
- What are the major steps in the decision-making process for healthcare consumers, and how do these steps differ from those in other industries?

HEALTHCARE PRODUCTS AND SERVICES

In developing a marketing initiative, a marketer's first task is to understand the product that is to be promoted. In healthcare, the product may be something as simple as a bottle of aspirin or as complex as heart transplant surgery. Whether simple or complex, the marketer must be able to conceptualize the product in a manner conducive to effective promotion. This chapter addresses the issues involved in defining the product to be marketed and explores the challenges marketers face in making this determination in healthcare. The implications of defining the product in various ways are reviewed, and the emerging retail aspect of healthcare is discussed.

Introduction

As stated in Chapter 3, *marketing* refers to the promotion of ideas, goods, or services. Although the term *product* is often used interchangeably with *service* in healthcare, for purposes of this discussion, goods and services will be considered two types of products. Unlike marketers in other industries, who tend to promote clearly defined products, healthcare marketers expend a great deal of effort determining exactly what they are marketing.

The first questions a marketer is likely to ask in developing a marketing initiative are: (1) What is the product? and (2) How is it being sold? In most other industries, these answers would be straightforward and relatively easy for the organization to provide because its product is its reason for existence; an executive who cannot specify the company's product is not likely to be successful in today's environment. The situation is not so simple in healthcare, and health professionals are not used to thinking in terms of products. A health professional's response to the question "What is your product?" is likely to be something like "quality care," "improved health," or "treatment and cure." Although healthcare organizations hopefully provide such benefits to their customers, these answers are not helpful to a marketer.

Product Mix

An organization's *product mix* refers to the combination of goods, services, and ideas that it promotes to consumers. Large healthcare organizations, like hospitals, may offer a wide range of goods and services. A major hospital performs hundreds of different procedures and dispenses hundreds of different tangible products in the course of its normal activities. In addition, hospitals sell a variety of goods (in the form of drug doses, supplies, and equipment) to their customers.

At the same time, healthcare organizations often promote ideas that are intended to create a particular perception in the consumer's mind. The organization's brand image, for example, is an idea that can be promoted through marketing. The organization may also want to promote the perception of quality care, professionalism, value, or some other subjective attribute. Ultimately, an organization's mix of goods, services, and ideas will determine the focus of marketing activities.

Goods Versus Services

A *good* is a tangible product that is typically purchased in an impersonal setting on a one-at-a-time basis. The purchase of goods tends to involve a one-shot episode, whereas the purchase of services may be an ongoing process. Although healthcare is generally perceived as a service, the sale of goods is ubiquitous in the industry. Consumer health products, such as toothpaste and soap, are common household articles, and virtually every household buys pharmaceuticals. Home testing kits and therapeutic equipment are becoming increasingly available to consumers, and the sale or rental of durable medical equipment is common.

A *service*, on the other hand, is defined as an intangible activity or process provided to customers to solve a problem. A physical examination, a flu shot, and open heart surgery are examples of healthcare consumer services. Although most people would recognize these activities as health services, the nature of services in healthcare is often difficult to describe.

The primary distinction between goods and services is their degree of tangibility, or the extent to which they can be examined, touched, or experienced before purchase. Secondarily, goods and services can be distinguished in terms of their durability. Services tend to be consumed at the time they are provided (e.g., an immunization), whereas many goods tend to endure for an indefinite time (e.g., a home blood pressure cup). These distinctions clearly determine the marketing strategy developed for each category.

Healthcare is unlike other industries in that different parties are likely to have different perceptions of the services offered. In the case of childbirth, for example, the mother is likely to see the event as a natural experience, whereas the physician is likely to see it as a medical episode, and the hospital administrator is likely to see it as an accounting event. Looked at differently, the mother is likely to see it as a unitary episode, whereas the physician is likely to see it as a series of discrete activities, and the accounting department is likely to see it as a grouping of billable and non-billable services. The healthcare marketer may see such an event as yet something else. The marketer's task is to conceptualize the product and package it in an appropriate way for marketing purposes. In doing so, the marketer has to conceive of the service in a manner to which the consumer can relate.

Consumer Goods Versus Industrial Goods

Goods can be classified by the types of users who buy them. **Consumer goods** are goods purchased by the ultimate consumer, or the person who will actually consume the goods. Consumer goods may be classified in terms of the amount of effort and type of search the consumer uses in selecting the product. Consumer goods in most industries are divided into three categories: (1) convenience goods, (2) shopping goods, and (3) specialty goods.

Convenience goods are products that consumers purchase frequently without having to think about them or search for them at length. Cold remedies, analgesics, and dietary supplements are examples of convenience goods. Because the consumer engages in little deliberation when purchasing such items, name recognition and product distribution are critical concerns for the marketer. The manufacturers of over-the-counter drugs, for example, expend considerable effort in establishing brand identity and ensuring their product is displayed prominently in retail outlets.

Shopping goods are products that require the consumer to search for and compare competing brands on attributes such as price, style, or features. Fitness equipment, computers, and cameras are common examples of shopping goods. Marketers of shopping goods must differentiate their brand from their competitors' brands by emphasizing features that are important to their customers. Salespeople often play a major role in helping consumers learn about alternative brands.

Specialty goods are specific items a consumer seeks. Often the consumer is loyal to a particular brand and will go to great lengths to find an item with that brand name. Common examples include exclusive brands of jewelry, perfume, and electronic equipment. Few goods in healthcare are included in the specialty category.

Industrial goods are products purchased for use in the manufacture of other products, which will at some point be purchased by the ultimate consumer. Although healthcare marketing is mostly concerned with consumer products, a distinction will be made in this discussion between personal consumer goods and goods purchased for professional or institutional use.

Industrial products are stratified into two broad levels. *Production goods* are those that become part of a final product. Raw materials (such as the chemical components of a pharmaceutical) fit into this category. *Support goods* are items used to produce other goods and services. Examples include a computed tomography (CT) scanner, an examination table, and the printer used to generate patient bills.

Nondurable Goods Versus Durable Goods

Goods can also be divided into two groups on the basis of their durability: nondurable goods and durable goods. A *nondurable good* is an item that should be consumed within a defined time frame—for example, food products, drugs, and bandages. A *durable good* is a product that lasts for an extended period, such as hospital beds, wheelchairs, and computers.

The differences between goods and services and between nondurable and durable goods are important considerations in any marketing initiative. Nondurable products, such as pharmaceuticals, are often heavily advertised because consumers purchase such products frequently. Retail store displays play a major role in direct marketing to the consumer. Durable products usually cost more than nondurable products and are often more complicated to use. For these products, a personal sales approach, which includes answering questions and explaining the intricacies of the product, is often used to appeal to potential customers.

Product and Service Lines

In the 1980s, following the lead of other industries, healthcare organizations began to develop *product* (or *service*) *lines.* Most industries think in terms of product lines, but in healthcare, service lines seem more appropriate. To establish service lines, a hospital's programs are organized into vertical groupings centered on specific clinical areas. Specialty areas frequently selected for service lines include women's services, cancer services, cardiology, orthopedics, and pediatrics. Each service line is considered semiautonomous, and the service line manager is charged with the vertical integration of the relevant clinical services and necessary support functions. Thus, the service line administrator has broad control over the range of activities (including marketing) that support the service line.

Some observers contend that service lines are little more than a packaging of services for marketing purposes. Although there are certainly cases in which the service line relates more to packaging than substance, in most cases a certain level of reorganization occurs around the specific clinical area. The use of the service line approach in healthcare remains controversial, and its merits are still being discussed today. See Exhibit 7.1 for a discussion of the service line approach.

EXHIBIT 7.1
Healthcare Service Lines and Marketing

Since the 1980s, many hospitals have adopted the service line management concept long established in other industries. Service line management appeared attractive to hospitals looking for ways to become
more agile, move closer to their customers, strengthen relationships
with physicians, become more profitable, and move beyond cost cutting and reengineering to develop more innovative and effective ways
of serving their patients (Ireland 2003).

A service line is a tightly integrated, overlapping network of
semiautonomous clinical services and a business enterprise that bundles
needed resources to provide specialized, focused care and value to a
patient population. The most common service lines include cardiovas-
cular services, orthopedics, rehabilitation, women's services, children's
services, and oncology services. Service lines can be "virtual" in that all
components may not be under one roof; some services are horizontal
and cross departments and disciplines. A service line may be created
around a business that is already well established, or the concept may
be used to focus on a new service or niche.

The product line concept was developed by organizations in
other industries, most notably Procter and Gamble, General Electric,
and General Motors, as a way to decentralize decision making, make
strategic planning more effective, improve cost management and productivity, improve communication and collaboration, and, most important, help its product line management teams better understand the
needs of their customers.

The product line management concept emerged in the healthcare industry in the 1980s as an organizational effort to deal with
prospective reimbursement, a tight economic environment, declining
revenues, and intense competition, all of which drove the need for
improving the way hospitals did business. In healthcare, this concept
has probably been carried furthest by pharmaceutical companies that
organize their business enterprise by product lines.

Many of the gains from service line management were erased
with the emergence of managed care and other innovative financing
structures in the late 1980s. Although many hospitals maintained their
service line orientation throughout the 1990s, the concept was latent
and reemerged only around 1997, when hospitals began to renew their

(continued)

EXHIBIT 7.1 (*continued*)

patient focus. This revitalized service line management model defines a hospital's clinical services, allocates organizational resources—human, financial, and strategic—to these service lines, and clearly assigns accountability for performance to a service line leader.

This new service line platform integrates clinical and support services on a matrix management grid. The idea was to create horizontal integration of clinical services along a traditional continuum of care and a vertical integration of support services. Also built into this platform are education and wellness programs, retail models, business development tactics, and a strong focus on physician relationships (administrative, economic partnerships, and service), all with an increased emphasis on creating enhanced quality and value for patients.

Because the service line is close to its costs and operational dynamics, its customers, and its competition, hospitals and health systems are able to decentralize accountability for strategic, operational, and financial performance from the corporate or executive office to the clinical service line. This shift in accountability to the service line maximizes hospital capacity by focusing on the best use of space and resources and provides more flexibility in managing growth.

Whether the service line concept is an effective approach to healthcare strategy development is still open to debate, and there is little hard evidence to document the merits of this approach. Service line management does facilitate the marketing of services in many ways, and the close relationship between operations and marketing that can develop is an advantage. Focusing marketing resources in this manner does have its benefits.

Around 2005 another wave of interest in service line management in healthcare emerged (Litch 2007). This renewed interest reflected a number of developments in healthcare over the previous years, including a growing emphasis on quality control, integrated services, and physician collaboration. From a marketing perspective, the growing need to establish an advantageous market position appeared to drive the revival.

The significance of service lines to customers is not clear. Ideally, service lines are designed to address consumer needs, but most consumers probably think about healthcare as a continuum of services that extend across clinical lines, not in terms of vertical silos of care. As service lines become more entrenched in healthcare, a better understanding of their meaning for consumers should be established.

Ways to Conceptualize Products

A marketer must be able to conceptualize the products offered by healthcare organizations, so an in-depth understanding of the distinctions between the various product categories is important. The marketing approach must reflect the nature and complexity of the product, and the marketer must understand who uses the product and how they use it.

Level of Care

Products might be categorized in terms of the level of care they reflect. *Primary care* refers to the provision of basic health services (i.e., general examinations and preventive services) and the treatment of minor, routine problems. For the patient, primary care may involve some self-care and the services of a nonphysician health professional (e.g., a pharmacist) or, for certain ethnic groups, a folk healer.

Formal primary care services are generally provided by physicians who have been trained in family practice, general internal medicine, obstetrics/gynecology, and pediatrics. These practitioners are typically community based (rather than hospital based), rely on direct first contact with patients rather than referrals from other physicians, and provide continuous rather than episodic care. Physician extenders, such as nurse practitioners and physician assistants, are taking on a growing responsibility for primary care. In the mental health system, psychologists and other types of counselors provide the primary level of care. Medical specialists may also provide some primary care.

Primary care is generally delivered in a physician's office or in some type of clinic. Hospital outpatient departments, urgent care centers, neighborhood clinics, and other ambulatory care facilities also provide primary care services. For certain segments of the population, the hospital emergency department is a source of primary care. In addition, the home has become a common site for the provision of primary care. This trend has been driven by the financial pressures on inpatient care, changing consumer preferences, and improved home care technology. Case Study 7.1 addresses the marketing of primary care services for an urgent care center.

In terms of hospital services, *primary care* refers to services that can be provided at a general hospital. Hospital primary care typically includes routine medical and surgical procedures, diagnostic tests, and obstetrics services, as well as emergency care (although not major trauma) and many outpatient services. Hospital-based primary care tends to be unspecialized and requires a relatively low level of technological sophistication.

Secondary care involves a higher degree of specialization and technological sophistication than primary care because of the increased severity of the health problems encountered. Physician care is provided by more highly

CASE STUDY 7.1
Marketing an Urgent Care Center

During the 1980s, some enterprising healthcare professionals believed there was a need for an alternative to the traditional physician's office. While they conceded that many patients desired a long-term relationship with a physician and were willing to accept the deficiencies of the typical physician practice to obtain it, they also thought there was a significant portion of the population that did not have an established physician relationship but occasionally required some type of care. Some of these consumers were new to the community and had not found a regular physician, and others had become disillusioned with their physician but had not found a replacement. Still others were dissatisfied with the conditions under which care had to be obtained—long waits for an appointment, hours spent in the waiting room, only five minutes spent with the doctor, and then, a big bill.

Out of this situation, the urgent care center was born. The concept involved the development of conveniently located (i.e., in the community) walk-in clinics staffed by the same quality of physician one would encounter in a typical doctor's office. The clinic would offer only basic services and refer patients with anything more than a minor problem to another facility. Although the urgent care centers would accept insurance, they charged a low fee to attract patients without insurance and even those with insurance who were turned off by the challenges involved in seeing a "regular" physician. The centers would not maintain medical records beyond the basics, assuming most visits were onetime events. They would have the advantage of quick service with none of the hassle associated with a typical physician's office.

Convinced there was a demand for this type of service in a highly mobile, convenience-oriented society, physician entrepreneurs in a middle-sized Southern city set out to establish a network of seven urgent care centers at strategically located sites. They chose fairly new suburban areas close to high-traffic commercial and retail centers, believing that this type of location would attract the customers they were seeking. Having taken something of a gamble in terms of site location, they faced the challenge of marketing a new concept. They brought in marketers to survey consumers to determine who made the best prospects for this type of service.

Upon reviewing the surveys, the physicians developed a fairly clear idea of their prospective customers. Research indicated that the best prospects for an urgent care center were 25- to 40-year-old men and women who were highly mobile (often new to the community), fairly well educated, and more often than not in two-income families without children. Whites appeared to be more open to the idea than nonwhites, and the best prospects in terms of income were those in the middle- to upper-middle-class income categories. The more affluent were not attracted to this type of service, and the downscale populations were intimidated by this innovative form of care and concerned about having to pay cash on the front end. In terms of lifestyle categories, the research showed that those who were progressive, innovative, highly mobile, and more focused on the present than the future were more likely to use this service.

This information confirmed the developers' intuition about locating the centers in newly emerging affluent suburbs, and they set out to market this service to the target population. Taking advantage of various sources of data, the developers were able to target the households that displayed the desired characteristics within a five-mile radius of each site. Of the seven urgent care centers established, five were successful and two significantly underperformed. The only discernable differences between the successful and unsuccessful ones were the lower visibility and lower drive-by traffic characterizing the latter.

The developers' ability to target the most likely prospects helped them launch a successful promotional campaign that quickly resulted in a high volume of business. Without knowledge of the most likely prospects, the marketers' efforts would have been ineffective and the growth of the urgent care center clientele much slower.

Discussion Questions
- What factors encouraged the entrepreneurs to develop an alternative to the traditional source of primary care?
- What characteristics did the urgent care concept have that might make it unattractive to mainstream healthcare consumers?
- What assumptions did the developers make at the outset about the demand for such a service and the type of consumers who might use it?
- From their market research, did the developers find that the urgent care model would appeal to the general population or that some segments of the population would find it more attractive than others?

(continued)

CASE STUDY 7.1 *(continued)*

- What was the profile of the best prospects for utilization of an urgent care center?
- How did knowledge of the characteristics of the best prospects contribute to an effective marketing campaign?
- Given the characteristics of the best prospects, what attributes of the urgent care centers should be highlighted in promotional material?

trained practitioners, such as specialized surgeons (e.g., urologists, ophthalmologists) and specialized internists (e.g., cardiologists, oncologists). Problems requiring more specialized skills and more sophisticated biomedical equipment are included in this category. Although much of the care is still provided in a physician's office or clinic, these specialists tend to spend a larger share of their time in the hospital setting. Secondary hospitals are capable of providing more complex technological backup, physician specialist support, and ancillary services than are primary care hospitals. These facilities can handle moderately complex surgical and medical cases and serve as referral centers for primary care facilities.

Tertiary care addresses the most complex of surgical and medical conditions. The practitioners tend to be subspecialists housed in highly complex and technologically advanced facilities. Complex procedures, such as emergency care for a heart attack and reconstructive surgery, are performed at facilities that provide extensive support services in terms of personnel and technology. Tertiary care cases are usually handled by a team of medical and/or surgical specialists who are supported by the hospital's radiology, pathology, and anesthesiology physician staff. Tertiary care is generally provided at a few centers that serve large geographic areas. Single hospitals are often not sufficient for the provision of tertiary care; a medical center may be required. These centers typically support functions not directly related to patient care, such as teaching and research.

Some procedures performed at tertiary facilities may be considered *quaternary care*. Organ transplantation—especially involving vital organs such as the heart, lungs, and pancreas—is one example of quaternary care. Complicated trauma cases are another example. This level of care is restricted to major medical centers, often in medical school settings. These procedures require the most sophisticated equipment and are often performed in association with research activities.

Level of care plays an important role in determining the type of marketing to use. Consumers often have more discretion in decisions about primary care than they do with regard to specialized forms of care. Consumers can typically choose their primary care physician (although their insurance plan may limit their choices), and they can obtain primary care through urgent care centers or emergency departments if the situation warrants. Specialists, however, especially those involved in tertiary or quaternary care, are more difficult to access. Specialists typically require a referral from another physician or health professional, and insurance plans are reluctant to reimburse for the services of a specialist if the proper procedures have not been followed.

Because of these factors, consumers are a more viable marketing target for primary care services than for more specialized services. Marketing tertiary or quaternary care to the general public is not likely to be effective because someone other than the patient typically makes the treatment decision. Nevertheless, consumers need to be made aware of all available services, even if they cannot access them directly. See Exhibit 7.2 for a graphic depiction of the levels of healthcare.

Level of Urgency

Health products can also be categorized by the level of urgency of the condition to be treated. Health problems are generally classified as routine, urgent, or emergent. Routine health problems make up the bulk of primary care episodes, and many, if not most, urgent care episodes involve routine care that is provided during off-hours. Emergency care typically involves at least secondary care, if not tertiary or quaternary care.

Although marketing can influence the use of all three categories of care, some are more amenable to marketing than others. In general, routine care, such as primary care, allows the most discretion on the part of the consumer. Therefore, marketing for routine care is relatively straightforward and typically focuses on promoting awareness of available services directly to potential customers.

In some ways, potential urgent care patients may be more amenable to marketing than even routine care patients. Potential customers of urgent care centers may not have a regular source of care and are thus likely to be responsive to marketing messages when the need for care arises. Marketing for urgent care is not as straightforward, however, as that for routine care. Although most consumers will need urgent care at one time or another, its unpredictable nature and the many segments of the population that prefer more traditional primary care services pose a challenge for healthcare marketers. A marketer charged with promoting an urgent care center must be aware

EXHIBIT 7.2
Levels of Healthcare in the United States

Procedures	Location	Practitioner
Quaternary Care		
Organ transplantation Complex trauma	Multi-institution medical center centers	Teams of super-specialist physicians
Tertiary Care		
Specialized surgery Complex medical cases	Large-scale comprehensive hospitals with extensive technological support	Physician subspecialists
Secondary Care		
Moderately complex medical and surgical cases	Moderate-scale hospitals, some freestanding surgery and diagnostic centers	Physician specialists
Primary Care		
Routine care, standard tests, simple surgery, prevention, counseling	General hospitals, clinics, physicians' offices, urgent care centers, counseling centers	Primary care physicians, extenders

Complexity
Severity
Specialization

Source: Adapted from Pol and Thomas (2001, 36).

of the attributes that lead consumers to choose an urgent care center rather than their private practitioner or a hospital emergency department.

Emergency services are perhaps the most difficult to market effectively to the general population. Emergency department use is a rare event, and most consumers do not have preconceived notions about emergency care. In situations where people choose the hospital emergency department, their physician's affiliations and/or health plan restrictions are likely to be considerations. If, for example, a patient is taken to an emergency room at a hospital not in her network, she would have to be transferred to an in-network facility for her insurance to cover the charges. The marketer's approach to the general public might include promoting the quality of the organization's emergency services and the different ambulance services available, as well as promising a high level of patient satisfaction. In most cases, someone other than the patient is likely to make the choice about emergency care when the need arises. For serious conditions, emergency medical technicians will make the decision on the basis of the proximity of an emergency department or the type of emergency services required. Thus, emergency services may be more appropriately marketed to ambulance companies, emergency medical technicians, police dispatchers, and other decision makers rather than to the general public.

Inpatient Versus Outpatient Services

Health services may also be classified according to the site of care, as either inpatient or outpatient services. Inpatient services require at least an overnight stay and are typically provided in hospitals. Outpatient (or ambulatory) services include care that involves less than 24 hours' stay in a health facility. Outpatient services typically afford more consumer discretion than do inpatient services. For many outpatient services, consumers may present themselves for care without a prior relationship or even an appointment. The use of inpatient services requires at minimum a referral and/or admission by a physician, and possibly authorization by the patient's health insurance plan. Although targeting the general public directly for outpatient services makes sense, the marketing approach for inpatient services should focus on establishing and cultivating a loyal medical staff and negotiating favorable contracts with health plans.

Medical Versus Surgical Services

Although healthcare organizations may refer to "med-surg" wards where medical and surgical procedures are both performed, the distinction between the two therapeutic modalities needs to be noted. Medical procedures involve treatments based primarily on drug therapy, and surgical procedures are therapies that primarily involve surgery of some type. Of course, when any surgery is performed, some drugs are administered, and when drug therapy is administered, some surgical procedures, however minor, may be required.

The two approaches to care are obviously different and are implemented by different specialists. Medical therapy is typically carried out by internists and internal medical specialists (e.g., nephrologists, gastroenterologists), and surgery is performed by general surgeons or, more frequently today, surgical specialists (e.g., ophthalmic surgeons, orthopedic surgeons). Although risk is inherent in both types of therapies, the general public usually attributes greater risk to surgical procedures. In either case, the marketer must emphasize the benefits and minimize the risks of the procedures involved.

Diagnosis Versus Treatment

Differentiation between diagnosis and treatment is also common. Diagnostic procedures are used to assess health status and to test for the presence of a pathological condition. Treatments (or therapeutic procedures) are used to treat a condition once it has been diagnosed. Many diagnostic procedures are routine and administered at regular intervals to asymptomatic individuals; these procedures are usually referred to as *screening tests*. Tests administered in response to observed symptoms are usually referred to as *diagnostic tests*. For example, there are screening mammograms and diagnostic mammograms. This distinction is important because the same test might be marketed in a different manner according to its use. Clearly, the approach to marketing differs on the basis of whether the product is a diagnosis or a treatment. With diagnostic procedures, the emphasis is on prevention and early detection, and the intent is to maintain health. With treatment procedures, the emphasis is on treatment and cure, and the intent is to restore health.

Clinical Versus Nonclinical Services

Marketers may also distinguish between clinical and nonclinical services. Clinical services involve the administration of a formal medical procedure. Examinations, diagnostic tests, and therapeutic procedures administered by a clinical practitioner are examples of clinical services.

Healthcare providers have added a number of nonclinical services to their practices. Hospitals, for example, may have valet parking, food services for non-patients, and senior discount programs. In addition, practitioners may offer social support services that complement their clinical services (e.g., support groups for patients of an oncology practice). Others may offer child care or transportation. As noted in Chapter 11, some healthcare organizations have developed "concierge" services to complement their clinical services.

Obviously, nonclinical services are marketed differently from clinical services. Although clinical services may seem to be the most important (they generate the most revenue), consumers are more likely to evaluate their experiences on the basis of nonclinical services. Thus, marketers need to give nonclinical services adequate attention.

Elective Versus Nonelective Services

Finally, a distinction may be made between elective procedures and nonelective procedures. Nonelective procedures are those considered medically necessary, although they do not always deal with life-threatening conditions.

Elective procedures are those that patients voluntarily choose to undergo, such as non-therapeutic abortions, laser eye surgery, face-lifts, and hair transplants. Some surgery (e.g., for tennis elbow) might not be considered medically necessary and thus be classified as elective.

Although elective and nonelective procedures may be marketed in much the same manner, there are significant differences to note. For one thing, the decision maker is likely to be different. Nonelective surgery is generally prescribed by a medical practitioner and, being medically necessary, is covered under a health insurance plan. On the other hand, the decision to undergo an elective procedure is generally made by the patient, perhaps on the advice of a medical practitioner. Because of their elective nature, these procedures are typically not covered by insurance. For these reasons, marketers have to promote nonelective procedures differently from the way they promote elective procedures. For nonelective procedures, demand cannot be influenced by marketing to as great an extent. Thus, the emphasis must be on influencing the choice of provider when a condition arises. On the other hand, a hospital seeking patients for nonelective procedures may target its marketing toward admitting and referring physicians to channel referrals into its system.

The marketing of elective procedures has a lot in common with the marketing of nonmedical services. Providers of these services are much more prone to advertise their services and often compete on the same basis as providers of other types of services. Thus, eye surgeons and plastic surgeons may advertise their low prices, convenient locations, and efficient customer service. In addition, it may be possible to create demand for these services. Most balding men probably suffered in silence with their hair loss until they saw promotions for hair restoration services. By introducing this new service, a market was essentially created where one did not exist before.

One additional way to categorize products is in terms of their point in the product life cycle. A product may be in the introductory, growth, maturity, or decline stage. A product's position in the life cycle is significant in that it shapes the marketing strategy that should be pursued. Exhibit 7.3 describes the product life cycle and its implications for marketing.

Common Healthcare Products

This chapter has established that healthcare products can take the form of either goods or services. The following sections elaborate on the types of products in these categories and the types of healthcare organizations that provide them. The marketing team generally focuses on a specific service for a marketing campaign rather than marketing the organization in general, so it is critical for marketers to understand how to classify healthcare products.

EXHIBIT 7.3
The Product Life Cycle

Healthcare products, like other products, experience a natural life cycle that includes four stages: introduction, growth, maturity, and decline. For marketers, it is important to understand a product's stage in the life cycle. If an organization is primarily involved in providing inpatient services, for example, marketers need to recognize where inpatient services can be placed in the product life cycle. Or, if a marketing plan is being developed for a specific procedure, the marketer must determine where that procedure resides in the life cycle.

For any product, the first stage in the life cycle is the introductory or market development stage. A new product is likely to be innovative, so most of the marketing effort is directed toward creating awareness and cultivating the early adopters in the market. At this stage, there are relatively few competitors, and goods and services are not standardized. The market is relatively easy to enter because there are few established players, although in healthcare, regulatory requirements often must be met (e.g., Food and Drug Administration approval). New pharmaceuticals are one example of a healthcare product subject to regulation.

The second stage in the life cycle is the growth phase. At this point, the product has become established, and the market has accepted the good or service. Expansion is rapid, as new customers are attracted and more competitors enter the arena. Products or services become increasingly standardized, although enhancements may continue to contribute to product evolution. Marketing planning at this stage emphasizes differentiation of the organization, product, or service. The rapid growth of cosmetic surgery during the 1990s is an example of this type of expansion.

By the third stage, the product has achieved maturity. At this point, most of the potential customers have been captured and growth begins to tail off. Because few new customers are available, competition for existing customers increases. Product features and pricing are highly standardized, and little differentiation remains between competitors. The number of competitors decreases as consolidation occurs, and it becomes increasingly difficult for new players to enter the market. Marketing activities emphasize retaining existing customers and/or capturing customers from competitors. Traditional hospital inpatient services are an example of a product that has reached the maturity stage.

When a product reaches maturity, it must adapt to its new state to remain viable. At this point, there are three strategies for stretching the lifespan of the product: (1) modifying the product, (2) modifying the market, and (3) repositioning the product. Hospitals have attempted to use all of these strategies by adding goods and/or services to the existing hospital product mix, promoting their services to new markets, and shifting some services from the inpatient to the outpatient setting.

In the final stage in the life cycle, the product experiences a period of decline. The number of customers decreases as consumers substitute new products or services. Typically, there is a shakeout among industry players as the dominant competitors squeeze out the less entrenched, and other competitors adopt a different strategic direction. Competition among the remaining players for existing customers becomes even more heated. Because no innovations are being introduced and the customer base cannot be expanded, the remaining competitors tend to emphasize cost reduction to maintain profitability.

The role of marketing will differ depending on the product's stage in the life cycle. The stage will influence the packaging of goods and services, promotional techniques, approaches to competitors, and relationships with other organizations.

During the introductory stage, when the product is an innovation, the marketer's primary task is to educate consumers about the product while facilitating a first-to-market approach. During the growth stage, marketers focus on differentiating the product from those of competitors by capitalizing on its attributes and penetrating new markets. During the maturity stage, the role of marketing shifts dramatically. There are few new customers for the product, so marketers focus on retaining existing customers and capturing customers from competitors. Market consolidation is likely to occur at this stage, and the marketer may be involved in enhancing the organization's image during this period of turmoil. During the decline stage of the life cycle, the marketer must focus on maintaining current customers and presenting the product in creative new ways to extend its life span.

Categories of Goods

Although healthcare is considered a service industry, healthcare organizations and healthcare providers sell a significant number of goods. For example, hospitals provide their patients with bandages, supplies, medication, food, and other nondurable goods, as well as home monitoring or treatment equipment. Hospitals also sell durable goods, such as crutches, braces, prosthetic devices, hospital beds, and wheelchairs. They may also sell goods through a gift shop, a resource library, or another retail-type enterprise.

Some hospital service line extensions may also sell goods on a retail basis. For example, the fitness center might sell nutritional supplements, athletic attire, and fitness equipment, and the cardiac rehabilitation program may sell videos, books, and other resources used in the rehabilitation process. Exhibit 7.4 describes the emergence of retail medicine.

Other types of institutions providing inpatient care may sell similar goods, although none is likely to match the range a hospital offers. Nursing homes, residential treatment centers, and assisted living centers typically provide supplies, medication, food, and other nondurable goods to their patients

---

EXHIBIT 7.4
The Emergence of Retail Medicine

The concept of *retail medicine*, or healthcare that is available to the masses outside a traditional institutional setting, is a relatively new niche in the elective outpatient healthcare marketplace. Retail medicine focuses on unique, personalized products and services that help patients manage their healthcare. Patients often pay for these products and services out of pocket rather than through their insurance company. In its broadest sense, retail medicine includes a range of activities, from selling products in physicians' offices, clinics, and hospitals to establishing comprehensive body imaging centers. Some of the more common goods and services sold include dietary supplements and programs, wellness programs, cosmetic medical products and services, and diagnostic and imaging tests (Woods 2007). By the turn of the twenty-first century, the trend toward retail medicine had gathered significant momentum as entrepreneurs sought to profit from high consumer demand—and traditional medicine's failure to meet this demand (Pyrek 2002).

A recent trend has been the development of walk-in primary care clinics in nontraditional settings. For example, many large retail stores have added primary care services to supplement existing optometry and even dental services. For example, the Walgreen's drug store chain has introduced quick, convenient walk-in clinics staffed by nurse practitioners. These clinics cater to customers who are not interested in long-time physician relationships, have an immediate need, and may not have the insurance to cover a more expensive visit in a traditional healthcare setting (Take Care Health Services 2009a).

By 2009, Take Care Health had established primary care clinics in 340 Walgreen's pharmacies and had become the nation's leading provider of workplace-based healthcare services. These services include on-site health, wellness, and fitness centers; on-site pharmacies; and health promotion and disease management programs. Take Care Health Employer Solutions operates nearly 370 workplace health centers and pharmacies for 180 clients in 45 states, including Washington, DC, and Guam (Take Care Health Services 2009b).

CVS/Caremark is Walgreen's primary pharmacy-based competitor. A number of other retail medicine chains have opened primary care outlets in shopping centers and major stores like Wal-Mart and Target. Even some hospital systems have set up branded clinics in retail stores in their market areas.

The retail medicine trend has also introduced new buzzwords and phrases in the healthcare community, including *medical entrepreneurs*, who market their services to consumers known as the *worried well* and the *worried wealthy*. As of mid-2009, the trend toward retail clinics appears to be leveling off, and the future of retail medicine in the primary care arena may well rest with the outcome of the current healthcare reform debate (Merchant Medicine 2009).

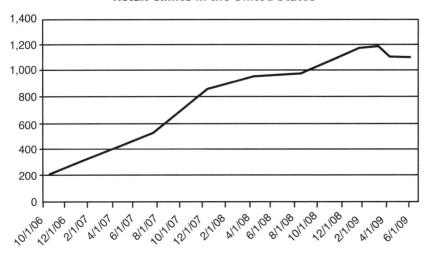

Retail Clinics in the United States

Source: Merchant Medicine (2009).

(continued)

EXHIBIT 7.4 (*continued*)

Aging baby boomers—the vast majority of those who consume retail medicine—are more concerned about their health than any previous generation, and they are driving a lot of the interest in retail medicine. One of the most sought-after components of the retail medicine trend is the full-body scan, which medical entrepreneurs say will reveal abnormalities in the body that can be addressed before they have a chance to become life threatening. CT scans promise to detect latent signs of conditions ranging from tumors and gallstones to clogged arteries and cancer.

Other examples of retail medicine include the variety of fitness and wellness programs that healthcare organizations are offering to the general public. There has also been a trend toward the retailing of goods through physicians' offices. Obstetricians and pediatricians might sell resource materials on childbirth and parenting. Dermatologists may offer a range of products for skin care, sun protection, and hair growth. A variety of different practitioners vend nutritional supplements and vitamins as a sideline to their practices.

or residents. Some of these goods are considered part and parcel of the room charge or surgical fee, and others are itemized on the patient's bill.

Many of the same procedures performed on hospital patients are carried out in physicians' offices, so physicians provide many of the same goods, such as wound dressings, casts, disposable supplies, and medications. These goods are typically not itemized separately but are included in the overall cost of the professional services. Some physicians have become increasingly involved in the retail aspect of healthcare, offering their patients a range of related goods. For example, a cardiologist may sell videos, audiotapes, and cookbooks describing ways to maintain heart health, or a family physician may sell nutritional supplements and vitamins. Although the American Medical Association does not encourage these retail activities, they are becoming entrenched in a number of medical practices.

Among other independent practitioners, some sell numerous goods and others sell relatively few. A major part of an optometrist's business (and, to a lesser extent, an ophthalmologist's) is the sale of eyeglasses and contact lenses. Likewise, although dentists and dental specialists primarily provide services, a considerable portion of their revenue may be derived from the sale of dentures, braces, and even high-end toothbrushes.

Categories of Services

The primary function of a healthcare provider is to offer services aimed at addressing a particular healthcare need. A hospital's fee schedule, for example, includes thousands of individual services. It would not be practical to itemize all of the services offered by a large healthcare organization; therefore, only the major categories will be noted in the following section.

One way of looking at these services is in terms of clinical areas. Services may be classified as obstetrics, pediatrics, cardiac, oncology, orthopedics, and so forth. The services provided to obstetrics patients, for example, are grouped together, as are those in the other clinical categories. The prospective payment system introduced by Medicare recognized these categories and made them the industry standard. Various clinical support services, such as radiology and laboratory services, are generally provided independent of a particular specialty and serve patients in all of the clinical categories.

Another way of classifying the services provided by hospitals (and certain other facilities) is to distinguish between facility-based services and professional services. Services associated with a hospital stay include room charges, nursing fees, technical services fees, and some overhead costs. Many of these services are bundled in the per diem room fee, but services that involve variable costs (e.g., breathing treatments) may be charged separately by the hospital as part of the facility fee. Hospital-based physicians (e.g., radiologists, anesthesiologists, hospitalists) also submit separate bills that may be combined with the facility fee. Professional fees are typically charged separately by attending and consulting physicians because they are not employed by the hospital but provide services (and bill) independently.

The services a hospital provides may also be divided into diagnostic and therapeutic categories with different coding systems. Routine diagnostic procedures (e.g., X-rays, blood tests, urinalyses) and specialized diagnostic tests (e.g., mammograms, CT scans, bone density tests) are offered in the hospital setting. Hospitals typically provide the widest array of diagnostic capabilities of any healthcare organization; other clinicians offer few diagnostic tests that are not available in hospitals.

Therapeutic procedures account for the widest range of treatments provided in hospitals. They take the form of simple treatments, such as administration of medication or intravenous fluids, or complex procedures, such as open heart surgery and organ transplantation. As noted earlier, these procedures are typically grouped into clinical categories and supervised by administrators dedicated to that clinical sphere.

Marketers need to have at least a basic understanding of the coding systems used in healthcare. Exhibit 7.5 provides an overview of these systems.

EXHIBIT 7.5
Coding Systems in Healthcare

It is impossible to develop an understanding of the bewildering range of diagnostic and therapeutic services without a working knowledge of the manner in which conditions and procedures are classified. The following is a brief introduction to the classification systems commonly used in healthcare; marketers will need to do additional research to gain a better understanding of them.

International Classification of Diseases
The most widely recognized and used disease classification system is the International Classification of Diseases (ICD) developed by the World Health Organization. The ICD system is used to classify conditions and procedures that occur in hospitals and certain other healthcare settings. The present classification system includes two components: diagnoses and procedures. A set of codes is assigned to each component. These codes are detailed enough that fine distinctions can be made among different diagnoses and procedures. (A different system is used for recording procedures in physicians' offices and other outpatient settings.)

The disease classification component comprises 17 disease and injury categories and two supplementary classifications. In each category, major specific conditions are listed in detail. A three-digit number is assigned to the major subdivisions in each of the 17 categories. These three-digit numbers are extended to another digit to indicate a subcategory within the larger category (to add clinical detail or isolate terms for clinical accuracy). A fifth digit is sometimes added to specify factors further associated with the diagnosis. For example, in the version currently in use (ICD-9), Hodgkin's disease, a form of malignant neoplasm or cancer, is coded 201. A particular type of Hodgkin's disease, Hodgkin's sarcoma, is coded 201.2. If the Hodgkin's sarcoma affects the lymph nodes of the neck, it is coded 201.21.

Current Procedural Terminology
Although the ICD classification system focuses on procedures performed under the auspices of a hospital or clinic, the Current Procedural Terminology (CPT) system relates exclusively to procedures and services performed by physicians. Physician-provided procedures and services are divided into five categories: medicine, anesthesiology, surgery, radiology, and pathol-

ogy and laboratory services. In the fourth edition of this classification system (CPT-4), each procedure and service is identified by a five-digit code.

Examples of coded procedures include surgical operations, office visits, and x-ray readings. The provider determines the most accurate descriptor from the CPT guidebook and assigns that code to the procedure. Modifiers may also be appended to the five-digit identifying code. Modifiers may indicate situations in which an adjunctive service was performed. Approximately 7,000 variations of procedures and services are catalogued.

Another set of codes has been developed to supplement the CPT codes. The Healthcare Common Procedure Coding System (HCPCS), administered by the Centers for Medicare & Medicaid Services (CMS), lists services provided by physicians and other providers that are not covered under the CPT coding scheme, including certain physician services as well as nonphysician services, such as ambulance, physical therapy, and the rental of durable medical equipment.

Diagnosis-Related Groups

In an attempt to contain costs under the Medicare program, the federal government introduced a prospective payment system as the basis for reimbursement for health services provided to Medicare beneficiaries. The Prospective Payment System (PPS) limits the amount of reimbursement for services provided to each category of patient on the basis of rates determined by CMS.

The basis for prospective payment is the diagnosis-related group (DRG). Using the patient's primary diagnosis as the starting point, CMS has developed a mechanism that assigns every hospital patient to one of 500+ DRGs. The idea is to link payment to the consumption of resources, assuming that a patient's diagnosis is the best predictor of resource utilization. To refine the 500+ diagnostic categories, the primary diagnosis is modified by such factors as coexisting diagnoses, the presence of complications, the patient's age, and the usual length of hospital stay. For situations in which DRGs represent too fine a distinction among conditions, the 500+ DRGs have been grouped into 23 major diagnostic categories (MDCs) based primarily on the different body systems.

Although introduced for use in federal healthcare programs, the DRG system was quickly adopted by other health plans as a basis for reimbursement. This system has become the standard classification

(continued)

EXHIBIT 7.5 (*continued*)

scheme for hospitalized patients in the United States and has been adopted by other countries around the world.

Ambulatory Payment Classification

In response to rising outpatient costs, CMS developed a system (similar
to the DRG system) for the outpatient environment, called the Ambulatory Payment Classification (APC) system. Like the DRG system, the
APC system focuses on the facility component of healthcare costs and
not on physician charges. The basis for the fee is the patient visit rather
than the entire episode of care, as in the case of DRGs. APC-specific
diagnosis codes have been developed, and CPT codes continue to be
used to classify procedures and ancillary services. Introduced in August
2000, APC codes are now widely used in outpatient facilities.

Diagnostic and Statistical Manual

The definitive reference on the classification of mental disorders is the
Diagnostic and Statistical Manual (currently in its fourth edition),
commonly referred to as DSM-IV. Published by the American Psychiatric Association, the DSM remains the last word in mental disease
classification despite long-standing criticism of its scheme. Its 17 major
categories of mental illness and more than 450 identified mental conditions are considered exhaustive.

The DSM classification system is derived in part from the ICD
system. Like the ICD system, it is structured around five-digit codes.
The fourth digit indicates the variety of the disorder under discussion,
and the fifth digit refers to any special consideration related to the
case. Unlike the other classification systems discussed, the DSM system
contains detailed descriptions of the disorders categorized therein and
serves as a useful reference in this regard.

Hospitals provide one other distinct category of services: emergency
care. The emergency department is designed to handle cases urgent enough
that they cannot be processed through normal admission procedures. Theoretically, this department handles serious injuries and health conditions that
require immediate attention. Emergency departments are staffed with physicians and nurses trained in emergency medicine and are backed up by a full
range of hospital personnel. Emergency departments maintain or have access
to diagnostic equipment that expeditiously determines a patient's condition.
Services provided in the emergency department are charged separately from

those for inpatients. Like inpatients, emergency patients are charged both a facility fee and a professional fee.

Hospitals are also likely to offer spin-off services related to their inpatient activities. For example, many hospitals have established occupational health programs and sports medicine programs to serve their patients and the community. Some hospitals offer home health, rehabilitation, and hospice programs as extensions of their core activities. Although these programs may contain some unique services, for the most part they are a repackaging of existing services. For example, a fitness program targeting the hospital's employees and community residents might combine existing services, such as physical examinations, stress testing, cardiac rehabilitation services, and recreational therapy, with services typically provided by nonmedical fitness centers, such as personal trainers and aerobics instruction.

Other categories of services that hospitals are likely to offer include prevention, education, and community outreach programs. Health educators may teach prevention to patients while they are hospitalized or provide educational programs outside the hospital to patients or the general public. Nurses may provide educational services to postsurgical and obstetrics patients, and nutritionists may offer guidance to a wide range of patient types. Some of these prevention and education services are built into the facility fee; others are charged separately to the patient. Community outreach programs involve information and referral, health education, and wellness training, generally geared toward the general public. They could also include home visits by hospital staff for purposes of monitoring health problems.

Categories of Service Providers

Marketers also need to be familiar with the different providers of health services to understand how the healthcare system functions. No other institutional setting provides the range of services of a *general hospital*, although some *specialty hospitals* may provide unique services. General hospitals treat the full range of services considered under primary, secondary, and tertiary care. Only the most advanced general hospitals, however, provide the most complex tertiary and quaternary care. Specialty hospitals may be dedicated to a particular population (e.g., women, children) or to a specific condition (e.g., substance abuse, mental illness). In the case of the former, services similar to those provided in a general hospital are likely to be offered, although the emphasis is on specialized services for the population in question. On the other hand, a psychiatric hospital is likely to provide services not found in other clinical settings.

Hospitals also provide support services of which patients are seldom aware, such as janitorial, landscaping, and parking services. Even less obvious, hospitals provide such services as medical records management, information systems operation, research services, and marketing services. Fees for these services are bundled into per diem or overhead charges. Other facilities that house patients on an inpatient basis include nursing homes and residential treatment centers. Assisted living facilities may also provide health services. The term *nursing home* is a misnomer in that nursing homes typically provide only a limited amount of medical care. Most of the services provided in a nursing home are custodial and involve the personal care of residents. As required, nursing personnel administer medication, monitor chronic diseases, and provide other forms of routine care in nursing homes. Physicians are on call but are not typically in residence. Unlike charges for hospital services, the charges for most services provided to nursing home residents are included in their monthly fee. Nonroutine health services are usually covered by a third-party payer, such as private insurance, Medicare, or Medicaid.

Residential treatment centers provide a narrower range of services than hospitals but typically a broader range than nursing homes. Unlike nursing homes, they are involved in the active treatment of most of their residents. Facilities for treating addictions or mental disorders, for example, provide services that are usually folded into the per diem charges of the treatment center.

Physicians are the most common type of practitioner the public encounters when seeking health services. The range of services physicians provide varies with the specialty involved, although most specialists provide a core group of routine medical procedures and diagnostic tests such as X-rays, blood tests, and urinalyses. Primary care physicians (i.e., family practitioners, obstetricians/gynecologists, pediatricians, and general internists) provide the bulk of routine care and, increasingly, are taking on the management of chronic patients. *Specialists*, as the term implies, focus on particular health problems. Patients are typically referred to specialists by their primary care physician, although some patients, depending on the health problem, may go straight to a specialist.

The services offered by *nonphysician practitioners* vary depending on the profession. For example, optometrists offer examination services and provide a limited range of therapies; chiropractors perform examinations and provide a narrow range of procedures aimed at spinal manipulation; and podiatrists perform examinations and offer a range of medical and surgical procedures for the treatment of foot problems.

Various *mental health* or *behavioral health providers* offer services geared toward the treatment of emotional and mental disorders, including counseling, psychotherapy, and drug therapy. The range of conditions for which treatment is available has expanded over time; mental health professionals may also treat such conditions as substance abuse, eating disorders, and Alzheimer's disease. Mental health services generally have been viewed separately from the treatment of physical health problems. This separation prompted the creation of a disease classification system unique to the mental health field. The most serious mental disorders are likely to be treated by a psychiatrist—a medical doctor with specialized training in mental disorders.

Alternative therapy practitioners offer services that take diverse therapeutic approaches to health problems. Chiropractors have already been mentioned. This category also includes practitioners of acupuncture, massage therapy, homeopathy, naturopathy, and other alternative therapies. Alternative (or complementary) therapies have grown dramatically in popularity in recent years. Although a growing number of insurance plans include alternative therapy benefits, many of these services are still considered elective and, hence, are paid for out of pocket. Alternative therapists have been some of the more aggressive marketers among healthcare professionals. Their efforts have raised consumers' awareness of—and created niche markets for—alternative products.

One other category of service providers that should be considered in this context comprises social service organizations. Although most of these organizations do not provide medical care, many do perform services that are health related and often reimbursable by third-party payers. For example, agencies addressing HIV/AIDS issues may provide diagnostic tests for HIV, and a family planning agency might provide physical examinations and perform clinical procedures. As the definition of *health* expands, the boundaries between healthcare providers and social service agencies can be expected to blur.

Summary

The first task of any marketer is to develop an understanding of the products being marketed. The healthcare industry, however, is not used to thinking in terms of products, and marketers often have to help health professionals define the goods and services they are offering to consumers. The complexity of the product mix in healthcare creates a challenge for marketers. Because of this complexity, healthcare organizations often market ideas, concepts, or images in addition to discrete goods and services.

Healthcare marketers must be able to distinguish between the variety of goods and services offered, recognize the relationship between various products and the relevant market segment, and develop marketing initiatives accordingly. Healthcare is complicated in that products may reflect different levels of patient need, different clinical settings, and varying clinical skills. The marketing approach will be dictated, for example, by whether the treatment is routine or urgent, is elective or medically necessary, or is performed in an inpatient or outpatient setting. Some healthcare organizations have adopted service line management to help organize the management of various types of care.

The operation of the healthcare system is complicated by a diversity of practitioners who provide an overwhelming variety of services. Physicians, other clinicians, and auxiliary personnel all provide care. In the hospital setting, the types of service providers are even more diverse. Traditional practitioners have also been joined by alternative therapists, further complicating the picture. Practitioners use a bewildering array of coding systems with which the marketer must become familiar. Furthermore, healthcare is provided in numerous different settings, including clinicians' offices, community clinics, mental health centers, hospitals, nursing homes, and residential treatment centers.

Key Points

- The healthcare field is characterized by a bewildering array of goods and services, resulting in a complex product mix.
- The product offered in healthcare varies with the type of practitioner and healthcare setting, and healthcare organizations use complicated coding systems to classify their products.
- Many goods and services in healthcare are marketed to the end user (typically the patient), but institutional customers in healthcare, such as clinics and hospitals, are also major purchasers of goods and services.
- Health professionals have not traditionally thought in terms of products, and marketers have to help them define what they are trying to market.
- The delivery of services in healthcare—and the marketing thereof—is complicated in that consumers may be characterized by differing levels of need, problems with differing levels of urgency, and a wide range of health conditions.
- Healthcare products are dispensed by a great diversity of practitioners in a wide variety of settings.

Discussion Questions

- Why were healthcare organizations not concerned about carefully defining their products in the past?
- What makes healthcare products difficult to clearly define?

- What are the distinctions between healthcare goods and services, and what are the implications of these distinctions for marketing?
- How do the challenges involved in marketing health services to consumers differ from the challenges involved in marketing products to healthcare organizations?
- In what ways is the complexity of the product mix of large healthcare organizations a challenge for marketers?
- Given the complexity of a hospital's service offerings, what dangers exist with regard to marketing services at cross-purposes (e.g., simultaneously marketing the urgent care center and the hospital emergency department, or the outpatient mental health center and the hospital psychiatric ward)?
- What is service line management, and what are the pros and cons of using a service line management approach in healthcare?

Additional Resources

Freedonia Group. 2008. *Cosmetic Surgery Products to 2012.* Cleveland, OH: Freedonia Group.

Kalorama Information. 2007. *Retail Clinics, The Emerging Market for Convenience and In-Store Healthcare.* Rockville, MD: Kalorama Information.

MarketResearch.com. 2008. *Sleep Aid Products in the U.S. Market: Non-Prescription OTC, Natural and Alternative Remedies.* Rockville, MD: MarketResearch. com.

FACTORS IN HEALTH SERVICES UTILIZATION

Marketing is all about identifying and responding to the demand for services and products. The decision to offer a service is generally predicated on the presumed level of demand for that service. Once a service is offered, virtually all decisions related to the continued provision of that service will be a function of the level of demand. For this reason, healthcare marketers spend a great deal of their time and effort trying to determine current and future levels of demand for aggregate health services or for the specific services offered by the organization involved in the marketing process. Calculating demand in healthcare is particularly challenging and requires an understanding of the many factors that influence the ultimate utilization of health services.

The factors influencing the level of demand for health services have become increasingly complex, and past utilization patterns are seldom predictive of future demand. The demographic, socioeconomic, and psychographic attributes of a population all play important roles. At the same time, managed care arrangements and other developments related to the financing of care artificially influence the demand for health services. These developments have made projecting demand for health services an increasingly challenging task at a time when the ability to do so is critical to the survival of most organizations.

The creation of demand—perhaps where none existed before—is an important function for marketers. While artificially creating demand for healthcare may seem inappropriate, there are plenty of situations in which the marketer might legitimately seek to create demand—for example, in the marketing of new drugs or the introduction of a treatment for a newly discovered disease to the public. Exhibit 8.1 illustrates the process through which demand might be generated for a healthcare product.

Defining Demand

In the context of health services, *demand* is an imprecise concept. The term is often used interchangeably with other terms, and no one definition of demand

EXHIBIT 8.1
Creating Demand for a Healthcare Product

Healthcare products are generally introduced to a market in response to a demonstrated demand, and providers of healthcare goods and services develop their products in response to an established health condition or other perceived need. Today, however, it is not unusual for health products companies to proactively identify new conditions that can benefit from an existing product. In this regard, marketers may be called on to create demand for a product in response to an identified health problem that did not previously exist.

Pharmaceutical companies have been particularly aggressive in their attempts to define new health conditions that could benefit from one of their products, and they subsequently promote that product to consumers and physicians writing prescriptions. To create demand, however, a healthcare organization must demonstrate to the public and the medical community that (1) an identifiable health problem exists and (2) the company has a product that can treat that problem.

Marketers create demand for a healthcare product in several ways, including classifying ordinary processes or ailments of life as medical problems, portraying mild symptoms as portents of a serious disease, defining personal or social problems as medical problems, conceptualizing risks as diseases, and maximizing disease prevalence estimates to enhance the perceived size of a medical problem.

A key strategy of pharmaceutical companies has been to target the news media with stories designed to create awareness of a condition or disease and draw attention to the latest treatment. Company-sponsored advisory boards often supply the "experts" for these stories, consumer groups provide the "victims," and public relations companies provide media outlets with a positive spin on the latest "breakthrough" medications.

For example, on the basis of research conducted in Australia, analysts identified a concerted effort on the part of a pharmaceutical company to create demand for products developed to treat irritable bowel syndrome (IBS). IBS is considered a common functional disorder and a "diagnosis of exclusion" covering a range of symptom severity, yet it is currently experiencing something of a global makeover. Without question, many people with the condition are severely disabled by their symptoms, but the arrival of new drugs has prompted manufacturers to seek to change the way the world thinks about IBS.

In this case, a communications company was engaged to formulate a medical education program to promote the perception of IBS as a "credible, common, and concrete disease." The educational program was part of the marketing strategy of the manufacturer of a leading drug for the treatment of IBS. The key aim of the educational program was to establish IBS in the minds of physicians as a significant and discrete disease state. Further, the campaign sought to convince patients that IBS is a common and recognized medical disorder for which there is a new clinically proven therapy.

The process for generating demand involved establishing an advisory board to provide corporate sponsors with current opinions about gastroenterology and best practice guidelines for diagnosing and managing IBS. In addition, the board produced a newsletter in the prelaunch period to "establish the market" and convince the medical specialists that the condition is a serious and credible disease. This newsletter was accompanied by a series of advertorials published in medical journals and distributed to general practitioners by pharmaceutical sales personnel. Other groups targeted with promotional material included pharmacists, nurses, and patients.

Although portrayed by the pharmaceutical company as a medical education plan, the intent was clearly to change public perceptions about IBS by establishing it in the public domain as a clinically identifiable condition, thereby creating a demand for a drug that could treat it. Although pharmaceutical companies may be particularly aggressive in attempting to create demand for a good or service, similar activities are becoming more common among other healthcare organizations.

Source: Adapted from Moynihan, Heath, and Henry (2002).

is universally accepted. Because it is so vague and used in so many different ways, the term is difficult to define operationally.

Part of the confusion in defining (and measuring) health services demand stems from a lack of agreement regarding *who* the customer for health services is. Customer identification is seldom an issue in other industries, but it is of paramount importance in healthcare. Typically, the end user's demand for services is the primary consideration and might be thought of as *consumer demand* (the end user is usually the patient). Other customer groups, such as physicians, health plans, and employers, may also play a part in determining demand. For a plan, the customer may be the manager of an employer-sponsored benefits package. For a medical supply or equipment company, the customer may be a retail distributor.

For these reasons, demand in healthcare may not be generated directly by the end user but by an intermediary. Thus, physicians may determine patient demand for hospital care and pharmaceuticals, insurance companies may influence the demand for services because of the treatments they cover, and so forth.

Perhaps the best way to approach the demand concept as it relates to healthcare consumers is to examine the component parts of demand. From a marketing perspective, demand can be conceptualized as the ultimate result of the combined effect of (1) healthcare needs, (2) healthcare wants, (3) recommended standards for healthcare, and (4) utilization patterns (Thomas 2003a).

Healthcare Needs

Healthcare needs can be defined in terms of the overall health status of a population or, more specifically, in terms of the number of conditions found in that population that require medical treatment. These health conditions would be those that an objective evaluation—for example, a physical examination—would uncover. The services required to address these conditions might be thought of as the *absolute* needs that exist without the influence of any other factors. The epidemiologically based needs that a team of health professionals would identify in a sweep through a community could be considered to reflect the true prevalence of illness in the population. All things being equal, the absolute level of need should not vary much from population to population.

On the basis of its characteristics, a population can be expected to experience a certain level of various health conditions. However, the existence of clinically identified health problems, at least in contemporary societies, does not translate directly into demand. In fact, the mismatch between these identified needs and the ultimate utilization of services is substantial. Many conditions go untreated (indeed, even undiagnosed) for various reasons. Many other conditions for which treatment is obtained would not be considered as absolute needs for that population. For example, no team of epidemiologists assessing the healthcare needs of a community is likely to identify sagging facial skin as a health problem. Yet tens of thousands of face-lifts are performed in the United States every year by medical doctors. Thus, demand for a health service might exist even though there is no clinical need for the service.

Healthcare Wants

Healthcare wants can be conceptualized as a population's wishes or desires for health services. Unlike needs, however, wants would not necessarily be uncovered by a sweep of public health investigators through a community. Desired healthcare services are determined less by the absolute needs of a population than by factors that influence the consumption of non-healthcare goods and services. Many health services that are consumed are considered medically unnecessary or elective; they are wants, not needs. Tummy tucks and laser eye surgery are examples of such services.

Healthcare wants are determined less by the level of biological morbidity in the population than by nonmedical factors. Wants may be determined by personal traits, such as fear and vanity; by social characteristics, such as group membership and family influence; or by cultural factors, such as societal trends. For this reason, the level of wants is likely to be elastic and subject to marketers' influence. The U.S. healthcare system has come to accommodate wants, and many healthcare organizations cater to people desiring elective services that might be considered medically unnecessary.

The type of organization and the services it offers will dictate whether needs or wants are the main consideration in marketing efforts. For example, a clinic for persons with HIV/AIDS deals with basic needs, and there are few elective procedures relevant to the treatment of HIV/AIDS patients. On the other hand, a plastic surgeon specializing in body sculpting is likely to focus on the want-driven demand generated by those motivated by vanity (see Exhibit 8.2 for a discussion of marketing approaches for an elective procedure). At the same time, if a plastic surgeon also maintains a reconstructive surgery practice for trauma victims, both wants and needs would be addressed.

EXHIBIT 8.2
Marketing an Elective Procedure: The Case of Laser Eye Surgery

Customer profiling is a common practice in most industries, but it has attracted limited attention in healthcare because the end users of health services did not historically choose the health services they used. These services were "ordered" by a third party. Expenditure of marketing resources on patients was seen as purposeless when physicians or health plans ultimately determined which health services they used.

With the resurgence of consumerism driven by the baby boom generation, emphasis on alternative therapies, and emerging interest in defined contributions, consumers have started making more of the decisions regarding health services and, thus, have become an increasingly important target for healthcare marketers.

One area ripe for the application of direct marketing methods is elective surgery. Elective procedures—that is, those not considered

(continued)

EXHIBIT 8.2 (*continued*)

medically necessary and thus not reimbursable under insurance—constitute a significant proportion of the procedures performed by medical practitioners. Everything from elective knee surgery to laser eye correction to face-lifts is included in this category. These procedures are elective in that the consumer, not the physician or health plan, usually chooses to undergo them.

Candidates for many types of elective surgeries are characterized by a particular profile and do not represent a cross-section of the population. In other industries, marketers typically define their best customers as those who use the company's services often, spend above-average amounts, pay promptly, and recommend the company's services to others. This information tells the marketer where to look for prospects. In the healthcare context, the best customers for elective medical procedures would be, for instance, people who respond to direct mail, are willing to attend a presentation on the procedure, and are able (and willing) to pay out of pocket for the procedure.

The most effective approach to developing a consumer profile involves gathering patient data that specify the characteristics of the best prospects for the service. Aggregate data on the patients obtaining face-lifts or elective knee surgery, for example, could be used to identify others in the population with the same characteristics. Even better, however, are actual names and addresses of patients who have obtained these services. This information can be used to link the patients to a variety of consumer databases to develop a more in-depth profile of the typical candidate for a procedure. Thus, patients for a particular service can be profiled in terms of their demographic characteristics, lifestyle orientation, and consumer behavior, among other characteristics.

Laser eye surgery has grown in popularity as new techniques have been perfected and outcomes improved. This procedure is almost always elective, requires out-of-pocket expenditures by the patient, is relatively expensive, and appeals disproportionately to certain segments of the population. Interest in laser eye surgery is particularly high today with the burgeoning population of nearsighted baby boomers and the search for new surgical opportunities on the part of ophthalmic surgeons.

For this particular analysis, patient data were obtained from a successful laser surgery clinic. Although information could have been obtained on the characteristics of the patients, only patient names and addresses were requested for those who had undergone the procedure, those who had presented themselves for surgery but turned out to be clinically ineligible, and those who had indicated an interest in laser eye surgery at some point but, as far as could be determined, had never undergone the procedure. The analysis involved approximately 700 laser eye surgery patients (and medically ineligible prospective patients) and another 1,200 prospective patients who had inquired about the surgery but never followed through. In addition, a random sample of 1,000 consumers was drawn from the zip codes that predominated the patient/prospect sample.

Analysts gathered the data necessary for the analysis by matching the compiled names and addresses to the consumer data maintained by Experian marketing services. The data obtained from Experian included

- individual-level data, such as age, marital status, and gender;
- household-level data, such as home ownership, estimated household income, and presence of children; and
- geographic data, such as the median household income of the census block group in which the consumer lived, the racial and ethnic profile of the block group, the median home value, and the MOSAIC lifestyle cluster assigned to each household (see Exhibit 8.3).

To ensure that the patient sample and the random sample represented the same underlying population, any consumer whose zip code fell outside the primary area served by the ophthalmic surgery practice was removed from the research database.

When the characteristics of the patients, prospects, and matched general population were compared, significant differences were found in the demographics and household characteristics of the three groups. Differences were found in age, gender, race, marital status, income levels, and rates of home ownership. Little distinction was found, however, between the patients and the other groups in terms of educational status or occupational characteristics.

When the groups were compared on the basis of MOSAIC lifestyle clusters, four of the clusters, typically assigned to neighborhoods of lower socioeconomic status, were determined to be negatively associated with a propensity for laser eye surgery. From these comparative data, a logistic regression model was derived to predict the probability that

(continued)

EXHIBIT 8.2 (*continued*)

a given consumer would fit the profile of previous laser eye surgery patients.

The model that was ultimately chosen demonstrated reasonable predictive validity. Overall, 63 percent of the sample was correctly classified as either a patient or non-patient. Although a logistic regression model yields both false positives and false negatives, this overall result, with 60 percent of the positives correctly classified and 66 percent of the negatives correctly classified, indicated that this model could be used to significantly increase the probability of identifying prospects for laser eye surgery within a defined population.

In the final analysis, the characteristics that had the most predictive power (in no particular order) were race, age, gender, marital status, and income. Although these factors all contributed to a person's likelihood of pursuing laser eye surgery, certain occupational statuses and lifestyle categories reduced a person's likelihood of becoming a patient.

The ability to predict classification of an individual as a patient versus a non-patient was improved dramatically using this approach. Careful use of this model as a basis for identifying targets for direct mail (i.e., targeting those who fall into the top three deciles in terms of customer potential) would increase the hit rate significantly and could drive up marketing effectiveness by 300 percent. As a result, the bottom-line impact on an ophthalmic surgery practice could be tremendous.

Source: Adapted from Barber, Thomas, and Huang (2001).

Recommended Standards for Healthcare

The third dimension of healthcare demand involves recommended standards for the provision of services. This component primarily involves diagnostic procedures and disease management activities that are recommended for patients who display certain symptoms or are at risk for a specified health problem.

The medical community has developed standards that recommend how often diagnostic tests should be performed, the time at which medical procedures should be performed, and the implementation of certain treatment plans for patients. These standards differ on the basis of health condition, age group, population segment, health risk, and so forth. For example, an annual mammogram is recommended for all women older than age 50, regular prostate exams are recommended for all men older than age 40, and regular cholesterol exams are recommended for persons at risk of certain conditions.

As healthcare professionals have become more attuned to prevention and health maintenance, the number of standards and recommended procedures has increased. For example, in the past, cholesterol tests were limited to patients under medical management. Today, regular cholesterol tests are recommended for everyone, along with Pap smears and breast exams for women, angiograms for men and women, and a growing number of other diagnostic and screening procedures. Many of these standards are considered important for public health purposes and, as such, may be promoted through social marketing efforts by such organizations as the American Cancer Society and the American Heart Association. The increase in the number of informally recommended diagnostic tests also reflects the trend toward "defensive medicine" on the part of physicians seeking to avoid malpractice liability.

Health Services Utilization

A fourth dimension conceptualizes demand in terms of the utilization of health services. The amount of services consumed is frequently used as a proxy measure for demand because utilization rates can be calculated for almost any type of health service or product. More data on health services utilization are available than on the other dimensions of demand, primarily because utilization data are routinely collected for administrative and billing purposes whenever a health service is provided. Utilization rates indicate the actual level of activity in the healthcare system as opposed to theoretical demand.

Because of the perceived relationship between demand and utilization, analysts sometimes work backward from utilization levels and use them as a proxy for demand. However, utilization does not equal demand, and, depending on the circumstances, the level of demand may exceed utilization or, conversely, utilization levels may exceed reasonable demand for services. For example, there may be less utilization than expected because of limited access to health services. On the other hand, some services may be overutilized for reasons (e.g., insurance coverage, physician practice patterns) unrelated to the level of demand.

Likewise, identifiable demand may not directly translate into utilization. Because marketers are concerned with what consumers actually do, situations in which the level of demand exceeds actual utilization may represent marketing opportunities. (See Pol and Thomas [2001] for a detailed review of the relationship between demographic characteristics and health status and health behavior.) Health services researchers commonly compare the assumed level of need with the observed level of utilization.

Factors Influencing Demand

Many factors influence the level of health services demand, and their interactions are complex. Although biological characteristics may predispose a person to certain health problems, other factors may ultimately determine the type and amount of health services utilized. Biological factors are comparable to the healthcare needs described earlier and may or may not translate into utilization. Nonmedical factors may be more of an influence on wants than they are on needs.

Knowledge of a population's cultural background, lifestyle patterns, and financing arrangements may allow a more accurate prediction of the type and level of services demanded than would knowledge of the actual level of morbidity. The following section describes some of the factors that influence the level of health services demand.

Population Characteristics

The population characteristics that influence the demand for health services can be categorized in terms of their effect on health status and health behavior. These categories include psychological factors, demographic factors, lifestyle and psychographic factors, and other (mostly structural) factors.

Psychological Factors

The *psychological factors* correlated with health services demand include personality types, attitudes, and the emotional responses evoked by health problems. The relationship between these factors and health behavior can be exceedingly complex, as in the case of a hypochondriac or in cases where fear pushes one person to seek treatment but prevents another from visiting the physician. In the contemporary U.S. healthcare environment, fear, pride, and vanity play a large role in the demand for many elective procedures (e.g., cosmetic surgery, stomach resection).

In industries where marketers pay more attention to psychological motivations, personality traits are often thought to drive consumer behavior. In healthcare, the individualized nature of psychological traits makes direct correlation with health services utilization difficult, and data on the correlation between psychological characteristics and health behavior are limited.

Attitude refers to a position a person has adopted in response to a theory, a belief, an object, an event, or another person. Attitude establishes a relatively consistent, acquired predisposition to behave in a certain way in response to a given object. When consumer attitudes are considered in healthcare, they typically refer to the attitudes that influence the preferences, expectations, and behaviors of the end user or purchaser of health services. Thus, consumers' attitudes toward the healthcare system, physicians, particular facilities, certain treatments, and so forth are believed to influence their decisions. A consumer's willingness to use urgent care centers rather than emergency departments, health maintenance organizations rather than traditional health plans, and chiropractors rather than orthopedic surgeons may be a function of his or her attitude.

Attitudes are not restricted to the consumers of health services; physicians and other health professionals also bring attitudes to the situation. The attitudes of physicians, for example, have been shown to affect the types of services that are provided to different communities and different groups within the population. These attitudes are reflected in the wide variation in medical procedure rates from community to community or in situations where practitioners will not perform certain services because of their religious beliefs.

Demographic Factors

Demographic characteristics exert a powerful influence on health services utilization. Of the various demographic attributes, age is one of the best predictors of health services use. Certain conditions are associated with specific age cohorts, and age influences the types of services used and the frequency of their consumption.

Utilization of health services in the United States has been shown to increase with age, primarily reflecting the heavy emphasis placed on hospital care. The rate of hospitalization for persons younger than age 45 is low, and the lowest admission rate to U.S. hospitals is recorded by the age 6 to 17 cohort. After age 45, however, admission rates increase dramatically; the rate for those aged 45 to 64 is more than double the 15 to 44 age group. In terms of emergency department utilization (for true emergencies), teens and persons in their early 20s (particularly men) account for a disproportionate share as a result of injuries and accidents. The elderly also account for a large share of emergency department utilization (NCHS 2009).

The *sex* of the consumer is another factor influencing utilization rates. In the United States, women are more involved than men in the healthcare system and are heavier users of health services in general. Women tend to visit physicians more often, take more prescription drugs, and use most other facilities and personnel more often. Women are also more aware of available health services and are quicker to turn to health professionals when symptoms arise. Perhaps more important from a marketing perspective is that women influence others' use of health services. Women often make healthcare decisions for their spouse and children and are thought to account for more than 80 percent of healthcare decisions (HCPro 2007).

Racial and ethnic characteristics also influence the demand for health services. The most clear-cut differences have been identified between African Americans and non-Hispanic whites. Certain Asian populations and many ethnic groups also display distinctive utilization patterns. Although differences in utilization may be traced to differences in the types of health problems experienced by these populations, many of the differences reflect variations in lifestyle patterns and cultural preferences. Perceptions and expectations of the healthcare system are also likely to differ among racial and ethnic populations (NCHS 2009).

In general, whites tend to use physicians at a higher rate than the rest of the population, but blacks are significantly more likely to use emergency department services. Some ethnic groups are more likely to use alternative types of care (e.g., folk medicine and acupuncture).

Marital status is related not only to level of demand but also to the type of services used and the circumstances under which they are consumed. Married people in the United States tend to have fewer health problems than the unmarried, widowed, or divorced, but, ironically, they use health services at a higher rate. The lifestyles associated with an unmarried status are believed to prompt a higher level of health problems (NCHS 2009).

A population's *income level* is probably one of the best predictors of health services utilization. There is a correlation between income level and the amount of health services used, as well as with the types of services used and the circumstances under which they are received. Despite the health penalty that accompanies low income, the unhealthy poor tend to use fewer services than the healthy affluent. This is true whether the indicator is for inpatient care, outpatient care, tests and procedures performed, or virtually any other measure of utilization (NCHS 2009).

The relationship between *education level* and utilization is similar to that for income. The distribution of health problems in a population is associated with educational status, making it one of the better predictors of the demand for health services. The rate of hospitalization for the least educated segments of the U.S. population is low, despite the higher prevalence of health problems in this group. The more educated segments, although less affected by health problems, have higher rates of health services utilization. This higher rate is thought to be a function of their greater appreciation of the benefits of healthcare and greater access to insurance coverage (NCHS 2009).

The relationship between *religious affiliation/degree of religiosity* and health behavior is probably the most idiosyncratic of any of the demographic associations. Research on this relationship is limited, so clear patterns are difficult to discern. Further, in the United States, religious affiliation and participation are associated with so many other variables that it is difficult to isolate the influence of religious involvement on utilization. Nevertheless, there is evidence that health status, and the subsequent use of services, is correlated with measures of religiosity. This factor may be an important consideration for marketers in some communities where faith-based healthcare organizations are common (Benjamins 2003).

Lifestyle and Psychographic Factors

Lifestyle and psychographic factors exert significant influence on a population's healthcare wants, needs, and behaviors. Health behaviors and the propensity to use health services may be more highly correlated with lifestyle characteristics than with other variables. If the lifestyle classification of members of a population can be determined, the types of health problems that group will experience, as well as likely utilization patterns, can be estimated. To a certain extent, lifestyles override, or at least refine, differences in health services utilization based on demographic traits. See Exhibit 8.3 for a discussion of lifestyle segmentation systems.

EXHIBIT 8.3
Lifestyle Segmentation Systems

Lifestyle segmentation systems have been used for decades in other industries but have never received wide acceptance in healthcare. For the most part, healthcare provider organizations depended on physicians or health plans to channel patients to them. For this reason, they did not need to know much about the characteristics of their patients.

Today's healthcare environment demands increased attention to customer segmentation. The market has become much more consumer driven, and individuals are taking a more active role in healthcare decision making. The pharmaceutical industry has led the way with a heavy investment in research on market segmentation. Healthcare providers who perform elective procedures, such as plastic surgeons, orthopedic surgeons, and eye surgeons, also need such information. As the health insurance landscape changes, growing numbers of health plans, health services providers, and other organizations are expressing an interest in customer segmentation and target marketing.

The first lifestyle segmentation systems—also referred to as *psychographic segmentation systems*—were developed in the 1970s. This approach to segmenting the population was developed in response to some of the perceived deficiencies in demographic profiling. Marketers realized that people in the same demographic category could be grouped differently on the basis of lifestyle. For example, all senior citizens used to be grouped into the over age 65 category. Lifestyle research discovered that within this demographic category, there were at least two major subgroups: active, financially secure seniors and frail elderly with limited resources.

The best-known early lifestyle segmentation system was developed by Stanford Research International in the 1970s. It was called VALS, for "values and lifestyle system," and inspired the development of a variety of lifestyle segmentation systems. VALS was never widely

(continued)

EXHIBIT 8.3 (*continued*)

used, but three systems—PRIZM (by Claritas), MOSAIC (by Health and Performances Resources [HPR]), and ACORN (by CACI Marketing Systems)—were subsequently developed. The systems were built using similar methodologies, but they differ in terms of the procedures used to create the categories.

The concept behind all segmentation systems is the use of geodemographic data in conjunction with data on consumer behavior, attitudes, and preferences to derive distinct lifestyle clusters that cover the entire population. A specific set of attributes can then be assigned to each cluster. Marketers and researches can then attach health characteristics to each cluster on the basis of these unique attributes.

PRIZM may be the best-known system, primarily because of the clever names assigned to its 62 lifestyle clusters. Individuals may be classified, for example, as "Patios and Pools," "Shotguns and Pickups," or "Executive Suites." The PRIZM system was probably the first to be used in the healthcare industry. This information, collected by means of a national sample survey, is proprietary and can be obtained only through subscription.

The MOSAIC system includes 60 lifestyle clusters grouped into 12 major categories. It has been used to develop a methodology for estimating health status and health behavior based on psychographic cluster. This methodology is based on data from the National Center for Health Statistics, supplemented by patient data drawn from a database of several million individuals compiled by HPR. This system has been used by Experian to assign psychographic clusters to over 130 million households.

A number of multivariate statistical methods were applied to create the ACORN system. The most pertinent consumer characteristics were identified from a wealth of data using principal components analysis and graphical methods. CACI carefully analyzed and sorted the country's 226,000 neighborhoods by 61 lifestyle characteristics, such as income, age, household type, home value, occupation, education, and other key determinants of consumer behavior. Next, the market segments were created by a combination of cluster analytic techniques. The techniques were selected to produce statistically reliable solutions and to handle an immense amount of information. This process assigned more than 220,000 neighborhoods to 43 lifestyle segments.

> These systems can be used to perform lifestyle analyses and, depending on the database, provide a wide range of demographic, socioeconomic, and consumer data linked to each psychographic cluster. Vendors of psychographic segmentation systems continue to expand the range of data, and the healthcare industry is slowly beginning to embrace a psychographic segmentation approach to market research.

Other Factors

Other, mostly "structural," factors, often operating independent of the characteristics of the population, also influence the demand for health services. Advances in technology usually lead to higher levels of utilization of the services supported by the new technology. Some operations, like laser eye surgery, never could have been performed without technological advances. Technological advances also have contributed to the shift from inpatient care to outpatient care and facilitated the emergence of home health care as a major aspect of healthcare delivery. The impact of technology has been particularly notable in the area of diagnostic testing. The variety of tests that can be performed has increased dramatically. The expanded use of home testing procedures is just one example.

Another factor unrelated to health conditions is the type and extent of health insurance coverage available to individuals and families. The availability of insurance has been identified as one of the best predictors of the demand for services. When insurers introduce copayments and/or higher deductibles into their insurance plans, the use of health services often declines in response. When insurance reimbursement for a service increases, use of that service tends to increase. The growing number of uninsured Americans has resulted in decreased demand for basic health services at a time when health problems are thought to be increasing.

Changing reimbursement arrangements also may influence practice patterns. Hospitals face restrictions on the services they can provide, imposed by health plans that are trying to limit claims payments. Changing reimbursement patterns and regulatory pressures are also forcing physicians to change their practice patterns.

The emergence of managed care as a dominant organizational structure in healthcare is yet another factor that has had an impact on utilization patterns. The very concept of managed care emphasizes health plans' ability to control their enrollees' service utilization. For example, health plans are increasingly encouraging their members to obtain certain services (e.g., chronic disease monitoring) while at the same time discouraging them from obtaining others (e.g., emergency room care).

The availability of health services in the form of facilities and personnel has an understandable impact on the level of health services utilization. In some situations, the demand for services is not being met because of a lack of facilities or personnel. In other cases, an oversupply of facilities or personnel may result in over-utilization of health services.

One final factor to consider is the practice patterns that characterize different health service providers. Far from being an exact science, medicine involves frequent value judgments on the part of physicians and other practitioners. Although there are individual differences among physicians within the same market area in terms of the volume and types of services provided to similar patients, there are even more striking variations from market to market (Fisher 2008). Local practice patterns may account for significant variations in utilization between groups of patients who have similar health problems.

The recorded level of health services utilization reflects a combination of a population's needs, wants, and recommended standards, as well as the impact of the structural factors noted in the previous paragraphs. Each category of demand poses a different challenge for health services marketers, but the real challenge is to be able to determine what combination of these factors is relevant for a particular situation. The determination of demand is clearly a multifaceted process that involves a number of different dimensions. Although it may be appropriate in a situation to use only needs, wants, recommended standards, or utilization as a proxy, ultimately some type of blended concept must be developed to more precisely specify the level of demand. Exhibit 8.4 discusses the elasticity of the demand for health services.

Measuring Health Services Utilization

Health services researchers have developed a number of indicators for measuring health services utilization. Commonly used indicators are discussed in the sections that follow.

Facilities Indicators

Hospital admissions is one of the most frequently used indicators of health services utilization because the hospital is the focal point for treatment in the system. The terms *admissions* and *discharges* are used to refer to episodes of inpatient hospital utilization. The hospital admissions rate is also a proxy for other indicators, as hospital admissions correlate with tests conducted, surgeries performed, and the allocation of other resources. Hospital care is both labor and capital intensive, so one admission represents significant

EXHIBIT 8.4
The Elasticity of Health Services Demand

Historically, economists considered medical care to be the one service for which demand was inelastic. The assumption was that, if an individual was sick, the individual would consume health services, and if an individual received health services, he must be sick. Today, we understand that this assumption applies only to rare, life-threatening situations for which treatment will almost invariably be received, regardless of other characteristics of the patient or the healthcare system. For every episode requiring life-saving efforts, there are thousands of situations in which healthcare is consumed, many involving individuals who are not technically sick. As a result of this realization, the demand for most health services is now considered to be relatively elastic.

A substantial body of evidence has been compiled about differences in demand for health services among people with similar health conditions. Indeed, one of the major factors driving healthcare reform efforts is the disparity that exists among various populations with regard to their utilization of health services. In reality, the demand for health services rises and falls in response to a variety of factors. In areas where there are few health services, for example, the demand for healthcare appears to be relatively low. On the other hand, in areas where there is an abundance of healthcare resources, the demand appears to be much higher. Similarly, a change in physician practice standards is also likely to affect the demand for health services. At one point, for example, it may have been "fashionable" among OB/GYNs to perform cesarean sections on a larger proportion of their pregnant patients; as more scientific evidence accumulated, a trend away from C-sections emerged.

Perhaps the best example of the elasticity of demand for health services is a situation in which the demand for care rises and falls commensurate with the availability of health insurance. Indeed, because access to insurance is one of the best predictors of the demand for health services, those who are adequately insured demand a greater number of services than do those who are poorly insured.

Healthcare marketers must be cognizant that the demand for health services is variable and affected by a wide range of factors. The marketer should be not only knowledgeable about the different levels of demand exhibited by various population segments but also able to anticipate changes in demand in response to trends affecting either the population or the healthcare system.

healthcare expenditures. Admissions may be measured for an entire community or for one facility, or they may be broken down into components of utilization (e.g., clinical specialty, demographic attribute, geographic origin, or payer category).

The term *patient days* refers to the number of hospital days a particular population spends in a facility and is calculated in terms of the number of patient days accrued per 1,000 residents. This measure refines hospital admissions as an indicator by reflecting the total utilization of resources on the basis of patient days to adjust for variations in length of stay. Like admission rates, patient days may be calculated by diagnosis, type of hospital, patient origin, and payer category. Changes in reimbursement procedures have made patient days a more effective indicator of resource utilization.

Another indicator used to measure hospitalization is the *average length of stay*. This measure is typically reported in terms of the average number of days patients remain in the facility during a specified period. This indicator is also a good measure of resource utilization. Medicare and many other healthcare plans reimburse hospitals at a per diem rate, making a facility's average length of stay an important financial consideration.

Several other facility indicators, each important in its own way, might also be used. Utilization rates may be calculated for nursing homes, hospital emergency departments, hospital outpatient departments, freestanding emergency centers, freestanding minor medical centers, freestanding surgery centers, and freestanding diagnostic centers, among others.

Personnel Indicators

One of the most useful indicators of health services utilization is the volume of physician encounters. This volume is typically measured in terms of *physician office visits*, although telephone or e-mail contact and physician visits to hospitalized patients are sometimes considered. The physician is the gatekeeper for most types of health services, and physician utilization is a more direct measure of utilization levels than hospital admissions, as most people avail themselves of a physician's services at some time. Physician utilization rates are often broken down by specialty because utilization among specialties varies dramatically.

Utilization rates also might be calculated for other types of personnel, typically independent practitioners who, like physicians and dentists, are not supervised by other medical personnel. Examples include optometrists, podiatrists, chiropractors, and mental health counselors and therapists. Other healthcare personnel, who generally cannot operate independently, but for whom utilization rates might be calculated, include home health nurses, physician assistants, and technical personnel. Physical therapists and speech therapists are other categories of healthcare personnel for whom utilization rates might be developed if, for example, the analyst were involved in marketing rehabilitation services.

Other Indicators

As the importance of home health care has increased, so has the importance of the volume of *home health care visits* as a utilization indicator. The scope of home care services has been expanded and now encompasses a broad range of services. Home care utilization is typically measured in terms of visits by various types of personnel. Thus, a population's utilization might be considered in terms of the number of home nurse visits or home physical therapist visits received. Alternatively, the number of residences (i.e., the rate per 1,000) receiving home care visits might be calculated.

Drug utilization is yet another indicator of health services use. Although patient care providers typically have limited use for information on drug utilization, analysts representing other entities, such as pharmaceutical companies, find it valuable. Their analyses typically focus on the consumption of prescription drugs because they (rather than over-the-counter medicine) are thought to more accurately reflect utilization of the healthcare system. Although the level of prescription drug consumption can be determined from physician and pharmacist records, rates of consumption of nonprescription drugs must be determined more indirectly.

Exhibit 8.5 presents some of the health services utilization rates discussed in this chapter and example calculations from which they might be derived.

The challenge for healthcare marketers is to increase utilization of the services provided by the healthcare organization. This endeavor, like much else in healthcare, is not always straightforward. As a general rule, increased volume results in increased revenue and, presumably, increased profit for the organization providing the services. However, healthcare organizations are often required by regulation, community standards, or consumer demand to provide services that may not generate enough revenue to cover costs. Furthermore, because the fee schedules adopted by insurance companies and health plans limit the reimbursement amounts healthcare organizations receive for many services, they may provide services for which the reimbursement is less than the cost of providing them. To further complicate the picture, a service that is profitable under normal circumstances may cause an organization to lose money if it attracts patients with poor ability to pay.

This situation has numerous implications for healthcare marketers. They must be familiar with the variety of services offered, the mechanisms for reimbursement, and the most desirable types of patients. In some situations, the sickest patients may be considered desirable, and in others, the target market will be healthy individuals. In some circumstances, a service

EXHIBIT 8.5
Commonly Used Health Services Utilization Rates

Hospital Admission Rate

Formula   *Example*

| Admission rate per 1,000 population | = | Number of hospital admissions in specified year ÷ Total population at midpoint of year | × 1,000 | 1,000 hospital admissions in 2005 ÷ 10,000 population estimate for midyear 2005 | × 1,000 = 100 |

Patient Days

| Hospital patient days | = | Hospital patients admitted in specified year × Average length of hospital stay | | 1,000 patients admitted in 2005 × Average length of stay of 5 days | = 5,000 patient days |

Physician Utilization Rate

| Physician office visits per 1,000 population | = | Number of physician office visits in specified year ÷ Total population at midpoint of year | × 1,000 | 30,000 office visits in 2005 ÷ 10,000 population estimate for midyear 2005 | × 1,000 = 3,000 |

Emergency Room (ER) Utilization Rate

| ER visits per 1,000 population | = | Number of emergency room visits in specified year ÷ Total population at midpoint of year | × 1,000 | 4,500 office visits in 2005 ÷ 10,000 population estimate for midyear 2005 | × 1,000 = 450 |

might be provided at a loss to establish a customer relationship, and in other circumstances, services may be offered at a loss because volume in this service area has implications for down-the-road profit in a related service. Clearly, healthcare marketers must be more intimately aware of the inner workings of their organizations than marketers in any other industry.

Predicting the Demand for Health Services

Knowledge about the current level of demand for health services, however measured, is important information for marketers. Even more important is the anticipated future level of demand characterizing the population under study. Important *predictors* of future demand (e.g., psychological factors, demographic factors, lifestyle and psychographic factors) were discussed earlier in the chapter. Now let's take a step further and discuss three of the *techniques* that have been developed for projecting future demand.

Traditional Utilization Projections

The simplest and most straightforward approach to projecting the utilization of health services involves straight-line projections based on historical trends. For example, in the past it was common to review several years' experience with hospital admissions and then extrapolate the observed trend into the future. This approach was intuitive in that, if the trend had been upward, the assumption was that it would continue to rise. On the other hand, if a downward trend had been recorded, the assumption was that the same historical pattern would persist into the future.

Few market analysts would use this approach in today's healthcare environment. Developments external to the healthcare arena have such an effect on the demand for services and subsequent patterns of utilization that extrapolating from the past to the future is not practical. This situation forced the development of more sophisticated approaches to the projection of utilization.

Population-Based Models

The most significant factor in terms of predicting health services utilization is the size of the population. The sheer number of people an organization serves has a greater effect on demand than any other factor. Because of the importance of population size, and because population projections are likely to be readily available and fairly reliable, population-based projections have become the most common technique used to forecast health services use.

The simplest approach involves multiplying the projected population by known utilization rates. Thus, population-based models depend on two components: (1) appropriate population estimates and projections and (2) accurate utilization rates. Various federal agencies provide population estimates and projections, as well as information on utilization rates. Commercial data vendors also provide population estimates and projections.

Although some benefit can be derived from basing the demand estimates on the total population, the analysis typically examines utilization in terms of various demographic factors. Changes in age distribution, for example, can have a major effect on utilization. Utilization patterns for males and females vary significantly and must be taken into consideration. To the extent that data are available, the population may be examined in terms of the influence of race and income on health services demand. In some cases, it may even be possible to conceptualize the population in terms of its health insurance status.

Projected utilization rates may be expressed, for example, in terms of hospital admissions or physician visits per 1,000 residents per year, patient days per 1,000 residents per year, live births per 1,000 women aged 15 to 44 per year, and so forth. These rates can be adjusted to account for regional differences when appropriate. The utilization rates of interest can be applied to different age and sex categories and adjusted for other attributes to the extent that the information is available.

Although population-based demand models, in all of their permutations, offer an intuitive, appealing approach to the issue, their usefulness is limited. The mobility of the population in contemporary America introduces an element of uncertainty into the projection process. The cohort effect (e.g., the changing characteristics of an age group as it grows older) also plays a role in determining differential utilization patterns. It is no longer safe to assume, for example, that the utilization patterns of 65-year-olds today will be the same as they were for 65-year-olds 20 years ago. Thus, applying an age-specific rate based on past experience to today's elderly may be risky.

Utilization rates themselves are subject to change for a number of reasons. Many of these factors have already been discussed, including availability of services, financing arrangements, and level of managed care penetration. Who could have predicted, for example, the decline in hospital admissions that resulted from the introduction of the Medicare Prospective Payment System and the emergence of managed care in the 1980s? Likewise, current discussions on healthcare reform certainly have the potential to establish a new paradigm. Further, the frequency with which paradigm-changing developments occur makes predicting levels of utilization even more challenging.

Econometric Models

Econometric models include a variety of different techniques for projecting future phenomena in complex situations. In their simplest form, econometric models are a type of time series analysis. They attempt to statistically improve on the aforementioned projection model that extrapolates past trends into the future.

Econometric models use equations that project utilization as a function of the interplay of independent variables. With a complex phenomenon like the utilization of health services, forecasting based on multiple factors makes more sense than forecasting based on a single factor. Theoretically, the more factors used in predicting future utilization, the more accurate the prediction will be. Econometric prediction addresses these factors in a series of mathematical expressions. The equation that is ultimately used is the one that best "fits the curve" in terms of historic demand. However, for this complex form of econometrics to work, projections are needed for numerous independent variables in the equation. Many analysts have attempted to apply econometric models to the prediction of health services demand. In today's environment, however, econometric models have limited utility because of the unpredictability and instability of the healthcare environment. See Case Study 8.1 for an example of the use of lifestyle analysis to predict the use of behavioral health services.

CASE STUDY 8.1
Using Lifestyle Analysis to Predict the Use
of Behavioral Health Services

During the last quarter of the twentieth century, behavioral health services emerged as an important sector in the U.S. healthcare system. This umbrella term covered many conditions, including psychiatric problems, emotional disturbances, substance abuse, hyperactivity in children, and other conditions considered treatable by mental health professionals. Behavioral health services were considered to be in a different category from services for the treatment of physical illness, and a separate industry developed for the management of behavioral health problems. Many health plans carved out behavioral health services, and, eventually, national managed care plans specializing in such services emerged.

By the late 1990s, the primary purchasers of behavioral health services—that is, major employers—were facing growing financial pressure as a result of increasing healthcare costs. Behavioral health services were particularly problematic because of the open-ended nature of many behavioral health conditions. At the same time, however, regulations that mandated parity between physical health coverage and

(*continued*)

CASE STUDY 8.1 (*continued*)

behavioral health coverage were enacted. Employers who wanted to offer behavioral health coverage to their employees were faced with a major cost-containment challenge.

ABC Health Services was a major player in the behavioral health arena, reporting an enrollment of more than 3 million members in its managed care plans. ABC was faced with the same issues other behavioral health plans had to address: customers who could not distinguish between plans and were shopping for the lowest price. As a result, ABC was losing clients to other, sometimes less capable, plans that quoted lower prices.

In response to this situation, ABC developed an innovative approach to the market using lifestyle segmentation analysis. On the basis of records maintained on enrollees who participated in its behavioral health plans, ABC believed the likelihood of using behavioral health services could be linked to different lifestyle categories among employees. ABC also thought that the type and intensity of services used could be correlated with lifestyle cluster.

ABC subsequently profiled existing clients in terms of its MOSAIC lifestyle clusters (see Exhibit 8.3). They found that approximately a dozen lifestyle clusters (of the 60 MOSAIC clusters) were associated with a high propensity to use behavioral health services. Another ten lifestyle clusters were almost never associated with the use of these services. The remaining clusters did not appear to correlate with use or nonuse.

For example, the cluster populated by middle-class suburban families tended to be characterized by high utilization levels, whereas the cluster populated by low-income rural families was characterized by low utilization levels. Furthermore, the older affluent suburban household cluster had a high propensity for using alcohol abuse services but not drug abuse services. On the other hand, the single, affluent, urban high-rise cluster had a high propensity to use drug abuse services but not alcohol treatment services. Some clusters were characterized by episodic use of services (e.g., in response to some stressful event), and members of other clusters were characterized by recurrent use of services, indicating deeper-seated problems.

ABC was able to use this information in marketing its behavioral health plan to existing customers and prospective clients. ABC representatives offered to profile the employees of existing customers, for example, to determine the extent to which the package of services offered by ABC was meeting their employees' needs. Profiling not only allowed ABC to more efficiently serve the existing client population but also helped the organization to predict future use of behavioral health services. The service mix could be subsequently adjusted to serve existing enrollees more efficiently and more cost-effectively.

To attract prospective clients, ABC distinguished itself from other behavioral health plans by determining a configuration of needs for the target group of employees. By serving in a consultative role, ABC demonstrated greater expertise than its competitors in the management of behavioral health clients. Further, ABC could offer a package of services tailored to the needs of its clients, rather than the one-size-fits-all plan offered by other firms. By developing an in-depth knowledge of the target population using lifestyle segmentation analysis, ABC was able to provide more effective services at competitive prices while raising the satisfaction level of employers and employees.

Discussion Questions

- What is the conventional wisdom with regard to the distribution of mental health problems in the population? Is it surprising to find that mental health problems are concentrated in different segments of the population?
- What are the implications of this irregular distribution of mental health problems for marketing?
- Are there sensitivities surrounding the marketing of mental health services of which the marketer should be aware?
- Does the fact that hospitals often lose money on mental health patients mean that they should not market to the affected population?
- Is this health problem one for which healthcare organizations might find social marketing useful?

Summary

Determining demand in healthcare is a complex task that requires marketers to develop an understanding of the many factors that influence the ultimate utilization of health services. From a marketing perspective, demand can be conceptualized as the ultimate result of the combined effect of (1) healthcare needs, (2) healthcare wants, (3) recommended standards of care, and (4) utilization patterns.

The demand for health services is surprisingly elastic. A number of factors influence the level of demand, including population characteristics, such as demographics, psychographics, and social group affiliation, and structural factors, such as availability of and access to health personnel and health facilities, financial arrangements (especially the availability of insurance), technological resources, and physician practice patterns.

A variety of indicators can be used to measure utilization rates. For hospitals, these indicators include use rates for admissions, patient days, and length of stay. Other indicators include use rates for physician office visits, procedures performed, and drugs prescribed. The utilization indicators chosen will depend on the type of organization and the product being marketed. In healthcare, increased volume is not always a desirable phenomenon, and marketers must have enough knowledge about the organization's operations to know which services to promote and which to discourage.

Information on the demand for a service is typically unavailable, so marketers must develop ways to determine potential demand. Similarly, data on utilization rates for various types of services may not be readily available. Marketers must also be able to generate estimates and projections of the demand for services and likely utilization rates to develop an effective marketing plan. A number of methodologies are available for this purpose, including population-based and econometric models.

Key Points

- In healthcare, the demand for services is viewed differently from the way it is viewed in other industries.
- The demand for health services reflects the combined effect of healthcare needs, wants, recommended standards, and utilization.
- Because the demand for healthcare is hard to quantify, the level of health services utilization is often used as a proxy for demand.
- The amount of sickness in a population influences the demand for health services but may be less important in determining demand than other factors.
- Because of the various factors influencing health services utilization, the demand for health services in the United States is elastic.
- Frequently, there is a mismatch between the demand for health services and actual service utilization; some needs go unmet, and some services are over-utilized.
- Besides biological factors, the demand for health services is influenced by psychological, demographic, sociocultural, and economic factors.

- Psychographic (or lifestyle) attributes may exert significant influence on health services demand by affecting health status and health behavior.
- In healthcare, demand for a service can be created where demand did not previously exist by introducing new procedures or drugs, modifying diagnostic criteria, or identifying new health problems.
- Extrinsic factors, such as availability of services, technological developments, physician practice patterns, and insurance reimbursement rates, also influence the demand for health services.
- A variety of indicators can be used to measure health services utilization, including use rates for hospitals, physicians, other practitioners, and pharmaceuticals.
- Health services researchers have developed a variety of techniques for predicting utilization of health services, including population-based and econometric models.

Discussion Questions

- Why is demand in healthcare a complicated issue, and what are some components that might contribute to the level of demand?
- What is the difference between healthcare needs and healthcare wants, and to what extent do the two overlap?
- Why is the correlation between health services demand and health services utilization imperfect?
- What are some demographic factors that influence the demand for health services?
- What role do psychographic or lifestyle factors play in influencing the demand for health services?
- Why may the mere presence of health services increase the demand for healthcare?
- Can demand for a service such as healthcare be created?
- What is the role of health insurance in determining the demand for health services?
- Why do patterns of health services utilization vary widely from community to community when the communities generally share the same characteristics?

HEALTHCARE MARKETING TECHNIQUES

Because marketing in healthcare encompasses a wider range of activities than marketing in most other industries, the topic is covered in the broadest possible sense in this book. This section reviews the marketing techniques used in healthcare, considers the advantages and disadvantages to their use, and assesses their relative effectiveness. The extent to which marketing techniques can be transferred from other industries is also considered.

Chapter 9 focuses on marketing strategy, describing the manner in which strategic options might be assessed and the need to interface marketing strategy with the organization's overall strategic plan. It emphasizes the importance of having an integrated strategy when developing marketing initiatives.

Chapter 10 provides an overview of the traditional promotional techniques healthcare marketers are likely to use, such as public relations, advertising, personal sales, and sales promotion. It provides an overview of media options and explains the modifications marketers must make to traditional marketing approaches to be able to apply them in healthcare.

Chapter 11 presents new and emerging marketing techniques, whether unique to healthcare or adopted from other industries. Two categories of techniques are discussed—those that involve programmatic changes and those that capitalize on contemporary technology. Numerous applications of innovative marketing techniques are illustrated, and the feasibility of their use in healthcare is considered.

Chapter 12, new to this edition, examines healthcare marketing from an international perspective. The prestige and perceived quality of the U.S. healthcare system has long attracted foreign patients, and health systems are aggressively seeking patients from overseas. At the same time, medical tourism has emerged as a significant phenomenon, and a growing number of American patients are exploring options for treatment in other countries. As the pace of globalization increases, international healthcare marketing is expected to grow in importance.

MARKETING STRATEGIES

Healthcare organizations are often tempted to rush a marketing campaign into the field, but few can be successful without first designing a well-thought-out business strategy to guide the organization's marketing initiatives. This chapter highlights the relevance of the traditional four Ps of marketing—product, price, place, and promotion—to strategy development. Factors influencing strategy development are reviewed, and the steps involved in formalizing marketing strategies are outlined.

Strategy Defined

The term *strategy* is used in a variety of ways by different students of marketing. For purposes of this book, it refers to the generalized approach taken to meet market challenges. A strategy sets the tone for any marketing activity (tactic) and sets the parameters within which the marketer must operate. The strategy influences the nature of the marketing plan that is ultimately developed and guides subsequent marketing initiatives.

Marketers often think of strategy in terms of the level to which it relates. For example, they might create a *corporate strategy* that deals with the overall development of an organization's business activities, a *business strategy* that indicates how to approach a particular product and/or market, or a *marketing strategy* that focuses on one or more aspects of the marketing mix. Marketing strategy is most relevant to this discussion and might be thought of as the marketing logic by which an organization hopes to achieve its objectives. The organization's marketing strategy is reflected in the initiatives it takes to target markets, the marketing mix it selects, and the marketing expenditures for which it budgets.

Ideally, strategies are carefully thought out and deliberately formulated through enterprise-wide strategic planning. The absence of an articulated strategy, however, does not mean that no strategy exists. Acts of commission or omission ultimately create a strategy, and even the absence of a strategy could be considered a strategic approach in a technical sense.

As a result, many healthcare organizations end up with de facto strategies that were not deliberately formulated. This situation may result from lack of a formal strategic plan, failure to link marketing to an existing strategic plan, or failure to articulate marketing strategies clearly. In most cases, this situation results when the organization neglects to engage in formal market strategy development.

Unplanned strategies are referred to as *emergent strategies* and are derived from a pattern of behavior not consciously imposed by senior management. They are the outcome of activities and behaviors that occur unconsciously but nevertheless fall into a consistent pattern. Although many healthcare administrators would concede that they do not have a strategy in place, some form of strategy, albeit unstated, usually exists. See Exhibit 9.1 for a schematic on the role of strategy in an organization.

Before discussing different types of strategies, let's review the reasons for developing a strategy. To a certain extent, strategies are developed for the same reasons any type of planning activity is carried out. All strategies should accomplish the following:

- *Provide direction for the organization or program.* The strategy should constitute the "how to" aspect of organizational development.
- *Focus effort on one of many possible options.* Because there will always be numerous strategic options from which to choose, focusing on a particular strategy prevents confusion of purpose and diffusion of effort.
- *Unify the organization's actions.* The strategy should give the organization a purpose and unify the actions of its members.
- *Differentiate the organization.* The strategy should solidify the organization's identity and distinguish it from competitors.
- *Customize the organization's promotions.* The strategy should guide the development of promotional material, and all materials should present a distinct, consistent image.
- *Marshall the organization's resources.* The strategy should guide the allocation of resources to focus them on one approach rather than many.

EXHIBIT 9.1
The Role of Strategy in an Organization

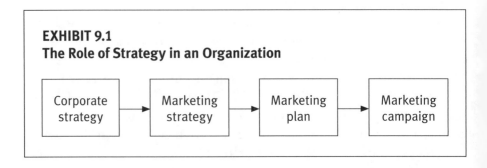

- *Support decision making in the organization.* The strategy should implicitly establish criteria to frame issues that require a decision.
- *Give the organization a competitive edge.* Ultimately, strategy development is about positioning the organization in relation to the market, capitalizing on the organization's strategic assets, and providing a strategic advantage.

The Strategic Planning Context

Strategic planning is a well-established activity in most industries and in many cases has become synonymous with corporate planning. The strategic plan is the primary mechanism through which an organization adapts to an ever-changing healthcare arena. The emphasis it places on market positioning underscores its central role in organizational development. A strategically oriented organization is one whose actions are aligned with the realities of the environment. The organization's strategic mind-set should ultimately spawn a marketing mind-set among the organization's members.

The strategic plan should guide the allocation of marketing resources, particularly when scarce resources are being dispensed. The plan should also provide a basis for relationship development in an environment that has become increasingly driven by provider networks, integrated delivery systems, and referral relationships. The strategic planning process should address the appropriateness of existing links and identify potential new relationships.

Most important, the strategic plan should be a call to action. Many healthcare organizations have spun their wheels for years, waiting for a clear direction to present itself. The strategic plan should not only embody the organization's strategy but also convey the organization's vision and lay out the scenario for the kind of organization it wants to become. This vision should help marketers picture the marketing activities they will need to engage in to support the organization's strategic initiatives.

Healthcare administrators tend to rush headlong into marketing campaigns without regard for the strategic implications. Because marketing challenges often provoke heated, high-pressure situations, the tendency is to address immediate marketing needs without concern for the broader implications of these actions. This all-too-common scenario underscores the need for a strategic orientation at all levels of the organization.

The Strategic Planning Process

The steps in the strategic planning process are summarized in the sections that follow. Although different authors have different perspectives on the steps and the sequencing of the planning process, the approach outlined here is a typical one. More detail on the strategic planning process is presented in Chapter 15. (See also Thomas [2003a].)

Step One: Plan for Planning

The first step in the strategic planning process involves planning for planning, and a good starting point for this phase is reviewing the organization's mission statement and corporate goals. Because the organization likely spent considerable effort in defining its mission and establishing its goals, the planning process should confirm the validity of these concepts or provide a rationale for their modification.

Much of the activity at this point in the strategic planning process is organizational in nature and focuses on identifying the key stakeholders, decision makers, and internal resources that should be involved in the planning process. A planning team should be established that includes representatives from all constituent groups, including stakeholders, key decision makers, and opinion leaders, as well as representatives from key departments in the organization.

Step Two: State Assumptions

One of the critical steps in developing a strategy involves the stating of assumptions. Assumptions might be made about the players involved in the local healthcare arena, the nature of the market area (and its population), the political climate, the position of other providers, and any other factors that might affect the strategic development process. Many of these assumptions are likely to have a marketing dimension. Assumptions stated during the strategy development process are likely to relate to the organization's position in the market, the nature of the competition, the distribution of the organization's facilities, and so forth. Although the team will undoubtedly refine its assumptions as the planning process continues, it should begin with some general ones—for example, "Managed care will continue to exert a major influence on the local market" or "We're number four in market share, and there is no way we will ever be number one."

Step Three: Gather Initial Information

The team begins the data collection process by gathering general background information on the organization, including reviews of available organizational materials, such as publications produced by the organization (e.g., annual reports); press releases; and marketing materials. The resumes of management and key clinical and technical personnel may also be reviewed. Other potential sources of information include reports filed with regulatory agencies, business plans that have been presented to funding sources, grant applications, and certificate-of-need applications. Internal documents such as executive committee minutes, planning retreat summaries, and evaluation studies may also be useful.

The team should also conduct an inventory and assessment of existing marketing activities. Marketing initiatives that are already under way need to be catalogued. Existing marketing themes or default strategic orientations should be identified. Healthcare organizations that are new to formal marketing efforts may have a lot more marketing initiatives under way than they realize, although they may not consider these activities as marketing. For example, an organization may offer perks to admitting physicians and conduct community health fairs without recognizing these initiatives as marketing activities.

Initial information should be gathered through interviews with knowledgeable persons in the organization who represent various functional areas, vested interests, and perspectives. In large organizations, these interviews may be restricted to key administrators and medical staff and perhaps one or more individuals who have a perspective on institutional history. In a smaller organization, such as a physician's practice, interviews with people further down the organizational structure may be necessary.

This stage of the process should also identify the *key constituents* of the organization. To whom does the organization report? Who does it have to satisfy? If it is a tightly held private organization, there may be few entities outside the organization that matter. On the other hand, a private, not-for-profit healthcare organization is likely to be accountable to board members, regulators, major donors, and other interested parties. In a publicly held company, the board of directors and the shareholders are also important constituents. Other constituents to consider include patient groups, referring physicians, employee benefits managers, insurance plan representatives, and political officials. The list should include the full range of constituents that would conceivably be addressed by any type of marketing initiative, including consumers (who need to be made aware of the organization's services), existing customers (whose loyalty needs to be strengthened), the medical staff (whose continued support must be ensured), and the media (who must be kept up to date on the organization's activities).

Information gathered during this phase should facilitate the conceptualization of the organization's *corporate culture*. The corporate culture defines the organization's character, sets the tone for employee interaction, affects the organization's operations, and determines the extent to which the organization is amenable to the planning process. The corporate culture will typically determine the ease with which a marketing mind-set can be established in the organization.

The planning team is not likely to have all the answers to every question raised at this point, and typically more questions than answers will be generated. Nevertheless, knowledge will begin to be accumulated and a sense of promising options and potential roadblocks should emerge as background information is compiled.

Step Four: Profile the Organization

The initial information-gathering activities should clarify what the organization is and what business it is in. Armed with the vision emerging from this knowledge, the planning team should review the organization's existing mission statement and goals. One critical turning point for any healthcare organization occurs when it comes to grips with what business it is in. For example, toward the end of the twentieth century, hospitals that continued to think they were in the hospital business rather than the healthcare business found themselves at a competitive disadvantage to hospitals that realized they had a broader mission. The redefinition of the mission of healthcare organizations that occurred in this period was a major contributor to the emergence of marketing as an essential healthcare function.

In profiling the organization, a couple of important questions must be addressed during the early stages of research. First, what is the organization's product or products? This question may seem easy to answer, but it is one to which few healthcare organizations can readily respond. Healthcare organizations historically have not had to think in terms of discrete products. Furthermore, healthcare organizations are often complex, and unless the organization's sole business is selling a healthcare "widget," the products and services it offers are likely to be difficult to classify. How does one conceptualize public health or occupational medicine, for example, in terms of goods and services? Regardless of the complexity involved, specifying the organization's products and services is an important step in developing both general strategies and marketing-specific strategies. (The nature of healthcare products is discussed in more detail in Chapter 7.)

Second, who are the organization's customers? In other words, who does the organization have to convince to purchase its services? The more multipurpose an organization is, the broader the range of customers it will have. For a hospital, the list of customers includes patients who receive services, family members and other decision makers who influence patient behavior, staff physicians, referring physicians, major employers and business coalitions, insurance companies, and managed care plans. In many cases, other care providers also are customers, especially with the emergence of provider networks and integrated delivery systems. The list does not stop there, particularly if the hospital is tax exempt as a result of its not-for-profit status. In this case, its customers may include consumer advocacy groups, policymakers, legislators, regulators, and the press.

Step Five: Collect Baseline Data

The initial information-gathering process sets the stage for a more intensive data collection agenda involving internal and external data audits. Although the primary driver of strategic development is the external environment, the process begins with a thorough organizational self-analysis. The intent of the internal audit is to determine who does what in the organization, when and where they do it, how they do it, and even why and how well they do it.

The internal audit covers a wide variety of organizational features and can be incredibly detailed. The following list includes aspects of the organization that might be addressed in an internal audit:

- Policies and procedures
- Existing services and products
- Nature, number, and characteristics of customers
- Utilization patterns for services
- Sales volume
- Staffing levels and personnel characteristics
- Management processes
- Financial situation
- Fee/pricing structure
- Billing and collections practices
- Marketing arrangements
- Location of service outlets
- Referral relationships

The internal audit for a strategic plan typically involves some type of operational analysis. This analysis is likely to include, at a minimum, an evaluation of patient flow, paper flow, and information flow. The operational analysis may also examine staffing patterns, physical space considerations, and productivity. Although this information might not apply directly to most marketing initiatives, it is critical to any internal marketing effort.

The scope of the external audit will be determined by the nature of the organization and the issues under consideration. Macro-level trends are more important for organizations involved in regional or national marketing initiatives. For most healthcare organizations, this analysis focuses on the local market because most marketing takes place there. The organization must consider the climate of the market area and determine what facets of healthcare make the community tick.

For marketers, the most important component of the strategic analysis is market identification and description. The organization's market can be defined in a number of different ways, and the definition used will depend on the purpose of the analysis, the product or service being considered, the competitive environment, and even the type of organization involved in the marketing effort. Markets may be defined on the basis of geography, demographics, consumer demand, disease prevalence, and so forth. (Issues related to the identification of markets are discussed in Chapter 5.)

In a typical strategy development initiative, the first task is to profile the market area population. The type of information that needs to be collected on the market area population varies with the nature of the project. Demographic data, including biosocial and sociocultural traits, are typically compiled first. At a minimum, the analyst would examine the population in terms of age, sex, race/ethnicity, marital status/family structure, income, and education. Insurance coverage is also typically assessed. Furthermore, the migration process has taken on increasing importance in community analysis, and information on the volume and traits of in-migrants and out-migrants is often collected.

The demographic analysis is often accompanied by an assessment of the psychographic characteristics of the market area population. Information on the lifestyle categories of the target audience can be used to determine the likely health priorities and behaviors of a population subgroup. Often a reflection of lifestyles, consumer attitudes are another aspect of the population that is typically considered at this point. The attitudes consumers display in a market area are likely to have considerable influence on the demand for almost all types of health services. Marketers must also consider the attitudes characterizing other constituents, such as referring physicians and policymakers. Exhibit 9.2 lists examples of data collected during the internal and external audits.

Step Six: Identify Health Characteristics

The salient health characteristics of the target market—fertility patterns and morbidity and mortality levels—will be identified during the course of the external audit. Information on these attributes provides insights into the *health status* of the population and, ultimately, into the types of health services it requires.

Historical *fertility patterns* exert a major influence on current patterns of health services demand, and a wide range of service and product needs revolve around childbearing. Childbearing also triggers the need for such down-the-road services as pediatrics. Health service demands in this area may also encompass infertility treatments and treatments for conditions related to the male and female reproductive systems.

The level of *morbidity* in a population is another major consideration in strategic planning. The incidence and prevalence rates that characterize a population provide a context for strategic development. To the extent possible, analysts must project incidence and prevalence rates into the future to anticipate service needs. The level of disability in the population should also be considered.

EXHIBIT 9.2
Data Collected Through Internal and External Audits

Internal Audit	External Audit
Organizational structure	Market area
Corporate culture	Target market
Decision-making process	Consumer characteristics
Key influentials	Consumer perceptions
Staffing patterns	Utilization patterns
Sales volume	Competitors
Customer characteristics	Market positioning
Price structure	Market shares
Sources of revenue	Reimbursement trends
Profitability by service	
Referral sources	
Existing marketing initiatives	

The level of *mortality* and the leading causes of death in the population of the market area should also be determined. Market researchers are typically less interested in mortality than morbidity because the latter is more closely linked to service demand. Nevertheless, mortality data are almost always examined in assessing a community's health status.

Once the population's health conditions have been identified, analysts need to determine what health services and products it requires. Healthcare needs can be conceptualized in terms of service utilization (e.g., inpatient services, ambulatory care), the performance of diagnostic and therapeutic procedures, the prescription of drugs, or other indicators.

Ideally, identified health conditions can be converted into demand for health services. The amount of goods and services actually consumed, however, will be determined by a variety of factors. For this reason, the actual health behavior of the target population needs to be considered. *Health behavior* refers to any action aimed at restoring, preserving, and/or enhancing an individual's health status. From a marketing perspective, information on health behavior provides insights into consumer behavior and the consumer decision-making process. Health behavior includes such formal activities as physician visits, hospital admissions, and prescription drug consumption, as well as informal actions on the part of individuals, such as wellness and fitness activities aimed at preventing health problems and maintaining, enhancing, or promoting health. Organizations involved in social marketing, for example, are likely to require information on unhealthy lifestyles or risky behavior inherent in the population. An understanding of the population's health behavior should supplement the information previously developed on the market area's need for health services.

Utilization data are often the best source of information on health behaviors, and healthcare organizations focus on indicators of health behavior that are most relevant to their operations. Hospitals are likely to consider information on most of the utilization indicators described throughout this book. Other organizations with operations of more limited scope are likely to focus on a narrower range of utilization indicators in their analyses.

Step Seven: Conduct a Resource Inventory

The resource identification process establishes an inventory of the facilities, personnel, and other resources available to meet the healthcare needs of the target population. Although there may be some situations in which the full range of available health services within the market area must be identified, emphasis is typically placed on the organizations and/or services that are likely to be in competition with the entity doing the planning. Given the role of marketing in countering the competition, the resource inventory is a critical piece of the strategy development process. Here are some examples of resources that may be included in the inventory:

- Healthcare facilities
- Healthcare equipment
- Health personnel
- Programs and services
- Funding sources
- Networks and relationships

The final category—networks and relationships—has become increasingly important in this era of managed care and negotiated contracts for health services. The importance of such connections cannot be overestimated, and many organizations have come to view relationship building and management of customer relationships as responsibilities of the marketing department.

An important aspect of this analysis involves referral relationships. As relationships grow in importance, so does the emphasis placed on them in the strategy development process. It can be argued that, in the future, patients will use a provider because of existing relationships (i.e., they will form a relationship with their health plan or provider before they become sick), rather than take the traditional approach involving relationship development *after* utilization (i.e., they don't see a doctor until they are sick and need care, and then develop the relationship after the encounter). The existence of networks, integrated delivery systems, and strategic partners in the community should be fully addressed during the strategic planning process.

By this stage of the strategy development process, the marketer has compiled a great deal of valuable data. On the basis of the information available at this point, the marketer should be able to determine the following:

- Overall societal/healthcare/service trends
- Market area delineation
- Market area population profile
- Market area population health characteristics
- Current position of the organization/product
- Customer profile
- Resources available in the service area
- Future developments that will affect the organization

A major component of the external audit is the competitive analysis. Organizations do not operate in a vacuum. Marketers must consider the healthcare environment and the other players in the arena. Any strategy must reflect the organization's position in the environment and in relation to its competitors.

After all of this knowledge has been accumulated, the state of the organization can be frankly described and its position in the market assessed. On these bases, all parties can develop consensus with regard to the assumptions stated in step two and choose those that will underlie the development of the strategic plan.

Developing the Strategic Plan

The effort expended to this point has returned a foundation for strategy formulation. The next question is when the strategy should be developed. Different strategists may sequence the development of strategy at various points in the process. From the author's perspective, the development of strategy should occur when adequate baseline data have been acquired and analyzed. The sequencing of the strategy development process as described in the next sections will depend on the nature of the organization and its particular circumstances. The actual process of specifying a strategy is discussed later in the chapter.

Set the Goal(s)

The goal(s) established in the strategic plan should reflect the information that has been compiled to date and should align with the organization's mission statement. The goal depicts an ideal state and serves as the target for future development. For example, the goal of a national medical products company might be to establish the firm as a low-cost provider of a certain product. For a local health services provider, the goal may be to position itself as a niche player to take advantage of market opportunities. For the purveyor of a specific service, the goal may be to become recognized as the provider of choice for a segment of the market.

Set Objectives

Objectives should support the stated goal(s). To many, objectives are the tactics that support the strategic initiatives. For example, in support of its goal of expanding its orthopedic product lines, a hospital might set an objective that its orthopedic practice will recruit a sports medicine specialist within the next 12 months.

For every goal, a number of objectives are likely to be specified. Multiple objectives for a single goal are common because action will likely be required on a number of different fronts to attain it. As the planning team establishes objectives, any barriers to accomplishing the organization's stated objectives should be considered, identified, and assessed.

The possibility that pursuit of the objectives will bring about unanticipated consequences should also be considered. For example, a successful marketing campaign may overwhelm the service providers or otherwise strain resources. If the organization cannot deliver on the marketer's promises, negative consequences will likely result. A marketing campaign may alert competitors to the organization's strategic direction, or the campaign might alienate a party that had been a strong supporter of the organization. Although negative consequences cannot be totally eliminated, conceding their existence is the first step toward minimizing their impact.

Strategic Options

In selecting a strategy, analysts must consider the organization's nature and mission, the market's characteristics (and, more specifically, those of the organization's customers), and the nature of the competition. The chosen strategy will influence the public's perception of the organization and will carry long-term implications. Unfortunately, there is no standard list of strategies from which the organization can choose. Each situation is unique and will call for creative design.

SWOT Analysis

One technique that can be used to determine an appropriate strategy is the SWOT analysis. A SWOT analysis examines markets, organizations, or products in terms of their strengths, weaknesses, opportunities, and threats. (See Exhibit 9.3 for more detail on the SWOT analysis.) A SWOT analysis simultaneously considers several dimensions of the situation, thereby establishing a basis for subsequent strategy development.

EXHIBIT 9.3
SWOT Analysis

The SWOT analysis has become a common technique for assessing the position of a healthcare organization in its market. A SWOT analysis involves an examination of the organization, the environment, and the way the organization and environment interact. It is an important tool for strategists and marketers and has numerous applications in healthcare. A SWOT analysis can be done for an organization's departments or for an organization as a whole. Factors in the macro and competitive environments should be included in the analysis.

A SWOT analysis examines the strengths, weaknesses, opportunities, and threats relative to the community or the organization.

- A *strength* is a distinctive skill or competence that the organization possesses and that will help it achieve its stated objectives. Strengths can include marketing capabilities, management skills, the organization's image, financial resources, and other assets.
- A *weakness* is an aspect of the organization that might hinder it from achieving its objectives. Weaknesses might include inadequate working capital, poor management skills, a lack of services, personnel shortages, and so on.
- An *opportunity* is any feature of the external environment that creates advantages for the firm in relation to an objective or a set of objectives. Opportunities may take the form of gaps in the market, new sources of reimbursement, demographic changes, weaknesses among competitors, and so forth.
- A *threat* is an environmental development that may present problems and hinder the organization from achieving its objectives. Threats may take the form of competitive activity, unfavorable demographic changes, anticipated reimbursement changes, and so forth.

The SWOT analysis should include input from quantitative research, as well as from interviews with key personnel (e.g., stakeholders, key decision makers, opinion leaders). Because the identified strengths, weaknesses, opportunities, and threats will guide further development of the plan, consensus needs to be reached on these attributes before proceeding with the planning process.

The assessment of the organization's strengths will indicate the attributes on which the strategist should capitalize. The weaknesses indicate aspects of the organization that should be minimized or ameliorated. The threats indicate aspects of the organization or environment that should be neutralized. Of the four dimensions, opportunities have perhaps the most salience for strategy development because an implicit goal of the chosen strategy should be to exploit opportunities that exist in the marketplace.

Ideally, the strategy used in any marketing initiative will support the organization's mission statement and reflect the strategies embodied in the organization's strategic plan. Thus, if the organization's strategy involves positioning itself as a caring organization, the organization's marketing initiatives should support this approach. In some cases, of course, a marketing situation may call for a departure from the established approach. For example, a hospital that has been content to live in the shadow of a more powerful competitor while adopting a "we're number two" approach may develop a world-class program in a particular clinical area and decide to take a much more aggressive approach in marketing this service than it would take for the organization in general. Thus, a "second fiddle" strategy may be displaced by a "flanking" strategy in light of the new developments.

Other approaches may focus on the market and concentrate on market-oriented strategies. Still others may focus on a product or service line and develop a product-oriented strategy. The approach may address an aspect of the marketing mix, as in the case of a pricing strategy, or it may cut across the marketing mix and be broader in its scope.

A *market penetration strategy* (existing market/existing product) focuses on efforts to extract more sales and greater usage out of existing markets by acquiring customers from competitors and converting nonusers into users. A *market development strategy* (new market/existing product) focuses on discovering new market sectors on the basis of different benefit profiles, establishing new distribution channels, developing new marketing approaches, and identifying underserved geographic areas. For example, a market niche strategy might be pursued by a healthcare organization that serves small segments of the healthcare market that other firms overlook or ignore.

A *new product* or *service development strategy* (existing market/new product) focuses on modifying existing services by introducing differing quality levels and/or developing entirely new products. A *diversification strategy* (new market/new product) involves such actions as horizontal and/or vertical integration, concentric diversification, and conglomerate diversification, all of which involve extending the organization's operations to encompass additional services not previously offered in-house.

The relationship between the product and the market can be depicted in five distinct configurations: (1) full service, (2) product/market specialization, (3) production specialization, (4) market specialization, and (5) selective specialization. This breakdown is illustrated in Exhibit 9.4.

Examples of each of these relationships can be found in the healthcare field, although the term *service* should be substituted for *product* in most cases. The *full-service approach* was typical of most hospitals in the past, particularly during the production era following World War II. General hospitals attempted to be all things to all people, and their strategies reflected this orientation. This strategy promotes all products to all markets. A *product/market specialization strategy* is typically adopted by an organization that supports a single service or service line for a defined market, such as in the case of a home infusion company that provides a discrete set of services to a narrowly defined market of home-bound pediatric patients.

Firms in the business of *product specialization* offer a distinct set of products that can be promoted to a number of markets in which consumers have one

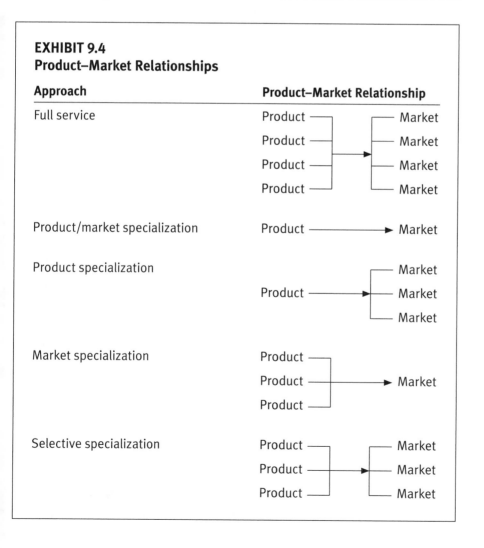

EXHIBIT 9.4
Product–Market Relationships

Approach	Product–Market Relationship
Full service	Product — Market Product — Market Product — Market Product — Market
Product/market specialization	Product ⟶ Market
Product specialization	Market Product ⟶ Market Market
Market specialization	Product Product ⟶ Market Product
Selective specialization	Product — Market Product ⟶ Market Product — Market

characteristic in common. For example, a firm specializing in assistive equipment (e.g., wheelchairs, walkers, home monitoring devices) promotes its products to consumers who have physical limitations that require assistive equipment. This firm's market would include the frail elderly, persons suffering from birth defects, injury victims, and those undergoing rehabilitation from surgery.

Organizations emphasizing *market specialization* typically develop a range of products geared to a certain market. Organizations that offer senior services or that specialize in women's healthcare goods and services are examples of enterprises focused on market specialization. Pharmaceutical companies are probably the best-known example of firms engaged in *selective specialization*. Each drug constitutes a product line that is targeted to a specific market. For example, ABC Pharmaceuticals' hypertension drug is marketed to the hypertensive market, its diabetes drug to the population affected by diabetes, its arthritis drug to the population of persons with rheumatoid arthritis, and so forth.

Another approach to strategy development examines the combination of market attractiveness and competitiveness found in the situation under study. For example, an area characterized by *high market attractiveness* and *high competitiveness* might call for a strategy involving investment and growth or, more likely, a strategy emphasizing selective growth that focuses on vulnerable areas. Different combinations of market attractiveness and competitiveness call for different strategies.

The following are examples of market-oriented strategies typically used in healthcare:

- *Dominance strategy*: The number one player in the market opts to focus on maintaining this position.
- *Second-fiddle strategy*: The runner-up in the market concedes its second-place status and acts accordingly (also called a *market-follower strategy*).
- *Frontal attack strategy*: The organization decides to confront the market leader or major competitors head-on.
- *Niche strategy*: The organization concedes that it cannot successfully compete for the mainstream market but instead concentrates on niche markets based on geography, population groups, or selected services.
- *Flanking strategy*: The organization outflanks the competition by entering new markets, cultivating new populations, or offering fringe products.

Strategy and the Four Ps

One approach to selecting a strategy considers the role of the marketing mix in establishing the strategic direction. The marketing mix is the set of controllable variables the firm uses to influence the target market. The mix includes the four Ps: *product, place, price,* and *promotion* (these terms were defined in Chapter 3). As noted previously, the strategy could focus on any dimension of the four Ps or could cut across all four. Strategic approaches based on the four components of the marketing mix are addressed in the following sections.

Product Strategies

As the name implies, a *product strategy* focuses on one good (or product line) or service (or service line). The strategy is built around the qualities of the product, and the marketing approach attempts to capitalize on product attributes (e.g., quality, durability).

One example of a product strategy is a *preemptive strategy*. A preemptive strategy would be used where there are only limited differences between the products in a product class. A preemptive strike attempts to convey something about a product that other competitors would be reluctant to repeat because of the risk of being labeled blatant imitators. Another product-oriented approach focuses on a *unique selling proposition*, in which an organization establishes and communicates a product benefit that competitors cannot make or refuse to make. Marketers might also adopt a *brand image strategy* that emphasizes psychological differences over physical differences between products. The aim is to associate the product with symbols and characters that resonate with the target audience.

A *positioning strategy* attempts to define the comparisons between one product and another in the consumer's mind. The organization's task is to identify weaknesses in competing products and strengths in its own that can be reinforced to gain a competitive edge. Positioning indicates to customers how the company differs from current or potential competitors. A positioning strategy can be created through the following steps:

1. Identify alternative competitors and competing products in the defined product category.
2. Establish consumers' perceptions of competing products.
3. Determine the relative position of competing products using a perceptional positioning map that graphically depicts the market.
4. Identify the gap within the market by assessing customer needs with regard to existing product offerings.
5. Select desired positioning.
6. Implement a promotional strategy.
7. Monitor and control the positioning process.

An example of strategy development is presented in Case Study 9.1.

CASE STUDY 9.1
Hospital Strategy Development

A hospital management company recently acquired a 150-bed general hospital in a medium-sized city in the southeastern United States. Although the company had little knowledge of the local market when it acquired the facility, its first thought was to continue to run the facility as a general hospital. However, given that the hospital had not been profitable in offering general care and that it faced competition from three large facilities that had access to almost unlimited resources, the new managers chose to perform a situational analysis to determine the most appropriate strategy.

The managers commissioned a study of the immediate market area—the five-mile radius surrounding the hospital. This market area was examined in the context of overall trends for the metropolitan area. The analysts reviewed demographic trends to determine the future size and composition of the population as well as trends in service utilization, and then developed projections of the future demand for health services in the urban area and the immediate market area. Particular attention was paid to the competitive situation to determine the services offered by other facilities, existing market shares for those services, and the nature of existing managed care contracts and other negotiated relationships.

The analysis determined that the immediate service area was not likely to support a general hospital. The payer mix was not favorable, and other facilities controlled significant portions of the local market. Further, most area employers were tied to the provider networks of the two dominant systems in the community. The hospital did not have a large or strong medical staff, and given the existing provider networks involving competing hospitals, attracting additional physicians to the facility would have been difficult.

Having conceded that it could not operate effectively as a general community hospital and that confronting large, established competitors head-on was not practical, the managers considered other strategies. After analyzing the data, the managers decided that, under the circumstances, a niche strategy was appropriate for the hospital. It would identify niche services, and corporate efforts would focus on exploiting those niches.

The hospital had previously developed an occupational health program that catered to the numerous employers in the area. Facilities were available, a basic program was in place, and adequate personnel were available to expand the program. Because no other entity was offering this service in the community, expansion of this program seemed like a logical next step. In addition, the hospital had a long-standing behavioral health program that had experienced some success in attracting patients, and some of the area's leading substance abuse experts were affiliated with the hospital. Thus, because a fledging program was already in place, key personnel were available, and the market was underserved, the hospital also identified behavioral health (including substance abuse treatment) as a promising niche. Finally, in view of the large Medicare population in the general area and the lack of geropsychiatric services in the community, the hospital decided to add psychiatric services for seniors to the behavioral health component. This niche strategy focused on services that were not being adequately provided to the community.

One other niche was considered but eventually rejected. Market research indicated that minority group members, primarily African American, made up a large proportion of the community. The Hispanic population in the area was also growing rapidly. Further, mainstream providers historically had neglected these populations. A niche strategy focusing on these target populations was considered that would convert the hospital into a facility specializing in minority care. Because of the many unknowns surrounding this concept and the potential controversy such a strategy might generate, this idea was rejected.

After carefully assessing the situation, the managers conceded that the facility could not successfully operate as a general hospital and therefore chose to pursue a niche strategy. The approach has, in the short run at least, been relatively successful. The hospital has maintained a significant share of the occupational health and behavioral health markets in the city and has earned a reputation as a facility that does not offer a lot of services but that does a good job with the services it does provide.

Discussion Questions

- What factors raised concerns among the hospital's managers about the viability of the facility as a general community hospital, and how did the market analysis validate those concerns?
- What steps were taken to determine the most appropriate focus for the hospital's services?
- How would one classify the strategic approach the managers chose, and to what types of services did it direct them?

Pricing Strategies

Healthcare providers have seldom used pricing strategies in the past. Historically, end users of health services have not known the prices of the services before receiving them, and the primary decision maker with regard to purchasing decisions, the physician, has seldom taken pricing into consideration. Further, the amount of reimbursement for services from third-party payers often has been established independently of the price set by the provider.

For these reasons, healthcare has had few opportunities to compete on the basis of price. On the other hand, more retail-oriented healthcare businesses, such as personal health product manufacturers, are likely to use pricing strategies in much the same manner as producers of other consumer goods.

Insurance providers are another sector of the industry in which price may be a factor. Although insurance premiums historically have been established according to the perceived risk to the insurer, the emergence of managed care plans prompted unprecedented competition. As managed care plans became more standardized during the 1990s, they were forced to compete in terms of price. Because their products were essentially the same, price became a rational basis for competition.

A major drawback to the use of pricing strategies in healthcare is that, historically, healthcare providers have not been able to determine the cost of providing a service. The development of an intelligent pricing strategy requires some objective basis. Further, restrictions related to price fixing have prevented healthcare providers from using the fee schedules of other organizations as models.

Despite these barriers to the use of pricing strategies, a growing number of providers are competing on the basis of price, particularly those providing elective procedures. Price can be used as a basis for competition for services that are discretionary and typically paid for out of pocket. Most cosmetic surgery would be included in this category, and as competition has increased among ophthalmic surgeons, ophthalmologists performing laser eye surgery have also begun to compete on the basis of price.

Place Strategies

Place focuses on the manner in which a good or service is distributed. In healthcare, *place* typically refers to the location where services are rendered. An important aspect of place is the channel of distribution, or the path a good or service takes as it travels from the producer to the consumer. Although this concept has traditionally applied to consumer goods, it is also applicable to health services.

A variety of distribution channels are used to deliver health services. Primary care centers are typically located near potential patients (e.g., in neighborhoods or heavily populated residential areas), whereas tertiary ser-vices are concentrated in medical centers, regardless of the proximity to popu-lation centers. (One of the major considerations at the end of the twentieth century was the movement of populations away from inner-city medical cen-ters.) Emergency services are delivered through a combination of distribution methods; ambulances travel to the patient but then take the patient to the hospital for treatment.

During the production era in healthcare, little emphasis was placed on the location of service outlets. Most care was provided by hospitals, and patients were expected to travel to where the hospital was located. Physicians (particularly specialists) had the same attitude. Although primary care provid-ers may have sought locations in the community that were close to patient populations, the overriding attitude was "if you build it, they will come."

The actions of some hospitals in the 1990s are an example of chan-nel management efforts. In the early 1990s, hospitals attempted to control the distribution of their primary care providers by purchasing and "control-ling" physician practices. However, hospital administrators failed to consider that the "product"—physician practice patterns—could not be so easily con-trolled. As a result, such attempts largely failed. Although hospitals controlled the distribution of the practices, they were unable to control the products and/or prices these practices offered, thereby failing to benefit from their control of the distribution outlets.

As the focus of healthcare shifted from the inpatient setting to the outpatient setting, healthcare providers were forced to pay attention to the location of services. Hospitals were largely immobile, but outpatient services could be established almost anywhere. Those who sought to compete with hospitals took advantage of their relative immobility and established facilities in proximity to target markets.

Furthermore, a new generation of healthcare consumers emerged with different expectations of healthcare providers. Led by the baby boom cohort, these patients brought a consumer orientation that demanded convenience of location and easy access to services. They placed a high value on their time and expected the same of service providers. The healthcare industry responded to this emerging consumerism by offering urgent care centers and freestanding diagnostic and surgery centers as convenient alternatives to tra-ditional sources of care.

The new emphasis on place has also been encouraged by the employers and business coalitions that are paying a large share of the healthcare bill. Em-ployers want their employees to have convenient access to services, not only to ensure patient satisfaction but to limit the time they are away from work using these services. In addition, one of the bases for competition among managed care plans is the convenience they provide their enrollees. To succeed, health maintenance organizations and other health plans found they had to establish networks of providers that were distributed in a manner that would meet the needs of their enrollee populations.

The combined influence of these developments has encouraged providers to take healthcare to the community. Expecting patients to come to the source of care is no longer a viable approach. The contemporary consumer demands convenient locations, and in cases where locations cannot be changed, healthcare providers are working to improve the value of an existing location through more efficient patient-processing methods or redesign to create more appealing facilities.

Promotional Strategies

The most visible type of strategy healthcare organizations use is promotion of the organization or its services. As healthcare marketing was coming into its own in the 1980s and 1990s, it focused on advertising, direct mail, and other traditional promotional strategies. The limitations of competition based on product, price, and place have encouraged healthcare providers to differentiate themselves through promotional strategies.

Promotional strategies should reflect the organization's overriding strategic orientation. If, for example, a hospital adopts a niche strategy, its promotional efforts should be focused on a narrow range of services and/or a targeted population. On the other hand, a hospital pursuing a full-service strategy should develop an approach that promotes the organization as the source of almost any service.

Similarly, a promotional strategy should reflect the organization's chosen approach to the market. If the organization has adopted an aggressive, hard-sell approach to the market, the promotional strategy should reflect it. Conversely, if the organization has adopted a soft-sell approach, it would be reflected in initiatives to educate the market.

A promotions-oriented strategy can take a variety of forms. A *resonance strategy* strikes a chord with the consumer. The intention is to portray a lifestyle orientation that is synonymous with the target group and easily recognizable. For example, this approach might be used to promote a hospital-based fitness center. An *emotional strategy* plays on (and to) consumers' feelings, as in the case of children's health services.

In the contemporary healthcare arena, promotional strategies involve far more than advertising. Increasingly, healthcare providers have turned to personal selling and sales promotions to compete more effectively. To develop an effective promotional strategy, marketers must understand the various media available to them and be able to craft a message with appropriate content and tone. (Promotional strategies will be addressed frequently throughout the remainder of the book.)

The marketing mix concept discussed earlier has been adopted from other industries and applied to healthcare. Critics suggest, however, that the four Ps of marketing have never fit comfortably in healthcare. As healthcare providers become more service oriented, they too are criticizing this concept. Some have suggested the need to revise the four Ps and replace them with some other set of attributes that are more appropriate for contemporary healthcare. These conflicting views on the importance of the four Ps are a source of ongoing debate among health professionals.

Branding as a Strategy

Branding as a strategy is a relatively recent phenomenon in healthcare. A *brand* is a name, term, symbol, or design (or combination thereof) that signifies the goods or services of one seller or group of sellers. *Brand identity* refers to the visual features that create awareness in the mind of the consumer. These features include the brand's name, image, typography, color, package design, and slogans. The intent of the brand image is to distinguish a company's product from competing products in the eye of the user (Mangini 2002). The brand image indicates what business the company is in, what benefit it provides, and why it is better than the competition. Thus, brand identity is the visual, emotional, rational, and cultural image that a consumer associates with a company or a product.

Branding is often confused with corporate identity or corporate image, but these three terms have different meanings. *Corporate identity* refers to a company's name, logo, or tagline. *Corporate image* is the public's perception of a company, whether that perception is intended or not. *Corporate branding* is a business process that is planned, strategically focused, and integrated throughout the organization. It establishes direction, leadership, clarity of purpose, and energy for a company's corporate brand. *Brand associations* are attributes of a product or company that come to consumers' minds when they hear or see a brand name. An effective brand name evokes positive associations with the company. Therefore, the logic behind branding is simple: If consumers are familiar with a company's brand, they are more likely to purchase the company's products.

A company's brand also has significant internal value. A strong corporate brand generates and sustains internal momentum. Employees have proven to be more committed to the brand's promise if it is understood and supported by every key player (Lake 2009). To maximize the effectiveness of its brand, a company must ensure that it is understood by all relevant audiences: consumers, prospects, business partners, the media, and employees. Corporate communication should reinforce the branding effort.

Branding was uncommon among healthcare providers in the past, although there were some notable exceptions. Branding is most effective for products that command a mass market, can benefit from advertising, and can be effectively evaluated by consumers. Few healthcare services have these characteristics. Because most healthcare is provided locally, few healthcare organizations need to develop national brand recognition. Furthermore, many organizations have been around for a long time, and efforts to rebrand them are often met with resistance. The national hospital chain HCA, for example, went through a period of renaming all of its hospitals with the HCA brand, only to have to revert to the hospitals' old names in some cases because of local resistance. The Mayo Clinic and Cleveland Clinic are examples of healthcare organizations that successfully established national brands, but few organizations are in their league.

The lag in adopting branding strategies in healthcare has had both negative and positive consequences for healthcare marketing. The negative consequences include a lack of expertise and success in today's healthcare branding efforts. The positive consequence is that there are lessons the healthcare industry can learn from other industries. The emergence of the new healthcare consumer has prompted increased interest in branding among healthcare providers. This revitalized consumerism is being driven by well-informed consumers who are demanding choices.

For established retailers of healthcare products (e.g., pharmaceutical and personal health product companies), branding has been an inherent part of their strategy. In these cases, consumers are more likely to be familiar with the brand (e.g., Claritin, Band-Aids) than they are with the corporation that created it. The development of branding strategies in this segment of the industry reflects the relative ease of branding consumer products.

According to Mangini (2002), several steps must be followed to establish a brand identity. First, an institution must decide what to brand. It must carefully consider the services it offers, the people who provide the service, the competition's services, and the population it serves. Branding can focus on the entire health system, outpatient services, a prominent department, or a particular medical group. In addition, an institution may choose to focus on products and services that are in high demand but difficult to emulate. No matter what the focus, effective brands are almost always linked to a target audience, such as women or senior citizens.

Second, a healthcare institution must define the brand message and decide what information it wants to communicate about the service it has decided to brand. For example, an institution may choose to focus on quality of care, convenience, or technology capabilities. Each of these approaches can be effective if the brand message relates to the target audience and the service being branded.

Third, the brand must be communicated both internally and externally. Internal communication is important to ensure the staff acceptance and enthusiasm necessary for brand success. Staff members can be brought on board by giving them ownership of the branding initiative and rewarding them for their involvement in the campaign. External communication can take place through such channels as business documentation and advertising. Most important, however, is that the overall message is clear, consistent, and continuous.

The true test of an institution's brand is performance. An institution must be confident that it will be able to fulfill the promise that its brand conveys. Every consumer interaction must reinforce the brand identity and be used to establish a relationship with that consumer. If consumers have a positive interaction with the organization and are satisfied, they are potential sources of new business. Thus, information is key in determining the performance of an institution's brand. The healthcare institution must develop a system-wide data collection, analysis, and reporting network so that it can continuously assess the success of its brand and make necessary changes.

Once an institution builds a brand, it must continuously update and revitalize it. Brand revitalization does not simply mean creation of a new logo or product repackaging but must focus on the company's point of differentiation. A successful branding process provides a framework that links the branding strategy to the business strategy. This linkage is essential because key components of a successful branding strategy are the commitment and involvement of executive management. Finally, once all key players understand the institution's brand identity and framework, documentation of the branding system can begin.

Past documentation efforts have imparted several lessons about the healthcare branding process. First, a branding strategy must build consensus and ensure concurrence between the branding identities and business strategy of an institution. Second, an institution's marketing department must be cautious about making changes to long-standing brand franchises. A strong brand, once tarnished, is difficult to reinstate. Next, an institution must remain flexible. A branding system should follow a set of guidelines, but there should also be room for carefully chosen exceptions to the rules. Fourth, an institution must consider its competitors. A successful brand strategy considers competitors' current and future brands. Fifth, to prevent inconsistency, an institution must secure commitment from every level, and all key players must reach consensus. Last, alignment of an institution's values with the values of its branding strategy is imperative to success. (See Case Study 9.2 for an example of a successful branding initiative.)

CASE STUDY 9.2
Establishing a Brand

One example of a successful branding initiative is the one developed by the Cleveland Clinic Foundation in Cleveland, Ohio. The outcome of its efforts demonstrates the potential of branding for healthcare organizations and illustrates how a small outpatient practice can be transformed into a national brand.

The Cleveland Clinic Foundation was founded in 1921 by four veterans of World War I medical units and is now a leading American healthcare organization. From its start, the clinic was highly regarded for the quality of its specialty care, basic science achievements, and medical research. The clinic's initial marketing approach, typical of healthcare organizations in the premarketing era, targeted the physician audience in an effort to increase patient referrals. Promotional activities consisted of developing and distributing fundraising brochures and disseminating press releases to the media.

In the 1990s, the clinic realized that healthcare consumers were looking for a trusted brand name and thus expanded its market research. Their research indicated that local consumers highly respected the name "Cleveland Clinic," so the clinic focused on maintaining and protecting its brand through an integrated marketing effort.

The 1990s also marked a period of hospital mergers and acquisitions in the healthcare industry, and the clinic played a significant role in this development. Over a two-year period, the Cleveland Clinic Health System was formed, building on the clinic's merger with ten local community hospitals. The formation of this system presented a challenge in that the clinic had to decide how much it could share its brand identity without diluting it.

To address this challenge, the clinic established a four-tiered marketing approach that applied to all organizations using the Cleveland Clinic brand. This approach is still used today. Tier 1 members represent the core organizations—the essence of Cleveland Clinic. These core organizations are the conservators of the brand and direct all marketing efforts. Tier 2 members include entities owned by Cleveland Clinic. These entities have their own brand equity, and in their advertisements, they are allowed to use only the words "Cleveland Clinic Health System" under their own hospital name in half size. Tier 3 includes Cleveland Clinic departments in hospitals the clinic does not own. Tier 3 entities are not part of the Cleveland Clinic Foundation or the Cleveland Clinic Health System, and the appropriate relationships are outlined in their advertising. Use of the Cleveland Clinic name, logo, or tagline by this tier is prohibited. Finally, Tier 4 includes organizations to which Cleveland Clinic belongs. In these relationships, the Cleveland Clinic logo may be used only in visual arrangements with the logos of other participating hospitals.

As this case study shows, Cleveland Clinic has been successful in supporting the integrity of the Cleveland Clinic brand while extending the brand's positive image to other entities without diluting existing brand equity. Although not all healthcare organizations can be expected to have the same success as Cleveland Clinic, this case illustrates how, with sound market intelligence and thoughtful planning, a successful branding initiative can be undertaken.

Discussion Questions

- What changes in the marketplace led Cleveland Clinic to reassess its marketing strategy?
- What challenges did Cleveland Clinic face in creating a viable brand?
- How did Cleveland Clinic adapt its marketing strategy to address the challenges of the new organizational structure?
- How was Cleveland Clinic able to preserve its commitment to its mission while at the same time address the challenges of marketing a complex organization?

Summary

A well-thought-out marketing strategy is essential for any healthcare organization that hopes to compete in today's environment. Strategies set the tone for marketing activities and establish the parameters within which the marketer must operate. The strategy chosen will influence the nature of the marketing plan that is ultimately developed and guide subsequent marketing initiatives. De facto strategies emerge in the absence of a formal corporate strategy. Strategies may be developed at different levels, from an overall corporate strategy to a specific marketing strategy.

The marketing strategy should be developed during the strategic planning process, thereby reflecting the overall corporate strategy. Strategy development follows a series of steps, from initial data collection through data analysis through the identification of strategic options. All key stakeholders should participate in the strategy development process.

Strategies are usually keyed to one of the four Ps of the marketing mix—product, price, place, or promotion. In healthcare, customer relationship development and management have become increasingly important. A SWOT analysis may be used to inform strategy development.

A number of different strategy options are available to healthcare organizations; the type of organization and environmental circumstances will determine the best option to use. The chosen strategy should reflect the organization's positioning in the market. Most strategies consider the product–market relationship; options range from matching a specific product to a narrowly defined market to dispersing a range of products to a broad market. Branding as a strategy has become increasingly important in healthcare, although many healthcare organizations still face challenges in applying this approach.

Key Points

- Every healthcare organization should choose a strategy to guide its marketing activities.
- The marketing strategy should support the overall corporate strategy and guide the development of the organization's marketing plan.
- The chosen strategy will perform a number of different functions, most important of which is to focus the entire organization on a common goal.
- If the healthcare organization does not proactively develop a strategy, a default strategy is likely to emerge that may not be in the best interest of the organization.
- Strategies can exist at various levels of the organization, from an enterprise-wide strategy to specific strategies for individual departments or products.
- As with any strategy, the development of a marketing strategy should follow fairly rigid steps.
- Both internal and external data must be collected to develop an informed marketing strategy.
- Marketing strategies may reflect the organization's desired position in the marketplace, emphasize one or more of the four Ps of the product mix, and/or focus on the relationship between the organization's products and the market.
- Branding as a strategic approach has become more common among healthcare organizations, although certain attributes of the healthcare industry militate against a branding strategy.

Discussion Questions

- What are some of the different functions that a strategy performs for an organization?
- What is meant by the statement "absence of a strategy is a strategic statement on the organization's part"?
- What are the steps involved in the strategic planning process?
- How should an organization's marketing strategy link to its strategic plan?
- What types of strategies might an organization use, and what determines the best type of strategy to use for a particular situation?
- What are some ways in which the product and market interface during strategy development?
- What is the relationship between strategy development and the four Ps of the marketing mix?
- What determines which of the four Ps is most relevant to strategy in a particular case?
- Why is a branding strategy not universally employed by healthcare organizations?
- Under what circumstances does a branding strategy appear to work best?

Additional Resources

Bashe, G. 2000. *Branding Health Services: Defining Yourself in the Marketplace.* Sudbury, MA: Jones and Bartlett.

Zuckerman, A. M. 2005. *Healthcare Strategic Planning,* 2nd edition. Chicago: Health Administration Press.

TRADITIONAL MARKETING TECHNIQUES: PROMOTIONAL MIX AND MEDIA

This chapter provides an overview of the application of traditional promotional techniques to healthcare. Established approaches to marketing are discussed, and direct marketing techniques are reviewed. The pros and cons to the use of these techniques are also presented. Finally, the communication model that underlies all promotions is described.

The Promotional Mix

The promotional component of the marketing mix could be considered the action component through which the marketing plan is implemented. *Promotions* refer to the techniques used to communicate with customers and potential customers for purposes of promoting an idea, an organization, or a product. Traditional promotional activities include public relations, advertising, sales promotion, and personal selling. For purposes of this discussion, direct marketing is also included. Each of these techniques is carried out through different means. The term *promotional mix* refers to the combination of techniques constituting a given promotional strategy. The following sections discuss these techniques and their respective applications to healthcare.

Public Relations

Public relations (PR) is a form of communication management that uses publicity and other forms of promotion to influence consumers' feelings, opinions, or beliefs about an organization and its offerings. PR typically involves "unpaid" promotional activities, meaning the organization's PR staff carries out these activities as part of their job without incurring additional out-of-pocket expenses. PR activities include distributing press releases, scheduling press conferences, preparing feature stories and public service announcements, and other promotional activities. See Exhibit 10.1 for a sample press release.

EXHIBIT 10.1
Sample Press Release

arGentis Files Patent on Nucleic Acid Sequences and Polymorphisms Predictive of Patient Responses to ARG201, an Immunotherapy for Late Phase Systemic Sclerosis

FOR RELEASE Tuesday July 1, 2008

Memphis, TN—arGentis Pharmaceuticals, LLC announced today that it has filed a patent application for Nucleic Acid Sequences highly associated with the inability of oral immune tolerance to be induced in some systemic sclerosis (SSc) patients. As explained in the patent application, the identified sequences predict which patients can respond to ARG201, an immunotherapy that induces oral immune tolerance in patients with Late Phase diffuse cutaneous systemic sclerosis.

Results from patient DNA samples from a 168-patient, double-blind Phase II trial indicate that 30% of systemic sclerosis patients have a specific nucleotide polymorphism (SNP). This same group of patients did not appear to respond to oral collagen therapy. Approximately 70% of patients did respond to ARG201 therapy. That group did not appear to carry the SNP. The results also demonstrate that there is a statistically significant difference in the changes in cytokine production by T lymphocytes necessary to induce immune tolerance between patients with and without the SNP.

Recently published Phase II results of ARG201 have demonstrated statistically and clinically significant reductions in modified-Rodnan Skin Scores (MRSS) in Late Phase SSc patients, a prospectively defined subpopulation in the trial.

"The SNP enables us to clearly define systemic sclerosis patients who can most benefit from the ARG201 therapy," said Tom Davis, CEO of arGentis. "Screening of Late Phase SSc patients for the SNP prior to Phase III clinical trial enrollment also greatly increases the likelihood of success of those trials." arGentis anticipates beginning Phase III trials in the first half of 2009.

Application of the SNP to identify patients susceptible to successful oral immune therapy in other autoimmune diseases is also being verified in a test group of rheumatoid arthritis patients. Preliminary results are very positive. arGentis researchers believe that the SNP maker may be applicable to achieving oral immune tolerance in many, if not all, autoimmune diseases, providing a platform for developing oral tolerance therapeutics for large subpopulations of those diseases.

About Systemic Sclerosis

Systemic sclerosis (SSc or systemic scleroderma), a type of Scleroderma, is an autoimmune disease causing widespread fibrosis of the skin, lungs and other organs. As SSc progresses, patients suffer increasing difficulties with digestion, breathing, joint pain and often develop pulmonary hypertension. Due to differences in immunologic function of the patient groups, SSc can be categorized as Early Phase, patients diagnosed for less than three years, and Late Phase, those diagnosed for more than three years. Median survival from diagnosis is eleven years (Mayes 2004). There are approximately 80,000 SSc patients in the U.S. with similar numbers in the European Union. No therapies are presently available to treat the underlying cause of the disease.

About ARG201

ARG201 is an immunotherapy designed to induce low-dose oral tolerance in Late Phase systemic sclerosis patients. A multicenter, 168-patient double-blind, placebo-controlled Phase II clinical trial has been completed. ARG201 has been granted orphan status by the U.S. Food and Drug Administration. Phase III trials are expected to begin in the first half of 2009.

About arGentis

arGentis Pharmaceuticals, LLC is a diversified specialty biopharmaceutical company seeking to license and commercialize therapies with demonstrated proof of concept for chronic diseases. Our pipeline consists of mid- and late-stage platform technologies in both autoimmunity and ophthalmology. ARG201, the company's lead compound for the treatment of systemic sclerosis, will enter Phase III trials in 2009. The ophthalmology pipeline includes three therapies for dry eye syndrome which are uniquely applied to the outer upper and lower eyelids for transdermal delivery to the affected glands.

Contact

Ted Townsend, Vice President and CAO, arGentis Pharmaceuticals, LLC, 901-448-2024

Reference

Mayes, M. 2004. "The Role of Genetics in Scleroderma: Is It in Your Genes or in Your Environment?" Originally published in *Scleroderma Voice* #2. www.scleroderma.org/medical/r&t_articles/Mayes_2004_2.shtm.

Source: arGentis Pharmaceutical, LLC. Reprinted with permission.

Publicity refers to any type of promotion that draws general attention to an organization without targeting a specific audience. Use of this traditional form of promotion predates the more recent emphasis on the use of advertising and other promotional techniques. Essential to the publicity efforts of any organization are the materials developed for the organization, program, or product. These collateral materials include brochures, letterhead, business cards, and websites. A potential customer's first exposure to an organization may be through such materials.

Collateral materials serve as a foundation for subsequent marketing efforts. Judicious use of collateral materials is an inexpensive means of generating and maintaining visibility and public awareness of the organization's activities. These materials also convey basic contact information about an organization, such as an e-mail address, a main phone number, and location.

Public service announcements (PSAs) are another vehicle through which publicity may be generated. A PSA is an advertisement or a commercial featured at no cost in an advertising medium as a public service to its readers, viewers, or listeners. PSAs may be aired on radio or television, printed in a newspaper or magazine, or featured on a billboard. Although the no-cost aspect is appealing, the downside is that the advertising organization has no control over the placement or timing of a PSA.

Publicity may also be generated through the mechanisms healthcare organizations establish to communicate with their publics (both internal and external). Communications staff develops materials to disseminate to the public and to the organization's employees, including internal newsletters, publications geared to customer groups (e.g., patients, enrollees), and patient education materials. Separate communication departments may be established for this purpose, or this function may overlap the PR or community outreach function.

Another form of publicity involves sponsorships on the part of the organization.

Corporate financial backing for a project or an event is expected to generate public awareness and goodwill. The sponsor typically does not run an advertisement but may be mentioned in a "brought to you by" message. An organization may sponsor a beneficiary for altruistic reasons or for purposes of gaining favorable attention and publicity. As sponsors, organizations often receive substantial media coverage. Sponsorships may also foster improved employee morale.

Some organizations use a campaign spokesperson to generate publicity. Depending on the type of organization, this spokesperson could be a national or local celebrity, such as an athlete, an entertainer, a community leader, or another person thought to influence the public. A well-known animated character, or a character created for the promotion, could also be a spokesperson.

By associating the organization with a recognizable person or character, the organization hopes to be perceived in a positive way.

Community outreach programs are yet another form of publicity. Community outreach is a form of marketing that presents the organization's programs to the community and seeks to establish relationships with other community organizations. Community outreach may involve episodic activities, such as health fairs or educational programs for community residents, or take the form of ongoing initiatives involving outreach workers who are visible in the community on a recurring basis (e.g., the "parish nurses" employed by some churches). This aspect of marketing emphasizes the organization's commitment to the community and its support for community organizations. Although the benefits of community outreach activities are not as easily measured as more direct marketing activities, the organization often gains customers as a result of its health screening activities, follow-up from educational seminars, or referrals by outreach workers.

As noted in Chapter 3, healthcare organizations are typically regulated by state and federal government agencies. Decisions related to reimbursement rates and adding, eliminating, or changing a service may be controlled by government agencies. Healthcare organizations often must cultivate and maintain relationships with politicians and other policymakers and various government agencies, as well as initiate lobbying activities. The PR department is typically assigned responsibility for these functions.

Advertising

Advertising refers to any paid form of nonpersonal presentation and promotion of ideas, goods, or services by an identifiable sponsor, typically using mass media as the communication vehicle. The objectives of advertising are to

- promote products, services, organizations, and causes;
- increase product usage;
- remind consumers of the organization or product;
- build customer loyalty;
- introduce new products;
- offset competitors' advertising;
- help sales personnel;
- alleviate sales fluctuations;
- educate consumers; and
- maintain visibility.

Not all of these objectives are relevant for every healthcare organization, and they are likely to be pursued selectively according to the type of marketing being undertaken.

Advertising is typically classified as institutional (or corporate) advertising or product advertising, depending on what is being promoted. *Institutional advertising* promotes an organization's image, people, ideas, political issues, or anything else not related to a specific product or service. Institutional advertising can take several forms. It may introduce or announce a new facility, present comparative information, or explain a public policy stance. *Product advertising* promotes specific goods or services.

Personal Selling

Another tool in the promotional mix is *personal selling*, or the oral presentation of information through a conversation with one or more prospective purchasers for the purpose of generating sales. The primary difference between personal selling and advertising is that the former involves two-way rather than one-way communication.

The primary objectives of personal selling are to (1) find prospects, (2) convince prospects to buy a product, and (3) keep existing customers engaged. These objectives involve providing after-sales service, forecasting future sales, and maintaining relationships with customers. Thus, the role of the salesperson involves more than selling; it includes communicating with customers in a wider sense and serving as the organization's eyes and ears in the marketplace.

One advantage of personal selling is that the salesperson can get direct feedback from prospects and existing customers. He or she can then refine or explain the message in greater detail to correct any misunderstandings or difficulties the customer had in interpreting it. Personal selling also has an advantage over advertising in that a company has more direct control over who receives the message. Hospitals that incorporate personal selling into their promotional mix report several benefits, including increased facility occupancy, improved medical staff relations, higher profitability, and increased market share (Powers and Bowers 1992).

Well-established personal-selling activities in healthcare include solicitation of physicians by pharmaceutical and medical supplier representatives, solicitation of consumers by insurance salespeople, and solicitation of hospitals by biomedical equipment representatives. More recently, healthcare providers have become active in personal sales, and hospital representatives may solicit referring physicians, employers, and other organizations to promote the hospital's emergency department, a sports medicine program, or a particular service line. These activities have become increasingly important as interaction between individual physicians and patients has been displaced by interactions between groups of providers and groups of purchasers.

As with any promotional tool, however, personal selling has its limitations. A major limitation is its cost. In addition to salary and benefits, sales staff costs include expenses for travel, promotional materials, and technical support. The number of sales visits a person can make in one day is limited, and sales visits to physicians' offices or corporate prospects can be time-consuming. Another limitation to personal selling is the variability in strength of the interpersonal communication. The message's "punch" may vary on the basis of the salesperson's training, disposition, or style.

The more technologically sophisticated the service, the greater the need for personal selling. For example, a salesperson might be needed to explain the intricacies of a diagnostic technique or program, or a health system might use a sales representative to introduce new diagnostic technology to potential referring physicians. Personal sales are also important when a variety of decision makers (especially with differing perspectives) are involved or when there is an element of risk in the decision (e.g., committing to a managed care contract).

The personal selling mix can involve a combination of sales presentations, sales meetings, incentive programs, sample distribution, and participation in fairs and trade shows. Regardless of the personal selling mix, the selling process involves specific steps (see Exhibit 10.2).

EXHIBIT 10.2
Steps in the Selling Process

Salespeople follow certain steps when promoting an organization or a product. These steps are presented in the following sections, with examples of the activities involved.

Prospecting and Qualifying
The first step in the selling process involves identifying qualified potential customers. In healthcare, for example, salespeople may identify potential referring physicians, organ donors, or purchasers of biomedical equipment.

Pre-approach
Once prospects have been identified, the salesperson learns as much as possible about them before making sales calls. If the salesperson is selling supplies to a hospital, he or she should find out the hospital's level of supply use and current suppliers. A pharmaceutical representative, on the other hand, must become familiar with a physician's prescribing practices and the drugs he or she typically prescribes.

(continued)

EXHIBIT 10.2 (*continued*)

Approach

In this step, the salesperson meets the buyer to establish a relationship. Healthcare sales are typically not characterized by the wining and dining that often accompanies promotional activities in other industries. Because of the variation in sales situations in healthcare, the industry has had difficulty establishing a standard approach to sales.

Presentation and Demonstration

In this step, the salesperson describes the product to the buyer, indicating its attributes and benefits. Many healthcare providers are not used to receiving sales calls, and salespeople may have difficulty meeting with the right person in a large healthcare organization. Exhibits at professional meetings are one way to gain exposure if other channels are not accessible.

Handling Objections

In this step, the salesperson seeks out, clarifies, and overcomes customer objections to buying. Because of the nature of healthcare, the sales representative is likely to take a consultative rather than hard-sell approach. Instead of trying to out-negotiate the customer, the salesperson is likely to address the customer's objections in a mutually beneficial manner.

Closing

To close, the salesperson asks the customer to order the product or otherwise consummates the sale. Establishment of an agreement among the various parties initiates the fulfillment process. Closing a sale is often less straightforward in healthcare than it is in other industries, as many parties may have to participate in the purchase decision.

Follow-Up

After the sale, the salesperson follows up to ensure customer satisfaction and repeat business. In healthcare, relationship management is likely to be more important than it is in other industries, and ongoing contact with the customer may be necessary.

An aspect of personal sales that characterizes many not-for-profit healthcare organizations is fundraising. Many healthcare organizations rely on donations to support their operations and fund capital improvements. These organizations must market themselves to potential donors to secure contributions. Although much of this effort may involve direct marketing in the form of direct mail or telemarketing, major contributors typically must be contacted in person. Thus, many large not-for-profit healthcare organizations maintain a sales staff dedicated to the solicitation of large donors.

Sales Promotion

Sales promotion refers to any activity or material that acts as a direct inducement by offering added value or incentive to the product or service for resellers, salespersons, or consumers. Enticements are offered to achieve a specific sales or marketing objective. The sales promotion mix includes health fairs and trade shows, exhibits, demonstrations, contests and games, premiums and gifts, rebates, low-interest financing, and trade-in allowances.

Although sales promotion methods have less application in healthcare than in most other industries, both "pull" and "push" incentives are frequently used. The *pull incentives* used to promote consumer goods also apply to personal healthcare products. Pull incentives include discounts on the customer's next purchase, cash refunds, coupons, buy-one-get-one-free promotions, consumer contests, loyalty cards, free trials (i.e., samples), free products, price reductions, and merchandising and point-of-sale displays. Manufacturers and service providers use *push incentives* to influence intermediaries to carry or deliver a product. Pharmaceutical companies use both pull and push strategies in promoting drugs to their target audiences. By using a pull strategy, pharmaceutical companies appeal directly to the consumer, recognizing that the consumer will create the demand for the product and "pull" the product through the channel. In other words, the consumer requests that the physician write a prescription for the product, which ensures that at least one intermediary is distributing the product. When the consumer asks the pharmacy to fill the prescription, the consumer is again pulling the product through the supply chain because the pharmacy must order the pharmaceutical from the manufacturer to fill the prescription. At the same time, pharmaceutical companies offer samples and make sales calls to physicians (push strategy).

For many provider organizations, participation in health fairs is a form of sales promotion. Providers may offer diagnostic tests and distribute health education materials at these fairs. Through these fairs, organizations attain greater visibility and interact with patients who might not be familiar with the organization. Consumers participating in health fairs can be enrolled in the organization's patient education or wellness programs, and those who test positive in screening tests can be referred for additional diagnosis or treatment.

Exhibition at trade shows, professional meetings, and conferences is also a form of sales promotion. Exhibitions give organizations an opportunity to interact with hard-to-reach prospects, such as physicians and hospital administrators. Where sellers cannot bypass the gatekeepers at the doctor's office to make a pitch, the exhibition hall brings the doctor right to the seller's booth. The decision to exhibit and the type of display developed depend on the nature of the organization and the product as well as the characteristics of the target audience.

An effective exhibit provides a unique opportunity to conduct market research, as many of the best prospects are assembled in one location. Many healthcare organizations are not accustomed to exhibiting at trade shows and professional meetings, but this form of sales promotion will likely become more common in the future.

A number of caveats must be considered when participating in an exhibition. Exhibit 10.3 lists ten tips for effective exhibit marketing.

EXHIBIT 10.3
Ten Tips for Effective Exhibit Marketing

Organizations that provide healthcare products and services frequently find themselves exhibiting at conferences, professional meetings, and trade shows, but little guidance is available for would-be healthcare exhibitors. Providing such guidance is a challenge given the variety of organizations involved in healthcare marketing. Nevertheless, some concerns are relevant for any healthcare organization that plans to exhibit. Following are ten tips for effective exhibit marketing.

Have a Formal Exhibit Marketing Plan
Having both strategic exhibit marketing and tactical plans of action is a critical starting point. To make trade shows a powerful dimension of an organization's overall marketing operation, there must be alignment between the strategic marketing and exhibit marketing plans. Trade shows should not be stand-alone ventures. Organizations should know and understand exactly what they wish to achieve at the show (e.g., shore up relationships with existing users, introduce new products/ services to new markets).

Have a Well-Defined Promotional Plan
An important component of exhibiting is promotion, including pre-show, at-show, and post-show activities. Most exhibitors fail to develop a plan that encompasses all three areas. The organization's budget will naturally play a major role in deciding what and how much promotional activity is possible. Developing a meaningful theme or message that ties into the organization's strategic marketing plan will help guide promotional decisions. Exhibitors should know whom they want to

target and consider developing different promotional programs aimed at the different groups they want to attract. Target audiences can be reached through direct mail, broadcast faxes, advertising, PR, sponsorships, and the Internet.

Use Direct Mail Effectively

Direct mail is still one of the most popular promotional vehicles exhibitors use. From postcards to multi-piece mailings, attendees are deluged with invitations to visit booths. Many of the mailings are based on lists of registrants, and as a result, everyone receives everything. To target the people they want to attract to their booth, exhibitors should use their own list of customers and prospects. Starting about four weeks before the show, exhibitors should mail materials to conference attendees at regular intervals. Distribution via first-class mail is recommended so that the mailing doesn't arrive after the show is over.

Give Prospects an Incentive to Visit Your Booth

Regardless of the type of promotional vehicles used, exhibitors need to give visitors a reason to visit their booth. Limited by time constraints and distracted by a hall overflowing with fascinating products and services, people need an incentive to visit a particular booth. First and foremost, visitors are primarily interested in new offerings. They are eager to learn about the latest technologies, new applications, or anything that will help them save time or money. If an organization doesn't have a new product or service to introduce, it should put a new twist on one of its existing products or services.

Have Giveaways That Work

Tied into giving visitors an incentive to visit the booth is an opportunity to offer a premium item that will entice them. The giveaway item should be designed to make the exhibit more memorable and communicate, motivate, promote, or increase recognition of the company. Developing a dynamite giveaway takes thought and creativity. The company should consider items that (1) members of its target audience want, (2) will help them do their jobs better, and (3) are not regularly available elsewhere. It should think about offering different gifts to different types of visitors. The company can use its website to tell visitors they can obtain important information, such as an executive report, if they visit the booth. Giveaways should be used as a reward or token of appreciation for visitors who participate in a demonstration,

(continued)

EXHIBIT 10.3 (*continued*)

presentation, or contest, or as a thank-you for providing information about their specific needs.

Use Press Relations Effectively

Press relations is one of the most cost-effective and successful methods for generating large volumes of direct inquiries and sales. Before the show, exhibitors should ask show management for a comprehensive media list to find out which publications are planning a special show edition. The company should send out newsworthy press releases focusing on what's new about its product or service or highlighting a new application or market venture. Press kits including information about industry trends, statistics, new technology, or production should be compiled for the press office. High-quality product photos and key company contacts should also be included in the kits.

Differentiate Your Products or Services

Too many exhibitors are happy to use the "me too" marketing approach. There is an underlying sameness about their marketing plans. In shows that attract hundreds of exhibitors, few stand out from the crowd. Because memorable exhibits are an integral part of a visitor's show experience, exhibitors should think about what makes their company different and why a prospect should buy its products or use its services. Every aspect of the exhibit marketing plan, including promotions, the booth, and the people working in the booth, should make an impact and generate curiosity.

Use the Booth as an Effective Marketing Tool

An organization's exhibit makes a strong statement about who it is, what it does, and how it does it. The purpose of an exhibit is to attract visitors so that the organization can achieve its marketing objectives. In addition to being an open, welcoming, friendly space, the exhibit needs to have a focal point and strongly communicate that the organization is offering a significant benefit to prospects. Displays that use large graphics are more effective than those that use reams of copy. Pictures paint a thousand words, and few attendees will take the time to read lengthy text. Presentations and demonstrations are critical parts of exhibit marketing. Exhibits should create an experience that gets visitors to use as many of their senses as possible.

Choose Exhibit Personnel Carefully

Exhibit personnel are a company's ambassadors. They should be carefully selected. Before the show, they should be briefed on why the company is exhibiting, what it is exhibiting, and what the company expects from them. Exhibit staff training is essential for a unified and professional image. The objectives of exhibit personnel should reflect the marketing plan, and staff should know how to close the interaction with a commitment to follow up. At the same time, the booth should not be crowded with company representatives, and specific tasks should be assigned to company personnel working the show.

Follow Up Promptly

The key to trade show success is effective lead management. The best time to plan for follow-up is before the show. Follow-up with show leads often takes second place to other management activities that occur after being out of the office for several days. The longer leads are left unattended, the colder and more mediocre they become. Exhibitors would be wise to develop an organized, systematic approach to follow-up. They should establish a lead-handling system, set timelines for follow-up, use a computerized database for lead tracking, make sales representatives accountable for leads assigned to them, and track the results of these efforts.

Source: Friedman (2009).

Direct Marketing

Direct marketing involves an interactive system that uses one or more advertising media to effect a measurable response or transaction. Categories of direct marketing relevant to healthcare include direct mail, direct-response advertising, mail order, telemarketing, computerized marketing, and home shopping television.

Direct mail is a means of promotion whereby selected customers are sent advertising material addressed specifically to them. Direct mail traditionally has been distributed through the postal service, but more contemporary approaches use fax or e-mail transmission. Junk mail, spam, and unsolicited faxes are all products of direct-mail promotion.

Although many people find these types of solicitations annoying, they are considered effective marketing tools. Marketers like direct mail because it can target specific audiences and be personalized to their needs. Even if a campaign is able to achieve only as little as a 2 percent response rate, marketers find direct mail to be reasonably cost-effective. Research has found that certain segments of the population are relatively responsive to mailed solicitations, and documents related to healthcare are less likely to be summarily discarded than others (Thomas 2008). Healthcare marketers find that direct mail works best when promoting an event, such as a patient education program or an open house. This approach probably does not work as well to stimulate action with regard to an activity that does not have to be completed by a certain date (e.g., an elective procedure). Marketers of some elective procedures (e.g., laser eye surgery), however, have had reasonable success with direct mail. See Case Study 10.1 for an example of direct-to-consumer marketing.

CASE STUDY 10.1
Using Direct-to-Consumer Advertising to Increase Drug Sales

After the U.S. Food and Drug Administration (FDA) relaxed its rules on mass media advertising of prescription drugs in 1997, the door was opened to direct-to-consumer marketing on the part of pharmaceutical companies. Rather than relying strictly on the prescription activities of physicians, pharmaceutical companies believed direct appeals to consumers would increase pharmaceutical sales in general and convince consumers to request particular drugs.

To take advantage of this opportunity, GoodDrugs, Inc., shifted a portion of its advertising budget to direct-to-consumer marketing. This advertising was intended to supplement existing approaches—visits by sales representatives to physicians' offices, advertising in medical journals, and the presentation of educational seminars to physicians.

GoodDrugs planned and implemented a six-month television campaign to promote its best-selling (and most profitable) drug for indigestion. Because it was available only by prescription, the intent of the advertising was to raise awareness of the drug among consumers with the hope that, once in the doctor's office, the consumer would request it.

At the end of the six-month advertising campaign, GoodDrugs conducted a telephone survey of consumers in the media coverage area. The results were encouraging. Consumers had become aware of the GoodDrugs indigestion drug: Half of the respondents remembered an advertisement for a prescription indigestion drug, and a fourth of them recalled the drug's name. About 25 percent of those who had seen the GoodDrugs advertisement said they had asked a doctor about using this drug for indigestion, and physicians wrote prescriptions for 71 percent of those who asked for one. Therefore, approximately 6 percent of the consumers who were exposed to the advertisement ended up with a prescription for the drug.

GoodDrugs marketers and sales executives were encouraged by the results of the television campaign. It had resulted in greater consumer awareness of their product, an increase in consumer preference for the drug, and an increase in desired prescribing behavior on the part of physicians. As a result, GoodDrugs reworked its marketing budget, shifting resources away from personal sales and journal advertising and toward direct-to-consumer advertising.

Discussion Questions
- What limitations were historically placed on pharmaceutical advertising, and what development opened the door to more aggressive action on the part of drug companies?
- What factors prompted pharmaceutical companies to shift the focus of their marketing efforts?
- According to the marketing team's evaluations, what were the results of the campaign?
- What did the GoodDrugs marketers do as a result of this campaign?
- How appropriate is it for pharmaceutical companies to market directly to consumers who may not be in a position to judge the merits of a particular drug?

Direct-response advertising involves promotions via print or electronic media that provide a call-in number, typically a toll-free number, to potential customers. People who want to order a product or service or obtain more information are instructed to call this number. This approach has been used successfully in other industries and is now being used in healthcare. Physicians performing elective procedures, for example, may have an answering service to field such calls and provide information on laser eye surgery, hair transplants, weight-loss programs, or whatever service the practitioner is providing. Fitness equipment is also commonly promoted through television advertisements taking this approach.

Telemarketing is another form of direct marketing. Direct-response advertising is a form of telemarketing that involves inbound calls, but most people are more familiar with outbound telemarketing in which people operating from a bank of telephone sets, often equipped with computer-assisted interviewing software, call people from a prospect list to offer a good or service.

This technique, however, has generated enough backlash among consumers that legislation has been passed establishing a do-not-call list.

Some telemarketing involves cold calls to individuals or households for which the demand for goods and services is unknown. More likely, the telephone numbers that are drawn from a sampling frame or randomly generated are keyed to certain characteristics of the target audience.

A more benign form of telemarketing in healthcare involves periodic contact with people who have expressed interest in a program or topic. Healthcare organizations assume that these people will be willing to receive calls describing such programs because of their implied previous interest and will not consider them an imposition. Hospital call centers frequently use this approach to follow up with prospects about the hospital's services.

Telemarketing is more expensive than direct-mail initiatives, but the costs are not unreasonable. Telemarketers' wages are relatively low, and the benefits gained by attracting a new patient are likely to be significant. Not all healthcare products lend themselves to this approach, but a surprising number do.

Distribution of *mail order catalogs* has been used to reach consumers directly since early in the country's history. It has not, however, been a traditional means of promoting healthcare goods and services. In recent years, however, as the market for alternative therapies and do-it-yourself healthcare tests and treatments has grown, catalogs have become an increasingly important vehicle for promotion. In many parts of the country, if a consumer wants to purchase herbal supplements, natural remedies, or other nonconventional treatments, mail order may be the only way to obtain them. People are also turning to mail order catalogs in search of better prices for prescription drugs.

Although mail order catalogs are never going to become a mainstream promotional medium in healthcare, use of catalogs does have advantages. It puts product exposure directly in the hands of targeted consumers and can be relatively cost-effective with economies of scale.

Venues for electronic marketing include *computerized marketing* and *home shopping television channels.* The Internet is a virtual marketplace attracting a wide range of buyers and sellers. A variety of healthcare products are available via the Internet, and aggressive e-mail marketing techniques carry messages about these products to everyone online. Healthcare consumers frequently turn to the Internet as a first resort when locating and pricing consumer health products. Home shopping channels try to capitalize on the fitness and wellness movement by selling fitness equipment, workout supplies, and skin treatments. Exhibit 10.4 summarizes the role of various promotional techniques in healthcare marketing and advantages and disadvantages to their use.

EXHIBIT 10.4
Matrix for Promotional Decision Making

Promotional Technique	Uses	Audience	Time Frame	Relative Cost	Advantages	Disadvantages
Public relations	Awareness Visibility Service rollout	General public Stakeholders Decision makers Influentials	Short term within a longer-term strategic context	Primarily staff time with low out-of-pocket costs	Broad reach Low cost Short lead time	Not targeted Short shelf life
Communication	Awareness Visibility Education Relationship development/ maintenance	General public Stakeholders Existing customers Employees	Ongoing with periodic flurry of activity	Primarily staff time with moderate out-of-pocket costs	Direct to target Low cost	Narrow focus Staffing costs
Community outreach	Awareness Visibility Education Relationship development/ maintenance	General public Targeted consumer groups	Ongoing with periodic flurry of activity	Primarily staff time with moderate out-of-pocket costs	Ongoing presence Personalized Localized	High effort Long lead time
Networking	Awareness Business development Relationship development/ maintenance Intelligence gathering	Key stakeholders Potential partners Potential referrers	Ongoing	Little additional cost	Ongoing Targeted	Time commitment
Direct marketing	Exposure Product introduction Call to action	Targeted consumer groups	Short term but with some lead time	Moderate costs	Focused Customized Multiple exposures	Low response rate High unit cost Short shelf life
Personal sales	Visibility Close contacts Relationship development	Influentials Potential customers	Regular periodic contact	Moderate to high costs	Face to face Ongoing Feedback on market	Sales force maintenance Cost
Advertising	Awareness Visibility Image enhancement	General public Targeted customer groups	Typically long term with long lead time	High costs	Many options Design options Easily targeted	Cost Negative connotation Short shelf life

Source: Thomas and Calhoun (2007).

Media Options

Because advertisers and other promoters typically use the media as their means of communication, the media options available to them are an important consideration. *Media* refers to any nonpersonal form of promotion. For this discussion, the media are divided into the categories of print media, electronic media, display advertising, and a residual category of other promotional venues. To capitalize on media options, marketers should have a *media plan*. The media plan outlines the objectives of an advertising campaign, the target audience, and the vehicles that will be used to reach that audience.

In many ways, the times are good for marketers in terms of promotional options. There has never been a wider variety of outlets for promotional material. Marketers also have an abundance of magazines, journals, and newsletters in which they can advertise. The advent of electronic media in the 1950s added an entirely new dimension to the information dissemination process, introducing unprecedented marketing efficiency.

The explosion of cable in the 1980s and the introduction of satellite television in that same decade allowed marketers access to almost unlimited transmission outlets. Now the Internet links up billions of people worldwide, creating an enormous opportunity for interaction with consumers. Marketers also have access to vast databases of information they can use to profile markets and target consumers.

Print Media

Print media is the most traditional form of promotion. Magazines, newspapers, journals, newsletters, and directories are common types of print media. *Magazines* include periodic publications aimed at the general public and trade publications geared to the interests of health professionals. A number of consumer-oriented health magazines are widely circulated. There are many advantages to the use of magazines for promotion. This format allows color production and ample space for health-related content, and marketers can use national readership survey data to target subscribers. Magazines have high potential readerships, and readers expect magazines to include advertisements. Magazines also have long life spans and can be read at the subscriber's leisure. Last, magazine advertising can be cost-effective, depending on the audience served. On the other hand, there are disadvantages to the use of magazines for promotion. Advertisements may appear in a magazine's "desert areas," where they are seldom noticed by readers or lost in surrounding clutter. Monthly magazine distribution is also a disadvantage in cases where marketers want to promote more frequently.

Newspapers include weekly or daily news publications, and they can be national, regional, or local in their distribution. Advantages to newspaper advertising include extensive market coverage, flexibility in terms of timing, and the use of illustrations. On the other hand, newspaper advertising is a mass marketing approach that attempts to reach all audiences and does not differentiate among groups of readers. Also, the format makes it difficult to get people to notice the advertising content. In recent years, newspapers have suffered a declining readership, with loyal readers concentrated in certain demographic groups. Depending on the market, newspaper advertising can be relatively expensive, so marketers need to ensure that the objectives of the marketing plan lend themselves to this medium.

Most cities now have *"alternative" newspapers*, usually weeklies that have emerged to cover aspects of the news neglected by the mainstream press. In some communities, readership of alternative newspapers approximates that of the conventional press, making them appropriate vehicles for the advertisement of many healthcare products. They are particularly suited for promoting progressive or innovative healthcare services that are likely to appeal to a population interested in holistic medicine or alternative therapies.

Many communities have also spawned special-interest newspapers devoted to some aspect of health. Some areas produce regular newspapers that chronicle developments in the local healthcare arena. Other newspapers deal with such topics as fitness and wellness, sports, and alternative therapies. These newspapers are advertising venues for many healthcare goods and services.

Professional journals are possibly more ubiquitous in healthcare than in any other industry. Every medical specialty and all allied health fields generate one or more journals. Most associations serving health professionals publish regular journals. Some journals are academically oriented and typically do not carry advertisements. However, some mainstream medical journals, such as the *Journal of the American Medical Association* and the *New England Journal of Medicine*, do feature advertisements. Journals are vehicles for professional advertising because they are geared to health professionals, not the general public. Pharmaceutical companies are heavy advertisers in these publications, as are medical supply, equipment, and information technology vendors.

Newsletters are yet another common source of information in healthcare. Change occurs rapidly in this field, and the lead time required to produce more traditional publications does not accommodate the needs of an industry in transition. Newsletters, therefore, have become a valuable source of current information. Although advertising opportunities are rare in newsletters, these vehicles do provide a venue for publicizing new programs, services, or organizational changes.

Most communities support one or more *shoppers' magazines* that are typically distributed to local consumers at no cost. Such magazines may provide opportunities to promote healthcare consumer goods and services. Ad placement in these magazines is relatively inexpensive but may not be effective in that these publications are considered "throwaways."

Directories have become an increasingly important means of gaining visibility. Some directories, such as state physician directories or hospital directories, are compiled for bureaucratic recordkeeping purposes. Such directories are generally not intended for commercial use, and an organization's inclusion may or may not be mandatory. Some directories are compiled for administrative purposes but subsequently shared with a larger audience (e.g., a health plan's provider directory).

Another category of directories includes those commercially produced for distribution. One function of these directories is to make their listed organizations more visible, and organizations may have to pay a fee to be listed. These directories are typically sold to customers who need the information. There are directories of physicians, hospitals, information technology vendors, and so forth. A number of publishers compile and distribute directories as their primary business activity, and many such directories are posted on the Internet.

Electronic Media

Electronic media is another ubiquitous venue for advertising and includes television (and its derivatives), radio, the Internet, cinema, and infomercials. Television is the prototypical electronic medium, and there are several advantages to its use in advertising. A company can build a high level of awareness of its offerings, reach large audiences, and demonstrate its products (using sound and visuals). In addition, television can be viewed at home in a casual atmosphere. Promotion via television has its downsides, too. First, viewers may find commercial breaks irritating. Second, the medium is considered transient. Third, audiences cannot be specifically targeted with network television as they can be with certain other media. Finally, television advertising time is expensive.

Historically, television advertising was concentrated on the national networks (ABC, NBC, CBS, and FOX). However, with the advent of cable television and satellite broadcasting, the situation changed somewhat. The fragmentation of viewers has resulted in the development of homogenous groups that watch particular cable channels. This development has enabled marketers to target television audiences much more precisely. For example, cable television subscribers who watch the travel or food channels are likely to be upscale innovators, so marketers seeking to target this population might choose to advertise on these channels. Advertising time is much less expensive in these venues than on network television, often costing as little as 10 to 20 percent of the cost for similar network placement.

Radio is a long-standing advertising medium that affords marketers many advantages. Radio is often considered a companion, more so than television and other forms of electronic media. The most important attribute of radio advertising is the greater precision with which an audience can be targeted, with regard to not only the station but also time of day. Further, radio advertising time and production costs are relatively low, especially compared to the cost of television advertising. On the other hand, the use of radio is disadvantageous in that radio has no visual attribute and is a transient medium.

In addition, the proliferation of radio stations has caused radio audiences to fragment and thus decrease in size.

Although most healthcare organizations, particularly those involved in patient care, were slow to warm up to Internet advertising, promotional "spots" (i.e., banners and pop-up ads) related to healthcare are now common on the web. The adoption of Internet advertising was spearheaded by consumer health products companies, which were eventually joined by healthcare providers seeking to capitalize on the many advantages of Web-based advertising. In addition to using banners and pop-up ads, many healthcare organizations pay a fee to be listed in Internet-based directories of physicians, hospitals, or other providers. Although the effectiveness of healthcare marketing via the Internet has not been thoroughly documented, any early reticence has mostly disappeared and a Web advertising presence is increasingly being taken for granted.

The cinema is sometimes used as an electronic form of advertising. Products often appear in film sets or are used by actors as props. This mechanism is seldom used for healthcare advertising. However, as healthcare becomes more consumer driven, cinema advertising will likely find a place in healthcare.

Infomercials are a popular form of advertisement among healthcare organizations. *Infomercials* are usually 15- to 60-minute television or radio commercials presented in a casual talk-show format designed to look/sound like an ordinary program. In some cases, they take the form of a standard 30- to 60-second commercial. Infomercials are usually framed as an educational piece, and the sponsor is only subtly noted. The intent is to soft-sell the organization or service by implying that the sponsor is the authority on that topic, thus attracting customers without having to overtly solicit them.

Display Advertising

Display advertising is a media form that includes outdoor advertising, transportation advertising, and posters. Outdoor advertising primarily involves billboards, although other types of signage (e.g., banners, portable signs) are also used. While billboard advertising has its critics, it is popular with hospitals, health plans, voluntary associations, and other healthcare organizations. Transportation (or *transit*) advertising consists of graphics, signs, or plaques placed on buses, taxis, and other commercial vehicles (e.g., trucks). Posters are bills displayed in public places to attract attention to an organization, a service, or an event.

There are many advantages to the use of display advertising. Marketers can reach large numbers of people and build a high level of awareness of a product or an organization at a relatively low cost. Display advertising can be short or long term, support local or national marketing campaigns, and be strategically located. On the downside, display advertising is often subject to the effects

EXHIBIT 10.5
Matrix for Media Decision Making

Medium	Uses	Audience	Resource Requirements	Relative Cost	Advantages	Disadvantages

Television	Exposure
	Service
	  introduction
	Call to action
			Production
			  skills
			Creative skills
				High	Consumer
					  appeal
					Multiple
					  exposures
						Cost
						Negative
						  connotation
						Short shelf life
						Competing ads

Network		General public			Broad reach	Diffuse impact

Cable		Targeted
		  consumers
					Targeted
					  reach
						Narrow impact

Radio	Exposure
	Service
	  introduction
	Call to action
		General public
		Targeted
		  consumers
			Production
			  skills
			Creative skills
				Moderate	Broad or
					  narrow reach
						Cost
						Short shelf life

Newspapers	Exposure
	Service
	  introduction
	Call to action
		General public		Moderate	Broad reach
					Low unit cost
					Frequent
					  exposure
						Cost
						Competing ads
						Short shelf life

Magazines	Exposure
	Service
	  introduction
	Call to action
		General public
		  (but higher
		  end)
				Moderate	Moderate
					  shelf life
					Design
					  options
						Cost
						Competing ads

Internet		General public
		Targeted
		  consumers
				Low	Appealing
					  medium
					Interactive
					Ongoing
						Incomplete
						  coverage
						Spam
						  annoyance

of weather and the criticism of environmentalists. Exhibit 10.5 compares the various media options in terms of their relative advantages and disadvantages.

Social Marketing

Social marketing in healthcare can be defined as the application of commercial marketing techniques to the development and implementation of programs that influence the attitudes, knowledge, and behavior of target audiences for purposes of improving individual and community health status. Social marketing is used most often by not-for-profit organizations and government agencies seeking to change consumer behavior. It is considered "social" in the sense that the organizations involved typically do not engage in these efforts for their own benefit but for the benefit of the general public or some subgroup of the public.

Social marketing also differs from other types of marketing with respect to the marketer's objectives and approach. In contrast to the top-down approach of traditional marketing, social marketers listen to the needs and desires of the target audience and build the marketing campaign from the bottom up. This focus on the consumer requires in-depth research and constant reevaluation. To sell healthy behavior, social marketers research their target audience and then segment it into groups on the basis of common risk behaviors, motivations, and information channel preferences. The marketing mix is continually refined on the basis of consumer feedback. Instead of a sales pitch, the target audience might be exposed to an "intervention" aimed at changing attitudes or encouraging healthy behavior (e.g., an educational program or a health screening initiative).

Social marketing takes advantage of contemporary technology (e.g., the Internet) to target audiences, tailor messages, and engage people in interactive, ongoing exchanges about their health. As the use of population-based approaches to healthcare becomes more common, the role of health communications is expanding. Community-centered prevention shifts attention from the individual to the group and emphasizes the empowerment of individuals and communities to effect change on multiple levels.

The functions of social marketing in healthcare include the following:

- Increase knowledge and awareness of a health issue, problem, or solution
- Influence perceptions, beliefs, attitudes, and social norms
- Prompt a desired response
- Demonstrate or illustrate skills
- Show the benefits of behavior change
- Increase demand for health services
- Reinforce knowledge, attitudes, or behavior
- Refute myths and misconceptions
- Coalesce organizational relationships
- Advocate for a health issue or a population group

Integrated Marketing

Given the number of promotional techniques available and the fragmentation of marketing approaches, determining the most appropriate marketing approach to take in a particular situation is a challenge. One approach that may help tie some of the parts together is integrated marketing. *Integrated marketing* or *integrated marketing communication* emphasizes the development of consistency in an organization's promotional strategy. The ultimate aim is to achieve synergy between the component parts to generate a more effective approach to communication.

Marketers coordinate advertising campaigns across varied media, increasingly supplementing television advertisements with marketing messages communicated via alternative media vehicles. A print advertisement might capture a frame from a television commercial and include a tagline that summarizes the 15- or 30-second message, or a radio station may air an excerpt of the dialogue and the announcer's product claims from that same commercial.

Integrated marketing involves the strategic choice of elements of marketing communications that effectively and economically influence transactions between an organization and its existing and potential customers, clients, and consumers. Integrated marketing ensures that all elements are delivered synergistically.

Many factors have encouraged the use of integrated marketing strategies. Tighter marketing budgets have squeezed available resources, and the fragmentation of the media demands some unifying force. The shift from mass marketing to target marketing and the rise of electronic media (especially the Internet) have contributed to this development. Although integrated marketing strategies appear to be an obvious step toward more effective marketing, there are those who would resist their use in that these strategies counter traditional patterns of behavior and are cumbersome to implement in some organizations.

If resistance can be overcome, an organization can derive major advantages from the marketing integration process. Its strategies will reinforce

CASE STUDY 10.2
Case Study on Integrated Marketing

Many people who might benefit from hearing aids do not wear them. Of adults with impaired hearing who are aged 18 years or older, 78 percent do not own a hearing aid. As the population ages, the need for hearing assistance will become nearly universal—but even today among the hearing impaired who are aged 65 years or older, 61 percent do not wear hearing aids. Research has found that although people would readily acquiesce to wearing eyeglasses to correct their vision, would have no problem taking pain relievers to alleviate aches, and would not mind having to walk with a cane, the prospect of having to wear a hearing aid would be difficult for them to accept.

The hearing and speech communications literature suggests that use of a hearing aid carries a stigma that implies the wearer is old, feeble, and incompetent. An article in the American Psychological Association's *Monitor* described the denial and depression people associate with hearing loss. In addition, hearing loss, if not addressed with hearing aids, can lead to greater dependence on a spouse and withdrawal from social events. People do not want to admit their hearing loss to themselves because it connotes aging; nor do they want to admit it to others for fear of being viewed as incompetent.

Given all these considerations, when *Business Week* featured a hearing aid manufacturer in its Annual Design Awards, the product receiving acclaim was tiny and said to "nestle discreetly in the ear canal." Hearing aid sales surged after President Clinton publicly acknowledged that he had begun to wear one, likely because they were perceived as more acceptable when they were associated with the relatively young and purportedly virile rather than the old and feeble.

A product with such a negative image as hearing aids clearly presents a challenge to marketers interested in stimulating sales. Around 2002, research was conducted to determine how to induce more favorable attitudes toward these personal, stigmatized products. In particular, the research assessed the applicability and effectiveness of integrated marketing communications, given their relative novelty and popularity at the time. In addition, the research looked at whether a stigmatized product might best be approached through multimodality approaches, thereby reinforcing the advertising message.

A panel of respondents was established as a test market. The researchers contacted 4,344 participants at time 1, before being exposed to the aforementioned marketing communications. The attitudes of 3,351 participants were then measured at time 2, after being exposed to the persuasive materials. Finally, the attitudes of 3,049 respondents were re-measured three months after being exposed to the marketing materials, at time 3.

Three advertising themes were tested in this study: warm and emotional, educational, and wedge of doubt. The warm and emotional print advertisement began with the question "Honey, can you pick up some nails?" A response of "Sure" was printed in the middle of the page, with a photograph of a can of escargot. The tagline printed at the bottom of the page inquired, "Is it any wonder hearing loss can frustrate those around you? Have your hearing checked. For you. For them."

The text in the educational message stated, "Use your head once a year" and was placed above a photograph of headphones. The advertisement's closing text read: "Annual hearing checkups help you spot changes in your hearing. Hear today. Hear tomorrow."

(continued)

CASE STUDY 10.2 (*continued*)

The wedge-of-doubt advertisement began with text that warned: "If you think it's difficult admitting your hearing problem, imagine admitting all the mistakes you've made because of it." At the bottom, the advertisement read: "When you can't hear clearly, it's easy to misunderstand someone. And before you know it, people start thinking you've lost your mental edge."

Once these messages had been tested with various audiences, they were adapted for delivery via other media vehicles: mass media (i.e., those that are standard in their appeal), namely print ads and television ads, and private media (which are customized to appeal to their target), specifically telemarketing phone calls and direct marketing mailings.

The analysis showed that consistent combinations of media (both private or both public) were more effective than mixed media; the two private media (telemarketing combined with direct marketing) outperformed any two mixed media (telemarketing and print, telemarketing and television, direct marketing and print, or direct marketing and television). In addition, the private media combination outperformed the public media combination, which makes sense for the hearing aid product category. Learning more about the product in a private setting appeared to increase acceptance.

Finally, the content of the message affected the impact of the particular class of media (private or public). The integrated private media (telemarketing and direct marketing) performed best, first with the wedge-of-doubt content and then with the warm and emotional content. The combination of two private exposures did not perform well in all cases—the combination with the educational advertising message was not effective. The wedge-of-doubt content, which worked best when delivered via the two private media, did not perform well in all cases, either; it performed the worst when delivered via a mass medium.

Marketing health services can be complicated. As this investigation demonstrates, rarely can a marketer choose a medium or an advertising message without considering the big picture. Media cannot be simply pasted together to achieve some seemingly critical threshold of ad weight; many mixed media can perform worse than fewer exposures of sensibly integrated media. Similarly, the choice of media outlets depends on both the product and the content of the ads. Thoughtful combinations of media and messages appear to have greater influence on consumers than haphazard collections of media and messages.

Source: Adapted from Iacobucci et al. (2002).

Discussion Questions
- What challenges are faced by those trying to promote hearing aids to the consumer market?
- How do marketers test the effectiveness of a promotional message?
- What type of message appeared to resonate most with consumers and why?
- Did mass media or private media fare better in terms of promotional results?
- What characteristics of integrated marketing contributed to the success of this campaign?

each other; its messages will be consistent and their delivery synergized; cost savings will ensue; and the organization will sustain a competitive advantage. See Case Study 10.2 for a description of an integrated marketing strategy.

Summary

A variety of established marketing techniques are available to the healthcare industry. All of these approaches are commonly used in other industries and have been adopted in varying degrees by healthcare organizations. Traditional approaches to reaching the organization's constituents include PR (e.g., publicity, communications, government relations), advertising, sales promotion, and personal selling. More recently, direct marketing was added to the healthcare marketer's arsenal of techniques.

The technique of choice depends on the type of organization involved and the product being marketed, among other factors. Of special importance is the objective of the promotional initiative. Objectives vary with the situation; different aims (e.g., to increase visibility, retain existing customers, change consumer attitudes, or increase market share) call for different marketing techniques. A common theme among all promotional objectives, however, is effective communication.

Likewise, different circumstances call for different types of media. Marketers have the option of using print media (e.g., magazines, newspapers), electronic media (e.g., radio, television, Internet), and display media. There are advantages and disadvantages to the use of each type. Display media, such as billboards, are not as applicable to healthcare as most other promotional techniques.

Healthcare organizations are recognizing the importance of integrated marketing. This systematic approach to promoting an idea, an organization, or a product instills consistency in the marketing initiative and facilitates the coordination of a potentially broad range of promotional activities.

Key Points

- Healthcare marketers have access to a variety of promotional techniques that have been used historically in other industries, although some have to be modified for use in healthcare.
- Long before most healthcare organizations embarked on formal marketing initiatives, they relied on various forms of publicity for promotion.
- Promotional activities that are not always recognized by health professionals as marketing include community outreach, networking, and government relations.
- Advertising has probably been the most visible form of marketing by healthcare organizations, although arguably not the most important.
- Although some health professionals have a negative view of advertising, this form of promotion can serve a number of positive functions.
- As healthcare organizations became more involved in ancillary endeavors (e.g., fitness centers) and business-to-business marketing, personal sales became more important.
- Sales promotion is not typically associated with the marketing of medical care but is commonly used to promote consumer health products.
- As the consumer has become more important in healthcare, use of direct-to-consumer marketing techniques has become more common.
- Direct mail and telemarketing techniques are often employed to deliver the message directly to the consumer.
- Healthcare marketers have a variety of media options from which to choose, including print, electronic, and display media.
- Print media include newspapers, magazines, catalogs, and other publications.

- Electronic media include radio, television (network and cable), and the Internet.
- Display media include store displays, posters, and billboards and other outdoor media.
- The promotional technique and medium a marketer chooses to use depend on the type of organization, type of product, and characteristics of the target audience.
- Integrated marketing involves the coordination of all promotional activities to communicate a consistent and uniform marketing message.

Discussion Questions

- What role does the nature of the product play in determining the promotional vehicle to be used?
- How important is the culture of the community when choosing a promotional technique?
- Why is PR often a preferred form of promotion for healthcare organizations?
- Can it be argued that a major function of promotional activities in healthcare is educating the healthcare consumer?
- Why do many health professionals and even members of the general public resist the idea of using advertising in healthcare?
- What steps are involved in the personal selling process, and under what circumstances is personal sales the most effective promotional technique?
- What is the difference between a "push" approach and a "pull" approach in the context of sales promotion?
- What developments in healthcare have encouraged the use of more direct marketing techniques?
- What are the pros and cons to using the different forms of print media?
- What are the advantages (and disadvantages) of using electronic media as opposed to print media?
- What factors are encouraging the growing emphasis on integrated marketing among healthcare organizations?

CONTEMPORARY MARKETING TECHNIQUES

The changes that the field of marketing experienced during its evolution eventually filtered down to healthcare. By the 1990s, healthcare marketing had adopted techniques from other industries and developed new healthcare-specific approaches. This chapter explores developments in healthcare marketing since the beginning of the 1990s and describes innovative and emerging marketing techniques in the field. The importance of customer relationship management, direct-to-consumer marketing, and other contemporary techniques is discussed, and the relative merit of these techniques is assessed. The shift in emphasis from mass marketing to micromarketing is also reviewed.

The New Marketing Reality

Historically, marketing trends outside healthcare have ultimately influenced the form healthcare marketing takes. Observers such as Scott (2009) contend that marketing has undergone a revolution so significant that marketers would do well to forget much of what they know about traditional marketing. The emergence of electronic modes of communication has led to a new paradigm that makes traditional marketing techniques—at least as employed in the past—obsolete. As Scott (2009) indicates in *The New Rules of Marketing and PR*, marketing is no longer about selling but about information dissemination. One-way "interruptive" marketing is no longer effective or even acceptable. Traditional media no longer control the playing field when almost anyone can become a new-media expert armed with what is essentially a free means of information dissemination. In today's environment, content trumps style, and information sharing replaces information hoarding. The following sections discuss current (and future) marketing techniques in healthcare in this context.

Emerging Marketing Techniques

Since the beginning of the 1990s, healthcare has experienced a number of trends related to marketing, including a shift in emphasis from image marketing to service marketing and a movement away from a mass marketing approach to a more targeted strategy. Healthcare marketing has moved away from a one-size-fits-all philosophy to one that emphasizes personalization and customization. Emphasis on the single healthcare episode has shifted to an emphasis on long-term relationships. These developments in healthcare, as in other industries, have benefited from the application of contemporary information technology.

The marketing techniques that have gained momentum in healthcare can be divided into (1) techniques that involve programmatic changes that support marketing and (2) techniques that capitalize on information management. The former implies an innovative approach at a conceptual level and the latter a technology-based approach that may be applied to traditional or innovative marketing techniques.

One factor common to both types of techniques is the emphasis on relationship marketing. *Relationship marketing* is the process of getting closer to the customer by developing a long-term relationship through careful attention to service needs and quality delivery. Relationship marketing succeeds by keeping existing customers happy, ensuring repeat business, and recognizing the revenue potential of long-term relationships.

Relationship marketing is characterized by

- a focus on customer retention,
- an orientation toward product benefits rather than product features,
- a long-term view of customer relationships,
- maximum emphasis on customer commitment and contact,
- development of ongoing relationships,
- multiple employee/customer contacts,
- an emphasis on key account relationship management, and
- an emphasis on trust.

All of the techniques discussed in the following sections incorporate at least some of these attributes.

Programmatic Approaches

Marketing techniques that involve programmatic approaches require a rethinking of the programs offered by the organization in the context of the new marketing reality.

Direct-to-Consumer Marketing

The direct-to-consumer movement is gaining momentum in healthcare as the industry becomes more consumer driven and the ability to target narrow population segments becomes more refined. Healthcare marketers are modifying their methodologies to consider the opportunity represented by over 300 million potential customers.

Toward the end of the twentieth century, the U.S. healthcare industry rediscovered the consumer. The consumer—the ultimate end user of health services and products—had long been written off as a marketing target. For most medical services, the physician made the decisions for the patient, and, for the insured, the health plan controlled choice of provider and the services that could be obtained from that provider. Choice of drug typically depended on the physician's prescription, and the supply channels for medical goods and services generally focused on intermediaries rather than the end user.

With the rediscovery of the healthcare consumer, these practices are undergoing dramatic change. Aided by access to state-of-the-art technology, consumers are now expressing their preferences for everything from physicians and hospitals to health plans and prescription drugs.

The direct-to-consumer movement was jump-started by the pharmaceutical industry. This industry has led the way in terms of expenditures and visibility in its attempts to attract consumers to its brands. Various health insurance plans have followed this trend, albeit at a safe distance, by offering their policies via the Internet, thereby increasing the number of insurance plans aimed at individuals rather than groups. The shift from defined benefits to defined contributions has made the ability to customize health plan benefits to the needs of specific groups—and, indeed, individuals—essential for any health plan that hopes to remain competitive.

This trend has not been lost on providers either, as hospitals, physicians, and other practitioners have established websites to maintain contact with existing customers and to entice prospective customers. Consumers can even bid online for elective procedures (e.g., a face-lift by a plastic surgeon). Such features have established a direct negotiating link between provider and consumer.

A number of factors have driven the trend toward direct-to-consumer advertising. Changed regulations in the pharmaceutical industry were a major contributor, at least for drug companies. The introduction of defined contributions, which allow increased consumer latitude in choice of products and services, has affected health plans, and managed care organizations have repositioned themselves by offering customizable menus of services. Providers are increasingly chasing discretionary patient dollars (e.g., for laser eye surgery), and product vendors use the Internet as a direct path to the hearts, minds, and pocketbooks of healthcare consumers.

Consumers have eagerly accepted this onslaught of direct marketing attention. Spearheaded by the baby boomers, a better-educated, more affluent, and more control-oriented consumer population is eagerly searching for information tailored to their needs.

The Internet has become a favored vehicle for engaging individual consumers, but television and print media expenditures have increased as marketers have found new ways to use these media. Direct mail also appears to be making a comeback as it overcomes its "junk mail" reputation. Although the pharmaceutical industry has driven much of this change, other parties chasing these same consumers are following suit.

This increasingly aggressive approach to the market has meant the end to any one-size-fits-all approach in healthcare. The challenge for marketers of health plans is to be able to offer unbundled services to a wide array of potential customers with highly specific needs, rather than a bundled program to all customers. Take, for example, a health plan that has historically offered a standard package of benefits to all enrollees. If the plan decides to shift its offerings and take a defined contributions approach, the marketer has to be able to promote a variety of unbundled services to a variety of consumers with different needs and preferences. In the past, an employer of a high school–educated, blue-collar workforce (Employer A) offered the same benefits as an employer of a college-educated, professional workforce (Employer B). In today's environment, the plan offered to Employer A is more likely to reflect the needs of Employer A's employees and will inevitably be different from the plan sold to Employer B, particularly in terms of the services offered to the respective employee groups.

For these reasons, healthcare marketers have had to go back to the drawing board in more ways than one. Marketers now must be more in touch with the end user than at any time in history if they are to develop an in-depth understanding of the wants, needs, and preferences of potential customers. To determine who wants particular products and services and the extent to which a population category wants standardization versus customization, marketers have to develop an understanding of consumer characteristics and behaviors at the household level, as they have historically done in other industries.

To succeed in direct-to-consumer marketing, marketers must understand the link between psychographics and consumer behavior to an extent never before necessary in healthcare. To link psychographic clusters to their unique needs, wants, and preferences, they need to develop an in-depth understanding of lifestyle traits and the linkages between lifestyles and services. See Exhibit 11.1 for the pros and cons of direct-to-consumer pharmaceutical marketing.

EXHIBIT 11.1
The Pros and Cons of Direct-to-Consumer Pharmaceutical Advertising

Pros	Cons
Meets increasing demand for medical information	Interferes with the physician–patient relationship and pressures physicians to prescribe
Informs consumers about new treatments	Confuses the patient
Encourages people to seek medical attention for conditions or symptoms that might otherwise go untreated	Emphasizes pharmaceutical treatments when other treatment options may be preferred
Decreases the cost of healthcare	Increases the cost of drugs
Promotes patient compliance	Results in unnecessary drug use

Source: Adapted from Craig (1998).

Business-to-Business Marketing

Although much of the discussion around healthcare marketing focuses on the patient and other end users, a significant amount of marketing in healthcare involves business-to-business transactions. The increasing corporatization of healthcare means that more and more relationships are between one corporate entity and another. The traditional doctor–patient relationship has been supplanted by contractual arrangements between groups of buyers and sellers of health services. Many hospital programs now target corporate customers rather than individual patients. The shift to a more business-like approach to healthcare delivery has also contributed to the growth of *business-to-business marketing*.

Clearly, business-to-business marketing in healthcare is nothing new. Healthcare organizations are major purchasers of a wide variety of goods, and large organizations do business with hundreds of vendors. Business-to-business marketing involves building profitable, value-oriented relationships between two businesses and their respective staffs. Business marketers focus on a few customers, and the sales transactions are usually larger in scope, more complex, and more technically oriented.

Business-to-business marketing has become integral to selling products or services to business, industrial, institutional, or government buyers. In past decades, innovative products, great engineering, or great salesmanship alone might have been enough to close a sale, but healthcare organizations no longer have the luxury of "build it and they will come" thinking. Statistical tools, data mining techniques, and marketing research techniques that work so well in the consumer product arena must be fine-tuned for business-to-business marketing in healthcare.

The factors involved in marketing to businesses are significantly different from those involved in marketing to consumers. Business customers and traditional customers do not buy in the same way; they are driven by different impulses, and they respond to different approaches. Business-to-business purchases are often considered group decisions, whereas business-to-consumer purchases are more personal.

Internal Marketing

Internal marketing refers to a service provider's efforts to effectively train and motivate its customer service and support staffs to work as a team to generate customer satisfaction. Internal marketing aims to ensure that everybody in an organization is working toward common objectives. It is based on the premise that the relationships between people who work together mirror the relationships between customers and suppliers. Internal marketing is a marketing effort inside a company that targets internal audiences. Its goal is to increase communication among staff members to maximize a marketing campaign's effectiveness.

Internal marketing is a combination of marketing, human resources, training, and behavioral science. It redefines employees as valued customers, with the rationale that anticipating, identifying, and satisfying employee needs will lead to greater employee commitment. In turn, greater commitment will promote improved quality of service to external customers.

The marketing department is a logical focal point for internal marketing because of its knowledge of the organization's overall strategy and its appreciation of external customers' needs. The marketing department has the expertise to deploy these tools with regard to internal customers and the budgets and financial resources to do the job. Internal marketing begins with communication, and communication is the marketing staff's primary responsibility.

For internal marketing to be successful, employees must be made fully aware of the organization's aims and activities. Amazingly, employees of large healthcare organizations are often unaware of the services or programs the organization offers. Although such lack of awareness is evident to some degree in any organization, it appears to be an inherent characteristic of healthcare organizations.

A great deal of training is required to instill requisite knowledge about internal marketing and ensure that all employees are working toward the same goal. Employees must also develop a basic understanding of the nature of their customers, especially as they are often isolated from the service-delivery aspects of healthcare operations. Employees may have little knowledge of the customer interaction process or, at best, only a partial understanding of service delivery.

Unfortunately, investment in internal efforts has always been a paltry fraction of most marketers' budgets and is probably even smaller in healthcare than in other industries. Lack of investment in internal marketing may also result from corporate distraction. Companies that are frantically trying to boost revenues and cut costs may not see why they should spend money on employees for this purpose. They end up missing the point that these people, their employees, will ultimately deliver the brand promises the company makes.

Lack of investment may also result from a conscious decision by executives who dismiss internal efforts as feel-good pseudoscience, even though research consistently demonstrates that poor service (people problems more so than product problems) is what pushes customers away and into the arms of competitors.

Internal marketing is also an important implementation tool. It facilitates communication and helps squelch resistance to change. It informs and involves all staff in new initiatives and strategies. Internal marketing initiatives are relatively simple to develop if the marketer is familiar with traditional principles of marketing. Internal marketing is based on the same rules as external marketing and is similarly structured. The main difference is that the customers are staff and colleagues from inside the organization.

There is nothing magic about internal marketing; most of it is common sense. Among the most common features of internal marketing programs are workshops, special events, company anniversary celebrations, appreciation dinners, brown-bag lunches, off-site/satellite office visits, internal newsletters, bulletin boards, e-mail newsletters, intranets, and broadcast e-mail.

Concierge Services

In the late 1990s, the healthcare field witnessed the emergence of *concierge services*. Some healthcare organizations have simply introduced practices borrowed from the hospitality industry, while others have restructured their practices to meet a broad range of health-related needs for a small, select patient population.

Some healthcare organizations have adopted concierge-type services as part of their customer service approach. Hospitals may offer valet parking, perks for family members of patients, or a menu of gourmet food options for hospitalized patients. Large physicians' practices may offer additional services at little or no cost to certain categories of patients, such as immediate Internet access to clinicians, help with insurance filing and referral scheduling, and transportation.

Concierge-type practices—usually involving one or a small number of physicians—accept only a limited number of patients who pay an annual fee in addition to the cost of care provided. The concept behind these types of practices is simple, if somewhat controversial. Participating physicians agree to accept only a small number of patients (e.g., 300 rather than the typical several thousand) in exchange for an annual fee (currently ranging from $1,500 per year for limited services for an individual to $7,500 per year for expanded services for a family). These services include access to the physician or other staff member 24 hours a day, seven days a week; immediate telephone response, same-day appointments, longer office consultations, and house calls. The physician may even accompany the client to visits with other healthcare providers to serve as an "interpreter." In most cases, existing insurance continues to pay for covered services.

The number of such practices is still small, but this approach appears to be gaining momentum. Most of these practices have been initiated by the physicians themselves, although hospitals are becoming increasingly involved in establishing concierge services. Since the first model was developed in Seattle in the 1990s, concierge practices have emerged mostly on the East and West Coasts. A handful of national chains of concierge practices have also been established.

This approach is not without its critics. Observers inside and outside medicine have condemned this approach as avaricious and likely to contribute to an already serious shortage or maldistribution of physicians. If large numbers of physicians reduce their patient loads from 5,000 to 300, many patients will be left without access to physicians. Indeed, established patients of physicians converting to a concierge practice must be among the first to sign up or face finding another doctor.

This new practice form reflects broader trends that are affecting society in general and healthcare in particular. Many observers point to managed care as a factor that has induced dissatisfaction and disenchantment among physicians. Features of managed care, such as the assembly-line approach, oversight imposed by nonclinical personnel, and limitations on utilization, have led physicians to take some radical approaches. The healthcare field already has seen the emergence of practices that do not participate in managed care and may or may not accept insurance. Similarly, direct-pay practices have been established that accept only out-of-pocket payments—but at half of the managed care rate.

Issues with current methods of reimbursement may not be the main factor in the emergence of concierge practices; the baby boomers may be. Born between 1946 and 1964 to parents who survived the Great Depression and World War II, baby boomers were destined to be America's golden children. With doting parents who wanted their children to have what they only dreamed of as youth—a carefree, prosperous life—boomers quickly became the target of mainstream marketing campaigns. Not all concierge members are upscale baby boomers, however; some Medicare managed care plans have added concierge services.

While there continues to be interest in concierge physician practices and the number of such practices continues to slowly grow, the public has not accepted this concept to the extent anticipated. It is a departure from the type of practice most patients are comfortable with, and the extent to which patients are dissatisfied with their existing providers may have been overestimated. In addition, some physicians have found that the 24/7 demands associated with a concierge practice were an unanticipated burden. As a marketing paradigm, the concierge concept makes a lot of sense, but whether it turns into a widespread form of medical practice remains to be seen.

Technology-Based Approaches

Technology-based approaches are considered "contemporary" in that they take advantage of the state-of-the-art technology now available to healthcare marketers. Pioneered in other industries, these techniques are increasingly being adopted by healthcare organizations that recognize the contributions technology can bring to the marketing endeavor.

Database Marketing

Database marketing is a well-established component of marketing in almost every industry besides healthcare. Although healthcare does not lend itself to the retail-oriented applications of this marketing technique, health professionals are increasingly recognizing the ways in which healthcare can benefit from some aspects of database marketing.

Database marketing involves collecting, storing, analyzing, and using information about customers and their past purchase behaviors to guide future marketing decisions. Ultimately, database marketing involves two main activities: (1) building a comprehensive database of customer profiles and (2) launching direct marketing initiatives based on those profiles. The resulting direct marketing must be response and outcome oriented to be considered database marketing.

Database marketing is closely linked to *customer relationship management* (discussed in the next section), which involves the creation of a centralized body of knowledge that interfaces internal customer data with external market data. This integrated data set can be analyzed to discern patterns relevant to the marketing process. The final step involves converting this knowledge into a communication vehicle that allows the healthcare organization to target relevant prospects and deliver the appropriate message.

A number of constraints are implicit in database marketing in healthcare. These constraints are legal or ethical and often relate to issues of privacy, confidentiality, and data security. The potential repercussions from disclosing the medical condition of a customer are much greater than those from disclosing grocery store purchases or even financial transactions. The enactment of the Health Insurance Portability and Accountability Act (HIPAA) in 1996 focused the spotlight on the issue of patient data confidentiality. (See Chapter 16.)

Database marketing is best suited to retail-type industries in which the consumer decision-making process is much different from that in healthcare. Products and services must generate adequate margins to be candidates for database marketing, and some health services do not qualify on this score. Healthcare is much more complex and includes numerous data collection points.

Adapting database marketing to healthcare requires a certain level of sophistication and the need for health professionals to buy into a relatively expensive high-tech solution capable of handling these complexities. With convoluted decision making and complex financing arrangements, the ideal system for database marketing in healthcare is difficult to conceptualize. The variety of coding systems alone will present challenges to the development of database marketing applications. Healthcare organizations must invest a lot of effort in the process, which is a challenge when many healthcare executives are not attuned to direct consumer marketing. Ultimately, the complexity of healthcare is the issue, not the technology.

A database marketing approach cannot be transferred from another industry without serious modification, and patients cannot be treated the same way as fast-food customers or car buyers. Nevertheless, the potential applications of customer relationship management to healthcare are almost unlimited. While the complexities of healthcare pose numerous challenges on this front, they also offer an opportunity to develop a structure for capitalizing on them. The data mining potential from a well-designed customer marketing information file is considerable.

Any choice-driven program—whether an affinity program (e.g., senior program), concierge-style services, or a fund-raising initiative—is a natural candidate for database marketing. Pharmaceutical companies already use a version of database marketing to target customers in their direct-to-consumer campaigns. Now health plans are beginning to use this approach to segment their enrollee populations.

Consumers' concerns about privacy can be addressed by having opt-in/opt-out capabilities and letting patients indicate their preferred means of contact. With these features in place, database marketing appears ideal for a number of areas in healthcare. Two obvious—but different—examples include the operation of wellness programs and the promotion of retail products and services on the part of healthcare organizations.

In other industries, database marketing is used for cross-selling, up-selling, follow-up sales, and so on. Healthcare organizations are starting to think more broadly about appropriate (and potentially profitable) applications of database marketing to their services and products.

Overt solicitation may be a turnoff for healthcare consumers, but if these opportunities are approached in the right way, they can be perceived as valuable. For example, if a patient registers for an educational program (and gives consent for subsequent contact), the patient may find that follow-up contact valuable. Likewise, many healthcare organizations promote ancillary goods and services (e.g., pediatric services to obstetrics patients), and patient data provide the basis for bundling services to the benefit of the patient.

The degree to which more aggressive database marketing will come to be accepted will depend on how it is implemented. Clearly, the call to action that pharmaceutical companies have issued through their direct-to-consumer marketing has been well received by patients (if not by physicians). If the database marketing initiative encourages or helps the customer to obtain more information, it will hopefully be seen as a positive outreach. Still, the potential for backlash exists, whether it is as mild and simple as a request to be removed from a solicitation list or as serious and complex as the anxieties engendered in patients with sensitive medical conditions.

Customer Relationship Management

Healthcare marketers are always searching for ways to have more impact and demonstrate value in their organizations. Customer relationship management (CRM) strategies may prove to be the next big thing in healthcare marketing, and for good reason. Well-thought-out and well-executed CRM programs are generating substantial returns for many businesses, and new technologies only add to the possibilities. Healthcare organizations are beginning to recognize the benefits of CRM, and increased spending on CRM activities is predicted.

At the same time, however, CRM is largely misunderstood by healthcare professionals, and the industry may not be ready to implement a flurry of customer-driven business strategies. Healthcare organizations need to significantly change the way they do business to realize the true benefits of CRM. The most important benefit of a CRM initiative is its contribution to the ways in which the organization defines its customers, identifies and segments their needs, and serves them. Healthcare organizations need to balance the value they provide to customers with the value CRM generates for the organization.

Marketers should first identify which of the organization's goals are most important. Subsequent internal planning and implementation efforts should be based on those goals. Some common goals and objectives of technology-driven customer relationship programs include

- improving customer service and satisfaction,
- reducing the number of negative customer experiences,

- allocating resources more efficiently,
- reducing expenses related to customer interaction,
- attracting prospects and retaining existing customers,
- anticipating customers' needs and building stronger relationships over time,
- improving clinical outcomes, and
- increasing profitability.

Most businesses use customer satisfaction as the key metric for defining CRM success. Given that most hospitals already use patient satisfaction as a key performance indicator, it should not be a big leap for management to see the value in CRM strategies that enhance customer satisfaction in all areas of the system. Marketers can then introduce more aggressive objectives aimed at patient volume, revenue, and profitability.

Existing businesses often have difficulty changing the institutional mind-set to one that is customer driven rather than driven by sales or operations. Healthcare organizations in particular seem to have difficulty making this shift. For this reason, most healthcare marketers will not be able to integrate every aspect of their organization into a CRM program, and they probably should not try. The success of these programs does not hinge on how comprehensive or complex they are but on how well coordinated and well orchestrated they are. Areas to which CRM strategies could potentially be applied (see Case Study 11.1) include the following:

- A disease management program for a chronically ill group of patients
- A physician-to-physician marketing program
- A community health screening or prevention program
- Specific product lines, such as cardiology, oncology, women's health, maternity, or sports medicine
- An urgent care clinic
- A website or an online community
- An organization's call center or customer service function
- Identification and servicing of the organization's top ten referring physicians
- Identification and servicing of the organization's top ten leading accounts or clients
- A frequent customer program or other affinity club

Internet Marketing

Although healthcare organizations were slow to jump on the Internet marketing bandwagon, some healthcare organizations came to lead the way with regard to certain aspects of online marketing. Hospital websites, for example,

CASE STUDY 11.1
Promoting Heart Health Using Customer Relationship Management

Health systems are increasingly turning to customer relationship management (CRM) for purposes of predictive segmentation. The Customer Potential Management (CPM) Marketing Group has been a pioneer in applying this technique to the cardiology market. CPM developed a program for three hospitals in the eastern United States that are part of a national healthcare system with more than 100 acute care hospitals in 17 states. The participating hospitals ranged in size from a small, local hospital to a large regional medical center. They are referred to as Hospital A, Hospital B, and Hospital C.

The overall objective of this program was to educate consumers about the early warning signs associated with heart attacks and encourage them to take a proactive role by determining their heart health. The program was also designed to build awareness of the healthcare system's local cardiology services and drive early intervention and service utilization.

This campaign used the Consumer Healthcare Utilization Index (CHUI), a predictive index developed by CPM, to select the top people in each market area most likely to benefit from the campaign information. Targeted people were referred for a heart health exam for which they paid a fee. The campaign also included a matched control group that was not involved in the marketing initiative.

Area referring physicians and providers were briefed on the campaign and encouraged to participate in screening patient results. This effort was designed to include physicians in the campaign, promote hospital cardiology services, and extend information to more patients. The following objectives were identified for the project:

- Identify people at risk for a heart attack and do an early intervention (promotion of low-cost heart health exam)
- Provide consumers with beneficial education (heart attack signs and symptoms)
- Strengthen relationships with primary care physicians and cardiologists
- Increase total charges attributed to cardiac-related services

The approach involved delivering segmented messages to male and female prospects drawn from the databases of the three facilities.

(continued)

CASE STUDY 11.1 (*continued*)

Solicitations were limited to one per household and targeted to persons aged 35 or older living in households reporting at least $30,000 income annually.

The package for the promotion consisted of a 7.5 × 5-inch, four-color informational piece with two versions—one for males and one for females. The primary offer was the heart health check, which included an electrocardiogram (EKG) screen with a free EKG wallet card, body mass index measurement, lipid screen, and cardiac education booklet. The secondary offer was a free take-home health risk assessment.

The cost per package, which included materials, lettershop services, and postage, differed for each hospital according to how many pieces were printed and how many were actually mailed, ranging from $.71 to $1.39. Package prices for Hospitals B and C were higher because they printed large quantities for future mailings.

A complete record was maintained of organization-initiated communications—outbound dialogues with customers and prospective customers through direct mail. These communication records were matched to individuals and households in the database to assess activities, behaviors, and service utilization with regard to the product line being promoted. Respondents were tracked through their appointment activity, and active responses were counted when members of the target audience scheduled heart health exams.

A 5 percent sample of the system's CRM database was flagged as a static market control group for each hospital. The control group was selected using the same criteria by which the organization-initiated communications group who received the mailing was selected. Members of the control group did not receive the mailing, but their activity was tracked in the database to compare activities, behaviors, and service utilization with those of the people who did receive the mailing.

The list of individuals with high predictive index scores compiled by Hospitals A and B returned significant positive results. Although Hospital C also reported positive results, fewer data were available for this site (e.g., EKG results were not available). At Hospital A, nearly half of those who signed up for the heart health exam had abnormal EKG readings. When combined with those whose EKG showed minor abnormalities, the percentage of people with some sort of abnormal reading rose to 54 percent. At Hospital B, 61 percent of those who signed up for the heart health exam had abnormal EKG readings.

The real measurement of success is a simple value proposition that demonstrates dollar for dollar the revenue received for revenue spent. Furthermore, an accurate calculation of return on investment (ROI) must account for utilization that might have occurred without the campaign—that of the control group.

The use of CHUI methodology to target potential cardiology patients benefited the participating hospitals. The combined response results for the first six months of this campaign indicated the following:

- Patient response rate: 5.36 percent; control group response rate: 1.61 percent
- Marketing response increase: 333 percent
- Net profit: $1,868,711
- Marketing lift after factoring out the control group: $1,684,643
- ROI: $44.78 for every $1 spent on marketing

Results for the first six months demonstrate that this health system was successful in identifying the most appropriate individuals for cardiology services and generating a high return on the marketing investment. The significance of these numbers illustrates that the CHUI enables organizations to target at-risk people for intervention by offering appropriate education, health maintenance, and wellness programs.

Discussion Questions

- What was the organization's objective in applying the CRM approach to its customer pool?
- In what ways did the initiative intend to change the knowledge, attitudes, or practices of the hospital's customers?
- What were the characteristics of the promotional package used for this initiative?
- How receptive were the organization's patients to this initiative?
- What tangible benefits did the organization derive from this initiative?
- How was ROI measured, and what did the evaluation reveal?

have become important sources of health information, and increasing numbers of healthcare consumers search popular online sites like WebMD. Patients and caregivers alike use the Internet as a resource both before and after the physician visit. Because they are seeking information, the message can be more customized than, say, a television advertisement.

Observers of the evolution of the Internet noted a progression in healthcare organizations' Internet marketing initiatives. The first stage involved simply a brochure site that identified the organization and described its work. The next stage introduced a deeper level of service line and health content and more interactive features and applications. Most websites are still far from being truly integrated with their organization's marketing efforts or other information technology applications in the hospital, but a growing number of health systems are pushing customized health information and medical records out to consumers, allowing e-mail communication with physicians and doing some level of actual disease management online. Some are now using their websites for the ultimate goal of establishing and maintaining customer relationships.

Today, many healthcare organizations' websites include unique, sophisticated features. The *Hospitals & Health Networks'* Most Wired Survey conducted by the American Hospital Association (www.hhnmostwired.com) is a useful indicator of what health systems are doing with information technology. Some of the early pioneers in this arena were Columbia/HCA, Kaiser Permanente, United Healthcare, and academic medical centers, such as the University of Alabama at Birmingham and the University of Iowa.

Most healthcare organizations devote part of their marketing budget to online brand promotion. To assess the value in providing information online, many are attempting to determine their ROI by measuring whether physician visits are increasing, more prescriptions are being written, more coupons are being redeemed, and more products are being sold. For most organizations, answering the ROI question will enhance the appeal of Internet marketing relative to offline marketing.

According to Scott (2009), the best websites focus on content that pulls customers, markets, media, and products together in a common location. A website should be the point at which all of an organization's online initiatives intersect, including podcasts, blogs, news releases, and other online features. A content-rich website should organize the organization's resources in a cohesive and interesting way that efficiently informs the audience. (See the section on social media that appears later in this chapter.)

The Internet is also a major channel in the direct-to-consumer movement. By providing information, education, advice, summaries of scientific studies, tools, and shared experiences, pharmaceutical companies use the Internet to better communicate with patients. Well-established sites include Sepsis.com, Schering Plough's Claritin.com, and Novo-Nordisk's Diabetes 4patients.org. In another notable effort, the National Headache Foundation and Astra Zeneca teamed up to create a Migraine Mentors at Work program (migrainementors.com). The site, which is an online extension of a workplace-based education/disease management program, provides users with information on how to manage their diseases.

Healthcare marketers are successfully using offline techniques to draw consumers to their sites to search for information or respond to specific offers. They invite consumers to their sites to find a physician, view photos of newborns, sign up for a health screening, or take advantage of other site features. Once consumers are online, marketers convert Internet surfers into prospects by capturing personal information in a customer database and having them sign up for interactive health news and medical reminders. This tactic enables hospitals to extend their marketing reach in a more personal way than just advertising on television or through the mail.

While healthcare organizations have typically not been on the cutting edge in terms of the adoption of social media, many are starting to take advantage of contemporary technology, such as Second Life. Second Life uses state-of-the-art technology to create a virtual world on the Internet. This application allows users to interact in cyberspace, create group activities, trade virtual properties and services, and socialize. Second Life also supports a three-dimensional modeling tool for "sculpting" objects and introducing animation. Case Study 11.2 describes a hospital's employment of Second Life for marketing purposes.

CASE STUDY 11.2
Hospital Takes Its Grand Opening to Second Life

In 2008, Palomar Pomerado Health in San Diego cut the virtual ribbon for a new facility not scheduled to open until 2011. In partnership with Cisco Systems, the health system was able to hold a "grand opening" three years early by creating a simulated version of the real-life Palomar West Medical Campus in Second Life. The health system claims that Palomar West Medical Campus was the first U.S. hospital to be unveiled in Second Life.

By entering Second Life, virtual visitors can tour the facilities and see some of the amenities of the $810 million, real-life publicly financed hospital, which will serve California's largest public health district. Under the direction of Palomar's chief innovation officer, the facility was designed from the ground up to be integrated with leading-edge technology, including medical technology. Its Second Life presence offers patients and the healthcare community a chance to explore these innovations in the virtual world years before the physical facility opens.

Virtual visitors to Palomar West are also helping Palomar Pomerado test some of its ideas regarding the use of leading-edge

(continued)

CASE STUDY 11.2 *(continued)*

technology at the new facility and the opportunities futuristic concepts present for the healthcare industry at large. The system is even using Second Life to test some technology proposed for deployment in the real-life hospital, such as radio frequency identification (RFID). Avatar patients taking the virtual tour can test out RFID-enabled bracelets that could not only track patients but also automatically guide them to the areas of the facility in which their services or treatments are scheduled to be provided. Thus, a virtual patient slated for day surgery could automatically have the hospital elevator land on the correct floor, according to the information programmed into the RFID bracelet. If this technology works in a virtual setting, it could be adopted in the real world. Some of the concepts being tested aren't considered feasible today, but these options can be explored in advance in this virtual setting.

Looking ahead, Palomar Pomerado will also use Second Life to host industry events and meetings with healthcare leaders, policymakers, and others on a variety of topics, including healthcare issues and the design, architecture, and technology that will be used in the real-life Palomar West.

Discussion Questions

- Why have hospitals and other healthcare organizations been slow to adopt contemporary technology for nonmedical purposes?
- What are the advantages and disadvantages of opening up development plans to the public and encouraging their feedback?
- By using Second Life technology for the hospital's virtual grand opening, is Palomar Pomerado in danger of creating unrealistic expectations among future customers?
- How do you think Palomar Pomerado's cutting-edge approach is likely to be perceived by the traditional healthcare community?
- How likely are other healthcare organizations to adopt this approach in presenting themselves to the public?

Source: Adapted from McGee (2008).

Many developments are anticipated with regard to healthcare Internet marketing. It is expected to

- better integrate online initiatives with more traditional marketing programs;

- leverage targeted marketing campaigns to generate new referrals and patient encounters for service lines like cardiology, oncology, and orthopedics;
- focus on online customer relationship management strategies;
- increase direct-to-consumer online marketing;
- increase multicultural marketing as the industry gains a better understanding of the healthcare needs of ethnic populations;
- better integrate the entire media mix; and
- position the Internet as the ultimate relationship management tool.

Social Media

In the past few years, a form of contemporary communication referred to as *social media* has emerged. Although there is no concise definition of this phenomenon, it is an umbrella term for a variety of communication modes that use technology to support innovative forms of communication. Forms of social media include texting and instant messaging, blogs, podcasts, Twitter, and other types of electronic communication. Social media are distinguished from traditional media in a number of ways. For purposes of distinction, the latter is often referred to as *industrial media*.

Social media were originally developed for purposes of social interaction and have been popularized by a new generation of young, technology-savvy consumers. With roots in cell phone and Internet applications, technological advances allowed individuals using social media to maintain contact with their friends and family at any time, no matter where they were physically located. This means of person-to-person interaction eventually expanded to create electronic "communities" of individuals who not only shared information but actively created "knowledge." Today, each form of social media provides a setting for forums for discussing social events, political perspectives, and consumer concerns.

Social media have been discovered by marketers who have found that they exhibit the characteristics considered important in an effective marketing medium. They can reach target audiences (assuming they are "wired") anywhere, at any time. They are highly accessible because, unlike traditional media, they are in the public domain in the sense than anyone can participate. Social media are user-friendly in that individuals (even children) can utilize them in their various forms without having to acquire specialized skills. They are timely in that information transfer can take place in real time, whereas industrial media may take days, weeks, or months to transfer information. Finally, social media are modifiable, in the sense that the message can be changed "on the fly" as new information emerges. Once printed or broadcast, traditional media are permanent—a disadvantageous characteristic in times of rapid social change.

Not surprisingly, social media have become popular with people interested in healthcare issues (Sarasohn-Kahn 2008). As noted previously, most people use the Internet to research health problems and find other health-related information; physicians and patients are increasingly communicating via e-mail; and online support groups for health problems have become common. Healthcare consumers are now adopting social media to interact, share information, and create online communities. Such sites as Google Health and MySpace's Cure Diabetes Group were created to capitalize on these interests. Online forums on health-related topics are burgeoning, and countless healthcare blogs have been created.

Although healthcare has lagged behind other industries in adapting social media for marketing purposes, innovative healthcare marketers have begun to appreciate the potential of this form of communication. If key functions of marketing are to inform and educate, it is hard to imagine a better vehicle for these activities than social media. Healthcare organizations are establishing sites for information dissemination and sharing, support group interaction, and customer feedback. Providers of healthcare goods and services are creating blogs to attract consumers concerned with a particular issue and are taking advantage of the exposure to promote their products. Pharmaceutical companies have been at the forefront of efforts to capitalize on the power of social media, and even government agencies have added social media to the set of techniques they use for social marketing. See Case Study 11.3 on the use of social media in healthcare.

CASE STUDY 11.3
Social Media—Virginia Blood Services

Before 2008, the legal age to donate blood in Virginia was 18. When the legal donation age in Virginia was lowered to 16 in 2008, Virginia Blood Services began to look for new ways to engage the population and drive donors to its blood collection events. In exploring new methods of communicating to potential donors, particularly first-time donors, Virginia Blood Services approached Neathawk Dubuque & Packett for more information on the use of social media to reach those audiences.

It quickly became apparent that utilizing social media was appropriate not only for reaching those as young as 16 but also for reaching college students. Upcoming blood drives on college campuses signaled an opportunity to market the events in a way that would be applicable to both demographics. With a scope target population that included late high school to college-age students, the challenge of drawing interest and engagement was greater.

Virginia Blood Services developed a strategy of using the Facebook Events feature to organize and promote a series of blood drives on campuses across the state. The event pages were built to take advantage of a newly launched Virginia Blood Services official Facebook page already being used to disseminate content and news. The Facebook Event strategy largely revolved around the measurement of ongoing interest through Facebook's built-in RSVP feature, through which invitees (and even non-invitees viewing the event page) could indicate whether they would be attending, might be attending, or would not be attending the event in question.

Another advantage to using Facebook Events is the public nature of the feature. People who have profiles on Facebook cannot see information on others unless they are "friends" or the information is specially made available to the public. Actions such as updating a profile or sharing a link to an interesting article, photo, or video are therefore visible only to those with whom a user chooses to share. However, if a person declares that he supports a service by becoming a "fan" of that service's official page, or, in the case of Virginia Blood Services, if he RSVPs to say he will participate in a blood drive, all of his friends will see that he plans on attending. If more than one friend is going to the same event, the homepage shows that both are attending. In the case of a community of friends, associates, and classmates that populates not only an actual campus but also an online one, this influence can be multiplied exponentially. If even 1 in 20 invited to a blood drive responds that she may or definitely will attend, it is likely that hundreds, if not thousands, of people who were not even invited will see that these people are considering, and in some way endorsing, the activity. In the case of Virginia Blood Services, these events could be promoted on college campuses via e-mail broadcasts that include the link to the Facebook Event page, and from there, the promotion would likely take on a life of its own. Once initiated, this experiment in new media established a pattern of response, endorsement, and awareness for little investment other than time.

The immediate effect was palpable when in just the first week, several hundred people had viewed each event online, and more than a third of those people had responded that they would attend—one of the first indicators that these events would attract a volume of donors never

(*continued*)

CASE STUDY 11.3 *(continued)*

before seen by Virginia Blood Services. In one instance, within the first week of posting a page on the Crimson War blood drive at the University of Virginia, Virginia Blood Services received RSVPs for 165 "confirmed" guests, 64 who said they may attend, 56 who indicated they would not attend, and 247 who had yet to declare an official response. More than 500 people had viewed the page in less than seven days.

The real results became evident at the actual events and afterward, when the initiative was evaluated. Data were compiled on individuals who actually attended the event, individuals who were viable donors, individuals who provided double-reds (i.e., particularly useful donations of a certain type of blood), and individuals who were new donors. Because people generally use their real names on Facebook, Virginia Blood Services was able to develop a small programming script that matched donors in the database with the Facebook Event log of names. The final tally was a remarkable 28 percent increase in new donors, all solicited through Facebook. For some of the events, the double-red total increased well over 20 percent.

Discussion Questions
- What demographic did Virginia Blood Services seek to penetrate, and why did it think an innovative method would be required to do so?
- In addition to Facebook, are there other forms of social media that the marketers might have employed?
- What characteristics of Facebook and other social media make them ideal for this type of campaign?
- How effective was the Virginia Blood Services campaign, and how do the results compare to what might be expected using traditional marketing methods?

The New Marketing Driver: Consumer Engagement

In previous chapters, the emergence of the consumer as a significant phenomenon in healthcare was noted. Redefining the patient as a consumer automatically attributes different characteristics to the healthcare customer. More important from a marketing perspective are the implications of this redefinition for the marketer's approach to the target audience. In particular, the manner in which a consumer is solicited differs from the manner in which a patient is solicited. This shift in orientation toward the consumer has led to a growing interest in consumer engagement in healthcare marketing.

Consumer engagement refers to the process through which a healthcare organization establishes a relationship with a customer or a prospective customer (or an employee or a health plan member) that involves the consumer's participation in bringing about a desired behavioral change. For example, a physician or other clinician might engage with a patient to encourage compliance; a health plan might engage with a plan member to encourage healthy behavior; and a wellness provider might engage with employees to encourage participation in a fitness program. In every case, the engagement process builds on an understanding of the background, needs, and motivations of the consumer; the most effective means of communicating with the consumer; and the type of relationship that will facilitate the consumer's movement through the phases of awareness, action, and maintenance. (See the discussion on Prochaska's work that appears later in the chapter.)

It has become increasingly clear that consumer actions are the key to reducing health risks and that, without consumer participation, the efforts of the healthcare system are likely to be wasted (Demchak 2007). Noncompliant consumers are not only detrimental to their own health but are also costly for the system overall. A not-for-profit community clinic fares much better managing a patient in the pre-diabetes stage; a much larger resource expenditure is required to manage a patient with full-blown diabetes. An uninsured patient can be managed much more effectively in a primary care office than in a hospital emergency department. A health insurance plan is much better off paying for a prevention visit, rather than for a hospital stay for an untreated condition. Even pharmaceutical companies complain about the billions of dollars of revenue lost annually as a result of patients who fail to purchase drugs that have been prescribed.

Implementing effective consumer engagement efforts involves considerable rethinking on the part of both consumers and healthcare organizations. Consumers have been told for decades that they should turn their health over to the healthcare system. Physicians have been trained to look at patients in isolation from their environments, to rely on laboratory tests rather than listen to a patient's story. Physicians and other healthcare providers historically have not been paid to provide preventive care but have been rewarded for heroic "downstream" clinical care. Health insurance plans have discouraged the use of services rather than ensure that each plan member receives the right care at the right place at the right time.

Healthcare experts now realize that consumer participation is fundamental to transforming the current health system into one that is more efficient. Consumers today are encouraged to engage by carefully selecting providers and health plans, working with their providers to ensure safe and effective treatments, adopting and maintaining healthy behaviors, and diligently managing their own health conditions. Healthcare providers, health plans, and employers are urging their patients, enrollees, and employees to become more involved in their healthcare by offering incentives and supporting consumer-directed health plans.

The most promising approaches to supporting consumer engagement are those that are participatory rather than didactic, involve family members, and have multiple dimensions. It is becoming increasingly clear that interventions tailored to the individual's level of initiative will yield good results. If members of the targeted populations are asked to take small steps that are realistic given their level of initiative, they have a greater chance of experiencing success and building confidence to meet their next challenge.

Segmenting consumers into groups to increase initiative could also prove beneficial, especially if the segmentation accounts for clinical risk factors. Segmentation would enable healthcare providers to customize their strategies to address the unique challenges associated with each stage of patient engagement in a particular group. If engagement strategies are implemented before risks increase or health worsens, patients could require less acute care as their self-management skills improve and they gain confidence. Other stakeholders, such as providers and employers, could use similar techniques. Together, insurers, providers, and employers can help increase patient engagement by addressing the specific challenges consumers face as they begin to manage their health. Outreach at the community level could help provide the local momentum needed to activate a specific population. Reaching out to those who are more motivated to become role models and opinion leaders may help to hasten change in the community.

An emerging theme in consumer engagement research focuses on the consumer's capacity to change. This capacity depends on the consumer's state of knowledge, the consumer's attitudes, the support resources accessible to the consumer, and other factors. The consumer's status with regard to change determines the approach an organization takes to consumer engagement. One such approach to consumer engagement was developed by Prochaska and colleagues (1995), who identified five stages of change: pre-contemplation, contemplation, preparation, action, and maintenance. These stages are similar to those of the consumer decision-making process discussed earlier. A consumer in the pre-contemplation stage is not ready to use a service and needs to be educated about it. A consumer in the contemplation stage may be aware of the service but needs to adjust his or her attitude toward it. A consumer in the preparation stage needs to be exposed to the service options available. A consumer in the action stage needs supportive services. A consumer in the maintenance stage needs reinforcement. Thus, the stage of change becomes

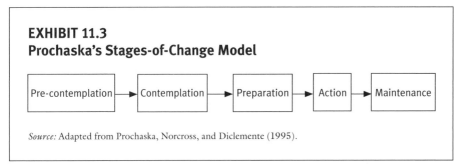

EXHIBIT 11.3
Prochaska's Stages-of-Change Model

Pre-contemplation → Contemplation → Preparation → Action → Maintenance

Source: Adapted from Prochaska, Norcross, and Diclemente (1995).

a major determinant of the type of marketing activity pursued. (See Exhibit 11.3 for a depiction of Prochaska's stages-of-change model.)

Effective consumer engagement requires meeting consumers where they are and progressively moving from a generalized approach to an individualized approach. As long as marketers continue to use a one-size-fits-all approach, they are likely to see little response from consumer audiences. Marketers need to recognize that consumers are unable to make these changes on their own and that the entire health system needs to engage them. An essential task in this process is educating providers on the different levels of engagement and how to tailor messages accordingly.

Marketers also need to understand what types of interventions have the greatest effect on outcomes, how various interventions affect consumers at each level of engagement and in the general population, and how populations with low literacy or without health insurance—which tend to have lower health status—can be engaged. Financial incentives are commonly used to motivate consumer behaviors, although different consumer segments are likely to respond differently to such enticements. Even more important, marketers need to determine whether responsiveness to incentives leads to sustained behavior change and increased engagement.

Although much more research will be required before the consumer engagement endeavor is thoroughly understood, some early conclusions can be drawn with regard to what makes a consumer approach effective. For a consumer to benefit from an engagement initiative, he or she must possess adequate knowledge about health problems and preventive measures, be motivated, have the capacity to change, be offered meaningful incentives, be provided appropriate pathways for action, and receive reinforcement for positive behavior. For those involved in fostering consumer engagement, the tools for change include an in-depth understanding of the target population, meaningful segmentation of the target population, a proactive intervention package, targeted communications, ongoing support, and regular monitoring of consumer activity.

Limitations to Contemporary Marketing Techniques

The contemporary approaches to marketing presented in this chapter have useful applications in healthcare. However, there are certain barriers to incorporating some of the more innovative and technology-based techniques.

The first of these barriers is the practicality of adapting these techniques to healthcare. Many healthcare organizations do not have the personnel or technical resources necessary to implement such techniques. They may lack the information technology infrastructure needed to support these approaches or may be unable to access the data on which these techniques depend. They are not likely to know how to implement database marketing or CRM without bringing in outside consultants.

Not only are the necessary data often lacking, but concerns about the confidentiality of the patient data used in some of these techniques always exist. The HIPAA legislation has made many healthcare organizations gunshy even when it comes to clearly legitimate uses of personal health data. Questions about the appropriateness of using patient data for marketing purposes reinforce these concerns. The conservative nature of health professionals poses a barrier to the use of data where people in other industries would have no qualms about doing so.

Contemporary marketing techniques are being slowly but surely incorporated into healthcare, particularly into areas that have fewer reservations about the use of data (e.g., pharmaceutical distribution). The demands of a competitive and consumer-driven system will need to be approached through new marketing techniques, and contemporary consumers are likely to insist on having more and more access to, and interaction with, healthcare providers. Ultimately, the challenge for healthcare is to use modern marketing techniques to establish and maintain customer relationships without violating or even giving the appearance of violating patient confidentiality.

Summary

The 1990s witnessed the adoption of marketing techniques from other industries and the development of healthcare-specific approaches. These contemporary approaches to marketing not only involve more sophisticated techniques but also in many ways represent the influence of a new marketing paradigm. These approaches generally emphasize organizational change or the application of technology to marketing challenges. Both types of techniques emphasize relationship development and management.

Among the emerging techniques that involve programmatic changes are direct-to-consumer marketing, business-to-business marketing, internal marketing, and the provision of concierge services. Emerging technology-based techniques include database marketing, CRM, Internet marketing, and the use of social media. Techniques that involve information technology and intensive use of data have tremendous potential for healthcare but remain controversial in many ways. The enactment of HIPAA legislation has made many healthcare organizations gun-shy even when it comes to legitimate uses of personal health data.

The Internet has changed the face of healthcare marketing, just as it has affected numerous other industries. In the future, the Internet is expected to facilitate the use of other technology-based marketing techniques.

Contemporary approaches to healthcare marketing emphasize customer relationships, the most recent of which is the consumer engagement movement. Experience has shown that promoting health services to consumers is becoming increasingly challenging. Consumers must be at a stage where they understand the importance of availing themselves of a service. Ultimately, consumers must be engaged to a point where they proactively participate in the management of their health. The task of engaging consumers will increasingly fall on marketers.

Key Points

- Healthcare, like other industries, has moved beyond traditional marketing techniques and adopted more sophisticated techniques that take advantage of information technology.
- Much of this shift in type of technique has been driven by the need to develop and maintain relationships rather than simply sell products.
- The ascendancy of electronic forms of communication has revolutionized the marketing industry.
- To employ contemporary marketing techniques, marketers require much more in-depth knowledge of the target audience than in the past.
- Direct-to-consumer marketing recognizes the importance of the consumer as the end user and targets identifiable segments of the population.
- The significance of business-to-business marketing in healthcare is often overlooked, but this form of marketing plays a major role in the industry.
- Internal marketing focuses on internal customers to create a culture that fosters customer service and turns all employees into marketers.
- Aggressive healthcare organizations are offering concierge services to cater to customers who desire special attention, and an increasing number of traditional health professionals are adopting a concierge-type approach.

- Database marketing takes advantage of information technology to create a repository of consumer data that can be used for relationship development and management and in follow-up sales efforts.
- Customer relationship management (CRM) is an approach that builds on database marketing to establish intensive relationships with customers.
- Internet marketing has become pivotal for many healthcare organizations, as a cyberspace presence serves as the interface for most of the organization's marketing activities.
- The emergence of social media is something of a revolution in communication and is beginning to have an impact on healthcare marketing.
- *Consumer engagement* has become the new buzzword in healthcare, as providers, health plans, and employers seek to proactively engage consumers in ways that positively influence their behavior.
- The nature of healthcare limits the application of certain contemporary forms of marketing, although most of these barriers are slowly being overcome.

Discussion Questions

- What marketing and/or healthcare factors are encouraging the adoption of more sophisticated marketing techniques?
- How has the discovery of the consumer influenced healthcare organizations' approach to marketing?
- In the pharmaceutical industry, why is direct-to-consumer marketing a radical departure from traditional approaches to marketing?
- What developments in healthcare have encouraged the growth of business-to-business marketing?
- In what ways can a healthcare organization use a customer database?
- What factors have influenced the trend toward establishing long-term relationships, as opposed to trying to secure an immediate sale from the healthcare consumer?
- What characteristics of healthcare call for a cautious approach to the application of technology-based marketing techniques?
- As Internet marketing has matured, how has this approach to healthcare marketing progressed?
- Why has consumer engagement become such a concern in healthcare, and what is the marketer's responsibility with regard to promoting this initiative?

Additional Resources

Bunik, M., J. E. Glazner, V. Chandramouli, C. B. Emsermann, T. Hegarty, and A. Kempe. 2007. "Pediatric Telephone Call Centers: How Do They Affect Health Care Use and Costs?" *Pediatrics* 119 (2): e305–13.

Herzenstein, M., S. Misra, and S. S. Posavac. 2005. "How Consumers' Attitudes Toward Direct-to-Consumer Advertising of Prescription Drugs Influence Ad Effectiveness, and Consumer and Physician Behavior." *Marketing Letters* 15 (4): 201–12.

Shankland, S. 2003. "To DTC or Not to DTC? Direct to Consumer Advertising Can Seem Like a Prescription for Futility." *Marketing Health Services* 23 (4): 44.

HEALTHCARE MARKETING IN INTERNATIONAL PERSPECTIVE

One of the emerging trends over the past two decades has been the internationalization of healthcare. This "movement" has involved adaptation of the U.S. healthcare system to the needs of immigrants and foreign nationals and expansion of American healthcare interests overseas. Despite world events that have caused many people to cut back on international travel, made visas more difficult to acquire in certain parts of the world, and put money transfer between countries under increased scrutiny, more people are seeking healthcare abroad than ever before.

For at least 20 years, U.S. policymakers have called for modification to the U.S. system to accommodate a growing immigrant population, and prestigious U.S. medical facilities have a long history of treating foreign notables. Now, reports from a variety of organizations reveal the extent to which U.S. healthcare organizations are serving immigrants inside the United States (Kaiser Family Foundation 2003), attracting patients from abroad (Van Dusen 2008), and establishing satellite facilities in foreign countries (Are 2009). More recently, "medical tourism" has prompted a growing number of Americans to seek care overseas (Smart Money 2007).

None of these developments should be surprising. For decades, the world has been shrinking as international travel has grown. The ability to receive news almost instantaneously from anywhere in the world has expanded everyone's worldview, and access to the Internet has made almost anyone in any country only a few clicks away. The explosion of international communication is a symptom of the globalization process that has been taking place for decades. This development has been spurred in some part by the expansion of international trade, but the emergence of multinational corporations that rival nation-states in their resources and influence has also been a major contributor. Their multinational character actually makes them more powerful than many countries because of their pan-national influence.

The internationalization of U.S. healthcare can be traced to the surge of immigration beginning in the 1980s. The growing immigrant population in the United States has raised sensitivity to the needs of non-Americans. Even more significant in the expansion of international medicine, however, are the forces of supply and demand. Population growth in the United States has been slow, and a variety of healthcare interests have sought to reduce the utilization of health services, particularly high-dollar inpatient services. As a result, some sectors of the U.S. healthcare industry have been left with unused capacity, leading health systems to cast a wider net in hopes of attracting patients from distant shores, particularly for hospital care and high-end elective surgery.

Changes outside the United States are also contributing to the expansion of international medicine. The economies of many foreign countries have been growing, and the demand for modern health services has outstripped the ability of some of these countries to provide them. This mismatch between an increasing demand for health services and dearth of local resources has led growing numbers of foreign nationals to seek health services in the United States. Conversely, U.S. health services providers have stepped up efforts to establish facilities in foreign countries. At the same time, some foreign countries have established health systems equal to or superior to those in the United States (usually with U.S.-trained medical staff) and as a result have attracted a worldwide following (including U.S. citizens). In many countries, issues surrounding centrally controlled healthcare systems have led to the growth of private-sector healthcare.

The growing middle class worldwide is also influencing the demand for health services. The increasing demand for high-quality and accessible health services is putting pressure on resource-constrained health ministries to improve services, even in some developing countries. With greater disposable income, individuals are more willing and able to pay for health services, or at least to share the cost of higher-quality and accessible care. For organizations seeking to expand infrastructure and services, the prospect of foreign investment is inviting.

Trends in International Healthcare

American Health Systems and Foreign Patients

Historically, U.S. medicine has been the standard that other countries have striven to achieve. Despite the obvious problems in the American system, hundreds of foreign healthcare professionals come to the United States every year to train; foreign governments routinely study U.S. models and approaches to medical care; and thousands of international patients seek care provided by U.S. healthcare facilities. More recently, foreign countries have been borrowing American ideas with regard to managing health insurance, applying new information technologies, and encouraging competition in healthcare. To many outside its borders, the United States maintains a sterling reputation for highly trained physicians, state-of-the-art medical equipment and facilities, high customer service standards, and expeditious access to treatment.

Canada and Mexico already provide a steady flow of patients to U.S. healthcare facilities. Canadians primarily enter the United States for routine care rather than for onetime major surgery. Now, many healthcare organizations are finding a rich source of patients in Europe, Asia, the Middle East, and other parts of the world. As mentioned earlier, the fast-growing economies and populations of developing countries such as China and India are creating a demand for health services that exceeds the ability of these countries to provide them. Given the growth of the global economy and the reputation of the United States for healthcare excellence, more and more healthcare businesses are expected to explore ways to market to international patients.

Healthcare providers in the United States can benefit in a number of ways by serving international patients. They can attain national and international recognition; inspire loyalty in certain countries, regions, and referral sources; gain experience by treating medical cases of greater severity and complexity; and receive maximum reimbursement. These factors create a strong incentive for healthcare providers to court foreign consumers and their interest in U.S. medical care.

U.S. Health Systems with Overseas Branches

Many U.S. hospitals and health systems have developed institutional affiliations with facilities abroad or established independent operations in foreign countries. The relationships that support such endeavors take a variety of forms, from U.S. investment in foreign facilities, to partnerships between U.S. entities and local entities, to the outright ownership of facilities on foreign soil by U.S. corporations. Other forms of interaction between U.S. medical interests and foreign healthcare systems include clinical consultation, organizational management consultation, architectural design and engineering, regulatory and accreditation support, and staff training and development.

In most cases, facilities are being established abroad by existing U.S. healthcare systems. For example, Johns Hopkins Medical Center in Baltimore, Maryland; St. Jude Children's Research Hospital in Memphis, Tennessee; and Harvard Medical School in Cambridge, Massachusetts, have attempted to replicate their domestic facilities in South America, Asia, and the Middle East. In addition to these not-for-profit organizations, many large healthcare corporations in the United States have become multinational corporations by expanding into countries around the world. Hospital Corporation of America (HCA), National Medical Enterprises (now Tenet Healthcare), Sun Healthcare, Integrated Health Systems, and many others have developed international holdings to some extent. When organizations are facing a flat U.S. market, foreign countries provide opportunities for expansion, and some U.S. companies have even been set up exclusively for the purpose of establishing U.S.-style health facilities overseas.

Other types of healthcare organizations are also discovering investment opportunities abroad. American health insurance companies, home health companies, and medical healthcare technology companies, for example, are all experimenting with exporting their expertise while importing new sources of revenue and growth.

Another area of expansion involves the administration of clinical trials for new drugs in foreign countries. The U.S. pharmaceutical industry is increasing the proportion of its clinical trials conducted outside the United States to lower costs, expedite approval, and test drugs in the countries where they will be sold. Nearly half of drug industry spending for human drug testing took place outside the United States in 2007, and the number of overseas clinical trials increases by about 15 percent each year (Gardner 2009). This figure does not indicate a decline in the number of U.S.-based clinical trials but an increase in the number of foreign trials. Pharmaceutical companies can reportedly reduce human-testing costs significantly by conducting trials in Eastern Europe, Asia, and Central and South America. Some nations even request that drugs be tested on their population before approving them for use.

Marketing U.S. Healthcare Products Abroad

American companies have a long history of selling domestically produced healthcare products overseas. With its strong manufacturing sector, the United States has produced the lion's share of industrial healthcare goods (e.g., medical equipment) and consumer healthcare goods (e.g., baby formula). The United States has also been the world's largest producer of pharmaceutical products. In 2008, U.S. companies' overseas sales for medical supplies and equipment were estimated at $20 billion (U.S. Department of Commerce 2009). The share of products produced in the United States is somewhat difficult to determine, however, given the trend toward establishing factories overseas to produce "American-made" goods.

Overseas markets for healthcare products are considered attractive because of their higher growth rates. For example, the demand for medical supplies in developing countries such as China and India is growing three times faster than the demand in countries with mature markets, such as the United States and most European countries. In the U.S. market, competition is fierce and cost-containment has driven down margins, but foreign markets are still relatively untapped and underserved.

Foreign Health Systems/International Patients

Although the U.S. healthcare system has a long history of treating foreign patients and selling healthcare products overseas, the emergence of modern, state-of-the-art healthcare systems in Central and South America, Asia, and the Middle East is a relatively new phenomenon. For the most part, these facilities have been established to meet the needs of increasingly affluent indigenous populations; international medical travel has been a long-standing practice, in fact, for the affluent in many countries. However, many facilities have found it profitable to serve "regular" patients from those countries.

Medical tourism pairs a medical experience with an opportunity to visit the attractions in a foreign country. This term is something of a misnomer, however, in that today, relatively few so-called medical tourists consider the recreational part of the experience to be as important as the clinical component. Thus, a more appropriate label for this activity might be "international medical travel."

Increasingly, U.S. residents who are uninsured or underinsured, or who want elective surgeries and procedures, are considering and often choosing doctors, surgeons, medical facilities, and hospitals abroad, where costs are a fraction of what they are at home and the quality of care is substantially the same or—some would argue—even better.

India is often considered the premier example of international medical care, known for its quality of care, relatively low prices, and the opportunity for a vacation for those who so choose. Private entities have established facilities to cater to foreigners, despite the fact that the country's domestic needs outstrip the system's capacity. Other countries attracting international patients include Singapore, Dubai, Thailand, and Malaysia, and, closer to home, Mexico, Costa Rica, Panama, and Argentina. The facilities in some countries may specialize in certain types of conditions or procedures, such as cardiac surgery, orthopedic surgery, and cosmetic surgery. See Exhibit 12.1 for the results of a Gallup poll on international medical travel.

Some important trends guarantee that the market for medical tourism will continue to expand in the years ahead. In the United States, an estimated 47 million people lacked health insurance in 2008, and this number is expected to grow (Johnson 2008). Patients in Britain, Canada, and other countries on waiting lists for major surgery have been just as eager to take advantage of foreign healthcare options. By 2015, the health of the 220 million+ baby boomers in the United States, Canada, Europe, Australia, and New Zealand will have begun its slow, final decline and will create a significant market for inexpensive, high-quality medical care.

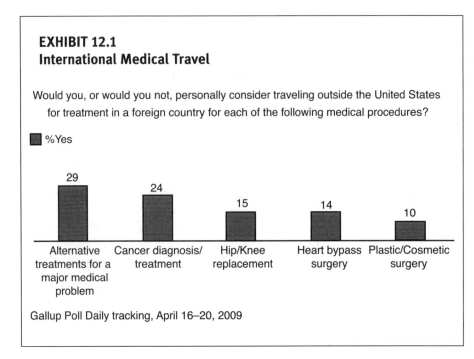

EXHIBIT 12.1
International Medical Travel

Would you, or would you not, personally consider traveling outside the United States for treatment in a foreign country for each of the following medical procedures?

■ %Yes

29 Alternative treatments for a major medical problem	
24 Cancer diagnosis/ treatment	
15 Hip/Knee replacement	
14 Heart bypass surgery	
10 Plastic/Cosmetic surgery	

Gallup Poll Daily tracking, April 16–20, 2009

Factors Contributing to the Growth of International Medical Travel

A number of factors will ensure that the volume of international medical travel will continue to increase for the foreseeable future, including

- massive investment in private-sector health infrastructure in certain developing countries, resulting in significant improvements in health standards and greater availability of the latest medical care technology and treatment;
- increasingly prohibitive medical costs in many European and American countries (see Exhibit 12.2 for comparative figures);
- the growing level of expertise of indigenous doctors and support staff who have trained in some of the best centers in the world, coupled with the continuing shortage of skilled medical care staff and specialties in developed countries;
- deficiencies in the public health systems in many countries, including long delays for services and bureaucratic hurdles to obtaining care;
- the positive experiences of patients who have received excellent care overseas and experienced a level of personal service unknown in the United States;
- a well-organized medical travel industry supporting the development of attractive packages of services and amenities and offering extensive support for those interested in traveling for healthcare; and

EXHIBIT 12.2
Comparative International Pricing by Procedure:
United States, Singapore, Thailand, and India, July 2009

Procedure	Comparative Pricing (in U.S. dollars)			
	United States	**Singapore**	**Thailand**	**India**
Heart valve replacement	$170,000	$13,500	$22,000	$1,200
Heart bypass	144,000	13,500	24,000	8,500
Angioplasty	57,000	7,500	7,000	8,500
Hip replacement	50,000	11,100	14,000	8,000
Knee replacement	50,000	10,800	12,000	7,000
Hysterectomy	15,000	4,000	5,000	5,500

Source: Medical Tourism Association (2009).

- for some patients, the opportunity to experience a foreign culture and visit tourist attractions.

Perceptions/Misconceptions About International Medical Travel

Marketers who promote international medical travel must address three common misconceptions. The first is that international medical travel is something of a gimmick, that the idea of obtaining health services at a 30 to 80 percent discount seems too good to be true. Many people think that either the care will not be as good or the surgery will be performed in a primitive setting. These misconceptions suggest that many Americans are not familiar with other cultures and have a hard time believing that care elsewhere could be comparable to U.S. healthcare, which they perceive to be the best care in the world.

A second common misconception is the fun-and-sun perception. In the early years, the Internet was filled with promotions from health travel brokers touting the notion that you can have your cosmetic surgery (e.g., liposuction) and then lie on the beach for ten days. This aspect of medical tourism is highlighted less today as the industry has matured, and the news media have begun to address some of the more important aspects of international medical travel, such as quality of care and personalized service.

A third misconception is that international medical travel is all about outsourcing U.S. services to overseas vendors—that is, foreign entities, in collaboration with U.S. interests, are establishing facilities overseas to siphon off patients from U.S. healthcare providers. In actuality, most of the hospitals that are attracting the international medical traveler in Asia, South America, and the Middle East were not built with the U.S. patient but rather international medical travelers from Europe, the Middle East, and Africa in mind.

People who become international medical travelers can be grouped into four categories—although the underlying consideration in most cases is economics. Among U.S. citizens who travel abroad for medical care, the largest group is probably those who lack insurance coverage for some major operation. Given the increasing cost of medical care in the United States, it is not surprising that those who need expensive operations are seeking cost-effective alternatives. As illustrated in Exhibit 12.2, a patient without medical insurance could save tremendous out-of-pocket costs on a variety of procedures performed overseas. By undergoing a total hip replacement in India rather than in the United States, the patient would realize nearly $42,000 in savings (minus the cost of the trip).

Another category of international medical traveler is the growing number of underinsured Americans who, despite having some level of insurance coverage, face high deductibles or are unable to pay for the portion of their medical expenses not covered by their existing insurance plan. As shown in Exhibit 12.2, if a coronary bypass graft costs $144,000 in the United States and insurance pays only 80 percent of the cost, a U.S. patient will still owe $28,800, so he or she would be better off undergoing this procedure in India, where the total cost for the procedure is $8,500.

Another major category of international medical travelers consists of those seeking elective surgery. In the U.S. healthcare system, such procedures are not considered medically necessary and include face-lifts, tummy tucks, hair transplants, and similar vanity services. Even some procedures that would improve mobility (e.g., correction of tennis elbow) may not be considered medically necessary if the person's functional limitation is not that prohibitive. The "pioneers" in this group were celebrities who went abroad for cosmetic surgery. They have since been joined by a growing number of average Americans who are concerned about their appearance but cannot pay out of pocket for expensive cosmetic surgery.

The final group of international medical travelers includes Americans seeking services that are not available in the United States. Perhaps the most publicized of these services are certain treatments for cancer. Some of these procedures may fail to meet U.S. standards (that some may consider unreasonable), while others may still be under review in the United States and are likely to be approved at some time in the future. Although there are risks involved in the use of such services (e.g., lack of recourse in the case of malpractice), the possibility of incurring them does not appear to have prevented thousands of Americans from taking advantage of these treatments.

Increasingly, health insurance companies and major employers are encouraging international medical travel on the part of U.S. citizens. Insurers that are at risk for the cost of care may profit from referring their plan members to overseas medical facilities; some have even entered into formal relationships with foreign hospitals. Some U.S. employers, concerned about rising healthcare costs, are using financial incentives (e.g., subsidizing the cost of travel) to encourage employees to utilize less costly services overseas. This practice is especially common in large firms that self-insure and pay directly for their employees' medical expenses.

Some level of backlash has occurred in the United States in response to the increase in international medical travel. Representatives of U.S. healthcare systems are concerned about patients being siphoned off to competitors in other countries. Realistically, the proportion of U.S. patients traveling overseas is still small, and U.S. medical facilities have enough of a challenge dealing with existing patients. Unions have raised concerns over the fact that their members were being encouraged by their health plans to go to foreign countries for care in apparent violation of "buy American" restrictions. These types of reactions are to be expected as the United States adapts to the increasing globalization of healthcare.

Limited definitive research is available on the factors that make a foreign health facility successful at attracting and effectively serving international medical travelers. However, consensus in the medical tourism industry points to four critical factors. Organizations must

- assure prospective patients that their facilities and the skill levels of their practitioners meet or exceed U.S. standards;
- partner with representatives in targeted countries who can provide assurance and support to prospective patients;
- develop as complete a package as possible that combines all aspects of the experience—travel, lodging, medical expenses, rehabilitation, touring, and so on; and
- offer the type of personal attention that is so often lacking in U.S. healthcare.

Market Research on International Healthcare

To date, limited research has been conducted on international aspects of healthcare, and few official statistics are available on the number of immigrants treated in U.S. hospitals or the number of foreign patients who travel to the United States for care. Some U.S. healthcare organizations have begun to track their international patients and carry out research on their characteristics and motives, but this information remains fragmented, and little progress has been made toward any national means of tracking these data.

Various organizations, including the federal government and certain trade organizations, track the export of medical products from the United States to other countries. Some research organizations also study trends in the sale of U.S. healthcare products around the world. Some organizations have emerged to promote international medical travel (e.g., Medical Tourism Association) and/or collect data from their member organizations (Joint Commission International). Much of this information is collected at the country level and does not necessarily provide a comprehensive account of the actual volume of activity. Even within a country, it is difficult to track all of the activity related to international medical travel.

Among the U.S. institutions carrying out research on international medical travel is Mayo Clinic. In a typical year, Mayo Clinic may treat 10,000 foreign patients from as many as 160 countries. Because serving foreign patients is such a significant part of its business, Mayo Clinic conducts research on its patients, international physicians, and international healthcare consumers to gain an understanding of why people leave their communities for healthcare, why some of them come to Mayo Clinic, and why others do not. See Case Study 12.1 on research on international patients at Mayo Clinic.

CASE STUDY 12.1
International Market Research at Mayo Clinic

One hundred years ago, the founders of Mayo Clinic began to research international medicine by traveling around the world to take notes and compare surgical approaches. This emphasis on international medical research continues today through the wide range of research initiatives conducted by Mayo Clinic staff. Several aspects of its international medical research are worth noting.

First, Mayo Clinic carefully tracks trends in its international medical business. To determine which countries are most predictable in terms of the behavior of their patients and where to anticipate an increase in patient volume, the clinic monitors its international data each quarter, carefully observing trends over time by country or region and tracking significant changes in volume, hospitalization rates, and percentage of new patients from any given market.

Second, Mayo Clinic gathers and analyzes feedback from its internal "salespeople"—that is, the physicians and support staff who deliver care to its international patients. Through carefully moderated focus groups, marketers identify barriers to providing excellent care as well as areas that are running smoothly.

Third, Mayo Clinic conducts quantitative and qualitative research on the international marketplace. It collects data from patients, international physicians, and international healthcare consumers to determine how healthcare decisions are being made so the clinic's marketers can better help decision makers, physicians, and staff understand their patients' needs.

As part of its ongoing research effort, the clinic conducts periodic and ongoing patient surveys that measure international patients' satisfaction with various aspects of the care they receive. To date, it has surveyed nearly 1,500 patients in 20 countries and in four different languages. These surveys have shown that the key driver of international patient satisfaction is excellent care, manifested by the physicians' willingness to listen and explain and the clinician's thoroughness. Other factors, such as the quality of language interpretation and waiting times, are also important to the international healthcare experience. To support the clinic's mission, the marketing staff also studies the wants and needs of Mayo patients as well as their preferences and behavior patterns.

Mayo Clinic will undoubtedly continue to be part of the international medical scene, and its physicians will continue to collaborate with colleagues around the world. International medical research can be expected to drive strategy development and marketing at Mayo Clinic for the foreseeable future.

Source: Adapted from Hathaway and Seltman (2001).

Discussion Questions
- Why is the topic of international medicine important to Mayo Clinic?
- What are some of the research techniques Mayo Clinic uses to develop a better understanding of the international medical travel phenomenon?
- Why are patient satisfaction studies important to Mayo Clinic?
- What are some of the research questions Mayo Clinic staff need answered for the clinic to be able to increase its share of international patients?

The Four Ps and International Marketing

As noted in previous chapters, the four Ps of the marketing mix (product, price, place, and promotion) do not apply easily to U.S. healthcare. The products (except for some elective procedures) are highly standardized. Price is so controlled by third-party payers that it seldom serves as a basis for differentiation between service providers. Place has become more of a factor in recent years, as the need to take services to the customer has become more important. The promotion aspect of the marketing mix has the most application in U.S. healthcare because most healthcare organizations must compete for customers.

The *product* dimension of the marketing mix is relevant in marketing to international patients. Obviously, U.S.-based healthcare systems want to package the product in a manner that reflects the high quality associated with U.S. healthcare. Product presentation should emphasize the use of state-of-the-art technology and assure patients that the most up-to-date procedures are followed. Foreign-based health facilities often develop a comprehensive package that includes travel arrangements, medical services, and, most important, the personal attention that may be lacking in U.S. healthcare. Large tertiary medical centers and teaching hospitals will always have a competitive advantage, as will healthcare systems that have built national and international reputations.

The *price* dimension is the most salient aspect of the marketing mix for international medical travelers. As noted, the primary draw for U.S. patients is the lower cost associated with the services provided in overseas facilities. Of course, the price differential is meaningless unless the services are equivalent. For patients in other countries, price is likely to be a consideration, but it is not as paramount as it is for American patients. For patients from countries that do not offer certain services, the mere availability of these services in the United States may be the most important factor.

The *place* dimension is intrinsic to the concept of seeking healthcare in another country. The cachet associated with the United States is an advantage to U.S.-based healthcare organizations. The location itself is attractive to many patients in other countries, and the high regard in which U.S. medicine is held around the world is a major asset. Major cities and ports in the United States are key geographic draws for international patients who find entering and leaving the country easier at these locales. Foreign nationals who seek medical care in the United States are often drawn to tourist areas and major attractions and, thus, are marketing targets for U.S. healthcare organizations. On the other hand, some foreign-based healthcare systems have highlighted the hospitable setting in which an international medical traveler will be able to recuperate.

With regard to the *promotion* dimension of the marketing mix (described in more detail in a later section), U.S. and foreign entities are more similar. Health systems in both areas prepare standard promotional materials and present their case at professional meetings and exhibitions. Beyond these basic promotional activities, foreign-based facilities appear to rely more heavily on word-of-mouth recommendations than U.S.-based facilities do. In addition, foreign-based health systems typically maintain offices or agents in other countries who serve as liaisons between the facilities and prospective patients in those countries.

International Marketing Strategies

Whether an organization already enjoys a large base of international business or is currently building an international program, its success depends on a detailed business strategy and a solid marketing plan. World-class institutions do not have to advertise aggressively but can rely instead on their reputation and brand to attract international referrals and patients. Smaller medical centers that are less well known (the bulk of the institutions in the United States) must make a greater effort to generate awareness and referrals to their programs and carve out a niche.

The marketing strategy that an organization decides to pursue will depend on the types of goods or services it offers and its location. The approach taken by U.S. health systems catering to international medical travelers will differ from the approach taken by those that solicit patients from the United States and other countries (Fell 2002). Marketers of U.S. health systems can capitalize on and promote the following attributes:

- *International brand reputation.* A good international reputation will help make a facility prominent in the minds of potential patients and, perhaps more important, opinion leaders in the target country.
- *Internationally known physicians.* Although prospective patients may not be knowledgeable about individual physicians, their local medical contacts might be, so their reputations will create momentum.
- *Internationally recognized clinical expertise in a specialty.* When someone is considering treatment for a particular condition, such as cancer, heart disease, or liver disease, that person will think first of a healthcare organization recognized for its expertise in that clinical area.
- *International reputation of U.S. medicine.* Marketers of U.S. healthcare organizations can capitalize on the premium placed on all things American. The worldwide reputation of U.S medicine and its history of innovation can be promoted to prospective customers who already have a high opinion of America.

U.S. healthcare organizations seeking to establish facilities in other countries might consider a different strategic framework. In this case, marketers might adopt one of the following strategies:

- *A relationship-based strategy.* This approach takes advantage of existing relationships between domestic health systems and foreign individuals, groups, and organizations. Ideally, a new facility in a foreign country could be presented as a tangible extension of an existing relationship between health professionals.
- *A needs-based strategy.* This approach focuses on gaps in existing services in other countries and seeks to fulfill an unmet need.
- *A product-oriented strategy.* This approach emphasizes the expertise, quality, and technological sophistication associated with U.S.-style medicine.
- *A partnering strategy.* This approach recognizes the importance of involving local entities to facilitate patients' entry into what they might perceive as an alien culture.

To attract international customers, foreign-based healthcare organizations may pursue one of yet another set of strategies:

- *A service-based strategy.* This approach emphasizes high-quality services that take advantage of the best specialists and the latest biomedical technology to provide a superior experience comparable to U.S.-style medicine in terms of skill and quality.
- *A price-based strategy.* This approach capitalizes on the significant cost differential between most foreign health systems and the U.S. system and promises a level of quality that is equal or better.
- *A patient-centered strategy.* This approach emphasizes the personal attention that will be accorded the patient who chooses to use a foreign-based health facility.
- *A collateral benefit strategy.* This approach promises not only a positive healthcare experience but also an opportunity to experience a different culture.

International Marketing Techniques

Regardless of the direction of flow of international medical patients, many of the same marketing techniques may be effective. Any international marketer, however, must recognize that, to be successful, a campaign of this type cannot just offer a little information in another language on the organization's website; it must follow an integrated marketing strategy. A healthcare organization catering to international patients, regardless of where they reside, should

- design a website that provides a point of first contact for international patients and engages them from first exposure through release from rehabilitation therapy;
- employ experienced call center and support staff who can coordinate all aspects of a patient's care, including travel, cross-cultural considerations, and personal needs;
- establish field offices and base sales representatives abroad to ensure continuity with marketing contacts and referral channel management;
- offer tours for international business, consumer, civic, and medical groups to showcase the facilities and services to potential healthcare audiences;
- maintain relationships with physicians and medical professionals who are active in international medical circles and support exchange programs, mission trips, and educational conferences;
- take advantage of relationships with medical schools and residency programs that train foreign physicians;
- cultivate relationships with U.S. companies that have international operations (and foreign companies that have U.S. operations) that could serve as venues for marketing to international patients;
- work with the ministries of foreign governments and, for U.S. firms, American embassies and other overseas government offices to gain access to referral lists and identify potential partners for overseas ventures;
- look for ways to partner with organizations involved in international programs (e.g., sister city programs) and consider partnering with the local chamber of commerce to promote hometown health facilities;
- initiate carefully thought-out international advertising as part of a coordinated marketing and communications effort;
- maintain ongoing public relations efforts to highlight recent successes, medical breakthroughs, new technology, and exceptional physicians; and
- maintain listings in international medical directories, both print and online, even if some cost is involved.

See Case Study 12.2 for an example of a country's international marketing efforts.

CASE STUDY 12.2
Marketing Medical Tourism in Asia

During the 1990s, Ballistan,* a small Asian country with a modern healthcare system and a strong economy, recognized the potential benefits of international medical travel. Its medical professionals and government officials felt that its healthcare system had features that would be attractive to medical tourists. The potential for revenue generation from this source was thought to be such that the national government had a vested interest in the success of the country's healthcare facilities.

To promote medical tourism, a government agency was established to attract international business. The agency was funded by the national government and operated with the full cooperation of the country's healthcare organizations. The agency was established at the ministry level, and the director of the medical tourism agency was a high-ranking government official.

One of the first steps the agency took was to assess the current situation with regard to the domestic need for health services and the availability of local facilities. It assessed existing capacity, took an inventory of medical equipment, and determined the number and qualifications of existing medical personnel. The agency also assessed the system's ability to meet domestic needs *and* serve an international clientele. Further, it estimated the size of the international market and calculated potential revenue.

Having determined that there was a large and growing market with substantial resources to spend on healthcare and that the system would be able to absorb a substantial number of international patients, the medical tourism ministry developed a multipronged marketing initiative. It embarked on a campaign to raise the awareness of medical tourism in the countries that had the most potential patients (i.e., elsewhere in Asia, in the Middle East, and in the United States). It followed up that campaign with another to promote the country of Ballistan and its healthcare resources. The communications media used in these campaigns included a series of newspaper, magazine, journal, and e-zine articles. These print materials were supplemented with promotional brochures and a state-of-the-art website that not only featured the country's health facilities but also served as a source of information on international medical travel. Although some paid advertising was used, the ministry felt that paid advertising was the least effective means of reaching the target population.

To facilitate international medical travel, comprehensive packages were put together in conjunction with the nation's travel and hospitality industries. These packages allowed blanket fees to be established for all components of the medical tourism experience. The all-inclusive package would cover travel expenses, medical expenses, rehabilitation as appropriate, follow-up care, and, if desired, options for visiting local attractions.

To facilitate patient access to the country's health facilities, liaison offices were established in several foreign countries to ensure that someone in-country was available to answer questions and coordinate arrangements for the international medical experience. In addition, relationships were developed with key medical practitioners in each of the targeted countries to establish legitimacy and ensure a source of referrals. Negotiations were carried out with health insurance plans that agreed to refer some of their cases to this country's practitioners.

In developing the case for international medical travel, the ministry highlighted the benefits of obtaining care in Ballistan. These benefits included state-of-the-art facilities staffed by English-speaking experts who had been trained in the United States; quality of care that was equal to or exceeded that found anywhere else in the world; personal attention to international medical travelers before, during, and after their medical experience; and the cultural opportunities available to visitors and their families. At the same time, these promotional materials attempted to neutralize the negative factors sometimes associated with traveling overseas for medical care.

The campaign to promote medical tourism in this country was highly successful, particularly with regard to the U.S. market. Patients who had never heard of the country began to flock to its cities to take advantage of its high-quality, low-cost facilities. A growing number of patients had commercial insurance that fully or partly covered the cost of care, but those who paid out of pocket were delighted to pay only a fraction of what they would have paid for the same procedures in the United States. Notably, research revealed an extremely high level of patient satisfaction with regard to the outcomes of care and the manner in which it was delivered—a critical finding, considering the importance of word of mouth in raising awareness and acceptance of medical tourism.

* Fictional country

(continued)

CASE STUDY 12.2 (*continued*)

Discussion Questions
- What prompted officials in Ballistan to consider entering the medical tourism business?
- What steps were taken to research the current status and future potential of medical tourism?
- What factors encouraged government officials to develop a marketing campaign to attract international medical travelers?
- What marketing techniques did the government agency use to promote medical tourism?
- What role did relationship development play in implementing the promotional strategy?
- How effective was the government-sponsored initiative in encouraging the development of a thriving medical tourism industry?

What Is Most Important to International Healthcare Consumers?

Both U.S- and foreign-based healthcare organizations have identified the following as prerequisites for attracting an international clientele:

- *Excellent care.* High-quality service is a must for those hoping to compete in this arena. Patients will travel to another country for services only if they are assured that they will receive the best services possible.
- *Physician thoroughness.* Most international patients are looking for a physician who will personally ensure that their needs are met. This factor may be less important to U.S. patients who are not used to receiving personal attention.
- *Word-of-mouth reputation.* Given that health facilities catering to an international market are of recent origin (except for some in the United States), they do not have the established reputation of an organization like Mayo Clinic or MD Anderson. Therefore, word-of-mouth recommendations are a critical factor in promotions.

- *Physician recommendation.* Most people are not likely to be familiar with the medical facilities in another country. Some may not even be familiar with the world-class organizations in other countries. For this reason, few people will travel overseas for health services without referral by a medical professional in their home country.

Summary

One of the trends over the past two decades has been the internationalization of healthcare. This movement began with the rise of "immigrant medicine" in the United States and continued with the expansion of U.S. healthcare organizations to meet the needs of international patients, the establishment of world-class medical facilities in foreign countries, and the increased flow of patients across international borders for medical care. Healthcare organizations in the United States have a long history of competing in the international healthcare market. Today, they are joined by providers of quality clinical services in (sometimes unlikely) worldwide locations.

To compete in a global healthcare environment, an organization must have more than just a desire to serve foreign consumers. The institutions and companies that are successful today have been working at it for decades and have learned what does and does not work. With a growing number of U.S. organizations (as well as other international healthcare groups) competing for the same business, U.S. companies will have to work harder to differentiate themselves. An organization that simply promotes quality or advanced technology will not stand out when ten other organizations are doing the same. Identifying and marketing attributes that make an institution or a medical program unique will be the key to future success in a crowded international healthcare marketplace.

The approach an organization takes to promote international medical tourism depends on its attributes and goals. For example, a U.S. health system seeking to attract foreign patients from a hospital in Singapore would employ a different strategy than that pursued by a hospital in Panama seeking to attract U.S. patients. A U.S. healthcare organization would attempt to capitalize on the cachet of all things American; a foreign facility, on the other hand, might tout its "American-style" facility while emphasizing the level of personal service its staff can provide. Packaging is clearly important for health systems seeking to attract international patients, and even successful U.S. operations must offer comprehensive services (e.g., travel, lodging, amenities, and perhaps even a package price) in addition to medical care.

The interest in international medical travel will likely continue to grow, and marketers will continue to support medical staff by studying patients' wants, needs, preferences, and behavior patterns and learning all that they can about the ever-changing, rich, and diverse worldwide healthcare market. Overall, provision of outstanding medical care and sensitive service to patients and families will be the most productive marketing strategy.

Key Points

- Healthcare has undergone globalization in much the same manner as other industries.
- The world is shrinking with regard to healthcare, and historical barriers to cross-national health services have been reduced.
- The populations served by U.S. healthcare organizations over the years have become increasingly diverse. Some healthcare systems have catered to foreign patients for decades.
- As long as the U.S. market for inpatient services remains flat, more attention is likely to be paid to the growing pool of patients in other countries.
- U.S. medical supply and equipment companies, as well as pharmaceutical companies, have a long history of selling U.S. healthcare products overseas.
- Foreign-based healthcare facilities have emerged primarily to address the needs of local and regional patients, but they also have a growing interest in international patients.
- Market research on international patients has been limited to date. There is a lot more to be learned about the subject. The more information marketers have, the more effective their promotion will be.
- Several countries in Asia, the Middle East, and Latin America have developed facilities to rival those in the United States and are attracting a worldwide clientele.
- Foreign health facilities compete in terms of price and quality and often distinguish themselves by emphasizing the personal service they provide.
- The attributes of product, price, place, and promotion have different implications for international medical services than for traditional U.S. healthcare services.
- Both U.S.- and foreign-based healthcare organizations should implement a multipronged marketing strategy that emphasizes personal interaction between health professionals and prospective patients.

Discussion Questions

- What factors are contributing to the increasing internationalization of healthcare?
- What role have U.S. healthcare entities historically played in international healthcare?
- What developments have allowed foreign-based health facilities to compete with U.S. facilities for patients, including U.S. citizens?
- What attributes of U.S. health facilities have historically attracted foreign patients?
- What factors have led to the dramatic increase in the number of U.S. citizens who are traveling to other countries for medical care?
- What concerns have been raised about medical services in foreign countries, and how have these concerns been addressed?
- Does the migration of U.S. patients to other countries negatively affect the U.S. healthcare system and economy? If so, how?
- What factors should marketers be sensitive to when seeking to attract foreign patients to a U.S. health system?

Additional Resources

Bookman, M. Z., and K. R. Bookman. 2007. *Medical Tourism in Developing Countries*. Basingstoke, UK: Palgrave Macmillan.
Medical Tourism website: www.medicaltourism.com

IV

MANAGING AND SUPPORTING THE MARKETING EFFORT

It is one thing to come up with a marketing idea but another to develop and implement a marketing plan or coordinate a marketing campaign. To carry out these activities, marketers must understand the entire marketing process and have process management skills. This section addresses the nuts and bolts of organizing, developing, and implementing marketing initiatives. The marketing initiative is described from beginning to end, and techniques for evaluating the effectiveness of marketing initiatives are discussed. Part IV also covers the support activities that make effective marketing possible, such as marketing planning and research.

Chapter 13 outlines the steps in the marketing process, from concept to marketing plan to project implementation, and breaks down those steps into activities. It discusses budgeting for marketing activities and the role of outside agencies in healthcare marketing. Techniques for assessing the effectiveness of a marketing initiative are also described.

Chapter 14 presents an overview of the different types of marketing research undertaken in healthcare and describes the techniques researchers use to study markets, products and services, locations, and pricing.

Chapter 15 introduces the reader to marketing planning and the role it plays in healthcare. Although presented late in the book, planning activities should occur early in the marketing process and guide the marketing initiative. The chapter guides the reader through the steps involved in the planning process, giving special consideration to the uniqueness of the healthcare environment.

Chapter 16 describes sources of marketing data. Marketing is a data-driven endeavor, and healthcare, unlike other industries, has not developed a clearinghouse of data for this purpose. Healthcare marketers must be able to determine the types of data they need for marketing planning and know where to access them. This chapter describes the methods healthcare marketers use to identify, access, interpret, and apply such data.

MANAGING AND EVALUATING THE MARKETING PROCESS

Numerous activities are involved in developing a marketing plan and implementing a marketing campaign. The process begins with a decision to carry out a marketing effort and ends with an evaluation of that effort. This chapter provides a guide through the steps involved in this process. It identifies the players involved in the marketing process and describes the manner in which the many components of the process come together to create a marketing campaign.

Organizing the Marketing Initiative

Although circumstances vary from situation to situation, all marketing campaigns operate under the assumption that the following conditions are in place:

- The organization is promoting well-defined products that lend themselves to marketing.
- The initiative fits within an established overarching strategic plan.
- Adequate information is available on the potential target audiences.
- The marketers have an in-depth understanding of consumer behavior.

Marketing is not an act, but a process. As such, certain steps must be followed, regardless of who is responsible for the marketing function. The sections that follow discuss each of these steps and consider their relevance to both plan development and campaign implementation.

The steps involved in the marketing process are as follows:

1. Organize the project.
2. Define the target audience.
3. Determine the marketing objectives.

4. Determine the resource requirements.
5. Develop the message.
6. Specify the media plan.
7. Implement the marketing campaign.
8. Evaluate the marketing campaign.

Organize the Project

The first step in any marketing process involves organizing for the effort or, in other words, planning for planning. An organization must lay appropriate groundwork before the campaign can be implemented. Whether the campaign is a long-term planning effort or a short-term promotional initiative, a campaign champion needs to be identified. A *champion* is someone who believes in the value of the idea or approach and supports it in the face of possible obstacles and even opposition from within the organization.

The planning phase is the foundation on which the rest of the process is built. To create an effective marketing program, marketers must understand the problem being addressed, the audiences being targeted, and the environment in which the program will operate. Market research is used to analyze these factors and to develop a workable strategy for effecting behavior change. As noted earlier, marketers are assumed to already have a body of relevant knowledge on the service area and its population.

Define the Target Audience

A marketing program has as its core the wants and needs of its consumers. As discussed earlier in the book, these wants and needs are determined through market segmentation analysis and market research methods that identify the target audience and its thoughts, feelings, and behaviors in relation to the service being offered. These methods include quantitative research, which generates objective data on the target population, and qualitative research, which provides insight into why people think what they think or do what they do. The actions taken to complete this step depend on whether a marketing plan or a specific marketing campaign is being pursued.

Determine the Marketing Objectives

The objectives of a marketing plan should be determined within the broad context of the organization's strategic plan. If the focus is on a specific marketing initiative, the objectives that are set should be in keeping with those of the overall marketing plan. Here, as elsewhere, the objectives established should be specific, should include quantifiable concepts, and should be time limited. The marketing objectives should be based on the stage at which the consumers are located in the purchase decision-making process.

Determine the Resources Required

A well-thought-out marketing budget is critical. The *marketing budget* is the section of the overall marketing plan or project plan that indicates projected revenues, costs, and profits.

The resources required for marketing include the dollars necessary not only for direct marketing (e.g., creative development, media time) but also for personnel, production facilities, and other resources required to carry out the project.

The marketing budget for a specific initiative should consider such direct costs as personnel expenses, market research costs, creative costs, production costs, media expenses, and a variety of other resource requirements. For initiatives built around advertising, media costs are likely to be the main expense and include the cost of advertising through various channels of communication, such as print, electronic, outdoor, and direct mail. Indirect costs may also be significant. Even if the campaign is outsourced, the marketing agency will require some time with internal staff, and there will also be some overhead costs. (Budgetary issues are covered in a later section.)

Develop the Message

This phase of the marketing program involves development of the marketing message and promotional materials. Concepts and materials are typically developed on the basis of the results of the research conducted in the planning stages of the project. The message is a combination of symbols and words that the sender wishes to transmit to the receiver. The message embodies the campaign theme—the primary topic, subject, motif, or idea around which a promotional campaign is organized—as well as the campaign slogan that the sender wants the receiver to identify with the product or service.

These concepts and materials are then tested on a group of target consumers to learn how well they resonate and to determine the best approach to use to achieve the program's objectives. Focus groups, consumer panels, and other methods can be used to test messages, materials, and proposed tactics on the target audience. Marketers may have to go back and forth several times between development and testing to make necessary changes to the messages, materials, or overall strategy.

Positioning concepts must be developed by the marketing staff and evaluated by members of the target audience. *Positioning* refers to the way the product is perceived by the target audience relative to similar products. Generally, positioning is based on the product's key selling point. Marketers typically select the best positioning statement that emerges after testing different concepts in focus groups or in-depth interviews.

Using the information obtained from concept testing, marketers create the "final" materials and then test them through different executions. These materials may include slogans, posters, news clips, videotapes, brochures, public service announcements, and product packaging. Members of the target audience can be used to test for memorability, impact, communication effectiveness, comprehension, believability, acceptability, image, ability to persuade, and other key attributes of the marketing materials.

With printed materials, the readability of the text is crucial, particularly for audiences with low health literacy. The readability of printed text may be assessed by checking sentence length and the number of polysyllabic words. Word processing programs with built-in readability calculators can simplify this task. Readability testing is generally recommended for materials that include a lot of text, such as long print advertisements, brochures, and information kits. It is often helpful to have health communication peers and representatives of intermediary organizations review them as well.

When the process reaches a certain point, it is customary to develop a *marketing brief* that presents the specifics of the campaign (see Exhibit 13.1). Development of a brief is essential if the organization is going to seek bids from several marketing agencies. Even if most aspects of the project are to be handled in-house, the brief should be fashioned so as to get everyone to buy in to the marketing project and its objectives.

EXHIBIT 13.1
Developing the Marketing Brief

In dealing with marketing agencies, clients commonly present a brief as a starting point for project planning. If the healthcare organization is in the process of selecting an agency, prospective agencies will base their presentations on the brief. The brief contains the specifics of the proposed campaign to the extent that they are known on the front end. The marketing sophistication of the healthcare organization will determine the sophistication of the brief. Even a bare-bones brief will give agencies something to which they can respond.

A brief typically includes the following components:

- A description of the product or service to be marketed
- Situational information on the company and the product
- The objectives of the marketing campaign
- The proposed strategy
- The anticipated budget

- Timelines
- In-house personnel and their potential contributions
- The means by which the campaign's effectiveness will be evaluated

The marketing agency or agencies will respond to the brief, addressing each of the issues presented. They will offer their interpretation of the marketing challenge, suggest creative and media strategies, indicate the control mechanism they will use, and show how agency responsibilities will be allocated. The agency will also present the terms and conditions under which it will carry out the project.

Specify the Media Plan

Projects will differ in the extent to which they emphasize the use of media. Few projects, however, will have no media component. Even those that do not involve advertising are likely to distribute press releases or other communiqués that end up in the media.

The steps of the media planning process are as follows:

1. Define the objectives.
2. Identify the audience.
3. Establish a media budget.
4. Evaluate media options.
5. Select the type of medium.
6. Determine the specific form of that medium.
7. Negotiate media relationships.
8. Develop the media schedule.
9. Implement the plan.
10. Evaluate the plan.

The media plan outlines the objectives of the advertising campaign, the target audience, the media vehicles that will be used to reach that audience, and the schedule for communication of the message. This step applies more directly to the marketing campaign than to overall plan development. For example, if the plan is to advertise, the marketer needs to consider whether print or electronic advertisement will work best. If electronic, will radio, television, or the Internet be used? If television, will the advertisement appear on network or cable channels? If cable, which channel(s) and time slots are appropriate?

In addition, the media plan must consider the reach, frequency, and waste involved, all of which must be balanced. *Reach* refers to the number of people exposed to an ad; *frequency* refers to the number of times a person sees the ad in a defined time frame; and *waste* refers to the number of people the ad reached but who were not part of the target audience. This last issue is particularly important in healthcare marketing, given that the healthcare organization may not want to encourage the patronage of some categories of patients (e.g., patients of a certain payer class).

Implement the Marketing Campaign

Marketing implementation turns marketing strategies and plans into marketing actions to accomplish marketing objectives. During the implementation phase, the program is introduced to the target audience. Preparation is essential for success, and implementation must be monitored to ensure that every element proceeds as planned. The process shifts at this point from the planning function to the implementation function and from the concept people to the operational staff. Planning in marketing is different from other types of planning in that the same people are likely to be involved in both planning and implementation.

To approach plan implementation systematically, marketers need to develop a detailed marketing project plan and an implementation matrix. The *project plan* systematically depicts the steps in the planning process and specifies the sequence they should follow. The project plan also indicates the relationships between tasks and the extent to which completing some tasks is a prerequisite to accomplishing others.

The *implementation matrix* should list every plan action and break down each action into tasks, if appropriate. For each action or task, the responsible party should be identified, along with any secondary parties that should be involved in the activity. In addition, the matrix should indicate resource requirements (e.g., staff time, money) and specify the start and end dates for each activity.

The resource requirements listed in the implementation matrix should be priced and combined to determine total project resource requirements. This information feeds back into the fourth step in the marketing process, where required resources are estimated. Once identified, the extent of the resource requirements may have to be addressed in relation to available funds and any other fiscal constraints. (See Chapter 15 for an additional discussion of marketing plan implementation.)

Evaluate the Marketing Campaign

Evaluation of the marketing initiative should be top of mind from the outset of the process and, in fact, should be built into the process itself. Project evaluation should include ongoing monitoring of the process, including the use of benchmarks and/or milestones for assessment along the way. Although evaluation is important for all types of planning processes, it is particularly important in marketing planning. Because the objectives of the marketing process are usually highly focused and there is likely to be concern over the return on investment, measures of marketing effectiveness are essential.

Techniques for evaluating marketing campaigns focus on two types of analysis: *process* (or *formative*) *analysis* and *outcome* (or *summative*) *analysis*. Both have a role to play in the project, although outcome evaluation is particularly important in the marketing process. Process evaluation assesses the efficiency of the marketing effort, and outcome evaluation addresses effectiveness. Campaign effectiveness can be measured in a variety of ways, and most projects will involve more than one means of evaluation—particularly in healthcare, where the intangible benefits of a marketing initiative may be as important as the tangible ones.

While the marketing initiative is under way, process evaluation should take place intermittently during each stage of the project. Process evaluation includes media monitoring and analysis, as well as evaluation of program activities. The key indicators to track include awareness of the product being marketed, advertising awareness and recall, knowledge level, attitudes and perceptions, images of the product and users, experience with the product, and behaviors (trial and repeat).

At this stage, the target audience should be asked specific questions about the product or campaign, in addition to the earlier, general questions about attitudes and behaviors regarding the marketing approach. For example, the penetration of the message within the target audience should be determined. How many consumers can recall seeing the television commercial or reading the newspaper ad? How often have they seen it? What image did the ad convey? While some of these factors will be revisited to determine the outcome of the campaign, they also serve as markers for evaluating the process.

Outcome evaluation judges whether the marketing campaign induced the desired change (e.g., an increase in consumer approval or greater patient volume). The impact of the marketing program is often difficult to assess accurately, however. For example, can one public service announcement cause a drop in morbidity and mortality from heart disease? Probably not, but several such efforts may combine synergistically to become a contributing factor in health status improvement. Because marketing campaigns are relatively short lived, the effect of a particular spot on overall trends cannot be determined. However, one can at least compare mortality and morbidity rates before and after implementation of, say, a social marketing program.

When marketers seek mass media coverage for their promotional activities, they need to be able to evaluate the outcomes of these activities. The most effective way to determine media "hits" is by subscribing to a clippings service. In addition, a media monitoring service, such as Arbitron, for example, may be used to track the frequency with which a program's public service announcements are broadcast. Today, access to the Internet makes tracking media attention much easier.

The most effective way of establishing a cause-and-effect relationship between healthcare marketing efforts and changes in behavior and health outcomes is to conduct an intervention study in one or more communities, using matched communities as controls. Assuming that there are no significant differences between the intervention and control communities, marketing activities may be linked with precision and reliability to changes in the communities.

The Players in the Marketing Process

The extent to which the staff of the healthcare organization is involved will be a function of the extent to which marketing is internalized in the organization. The nature of the organization's marketing arrangement will influence the manner in which the process is carried out. A number of options are available to a healthcare organization in terms of marketing arrangements, each of which has different implications for the organization.

One option is for the healthcare organization to outsource its marketing function. Outsourcing was typical of many organizations in the early years of healthcare marketing and is still common among smaller organizations, such as physicians' offices, that cannot support an in-house marketing function. In this case, all of the activities related to the marketing process are handled by an entity or entities outside the organization. The process can never be fully outsourced, however, because the client organization must provide information on the product to be marketed, offer feedback on marketing strategies, and approve the materials that are developed.

The second option is for the healthcare organization to outsource most of the marketing function but still carry out some activities in-house. Organizations that choose this option typically have a marketing professional on staff but no one else capable of fulfilling required tasks. In this case, the in-house marketing director would coordinate the process but leave most of the tasks to contracted agencies outside the organization. Conversely, a large organization such as a hospital may have the staff it needs to fulfill required marketing tasks in-house but no formal marketing function. It might have copywriters, graphic artists, printing facilities, website developers, and other personnel who could contribute to the marketing function, but no one to direct it.

The third option is to keep administration of most aspects of the marketing process in-house, although even healthcare organizations that have an internal marketing department are likely to continue to outsource some aspects of the process. The organization may not have personnel with certain specialized skills or the ability to handle certain activities. For example, the department is not likely to have the contacts and skills necessary to negotiate media purchases or implement a direct-mail campaign.

A small number of healthcare organizations are able to support nearly all of the functions required for marketing. Most multi-facility health systems, for example, have a centralized marketing department. This department coordinates the marketing activities for the system and ensures that all corporate entities convey a consistent message. Even these organizations, however, may rely on outside parties for a handful of functions.

Obviously, the extent to which the marketing process is incorporated into the client organization's operations will determine the extent of its control over and responsibility for the marketing function. Even with totally outsourced marketing functions, time, energy, and money will be required of the client organization. For example, if key staff members have to spend two person-days explaining a complicated service to external marketers, the organization will incur considerable direct and indirect expenses. Diverting resources from other functions to the marketing campaign may also involve unanticipated opportunity costs.

The planning process can involve a variety of personnel and departments or organizations depending on the extent of outsourcing involved. If marketing is fully internalized in the healthcare organization, most of these components will be found in-house. If the process is partially outsourced, some will be found in-house and others will be contracted out. If the process is entirely outsourced, nearly all of these components will be external to the organization. Following are some of the entities that may be involved in the marketing process.

Agencies

The term *agency* covers many different entities in the marketing industry. It could refer to a full-service marketing agency, creative shop, media independent, à la carte operation, or other entity. The term could even be applied to an in-house entity that carries out agency functions. Although agencies may be referred to informally as *advertising agencies*, they usually provide a wide range of services beyond advertising support. A *full-service agency* is an organization that can offer start-to-finish services to its clients. An *à la carte agency* is a specialty shop that offers custom services. In an à la carte agency, different services are handled by separate specialized sub-agencies.

Some of the functions that marketing agencies perform are as follows:

- Plan marketing campaigns
- Design creative components
- Schedule and buy media

- Buy and integrate other promotional materials
- Provide administration and accountancy functions for the process
- Implement marketing campaigns
- Monitor and evaluate the results of marketing campaigns

For healthcare organizations that intend to outsource some or all of their marketing functions, choosing an appropriate agency is an important step. This decision should not be taken lightly, and it requires organizations to do some meaningful research on available options (see Exhibit 13.2.)

EXHIBIT 13.2
Selecting a Marketing Agency

Any healthcare organization involved in marketing will have to search for an agency at some point, unless the organization has a professional in-house marketing staff. Many organizations have limited experience dealing with marketing agencies, and the people involved in the search for an agency may be relatively unfamiliar with this task. Many of the decisions involved in selecting an agency are a matter of common sense, but even so, the issues associated with marketing health services make this decision a critical one.

As in selecting any type of consultant, the client organization should have its requirements well defined before engaging in discussions with prospective agencies. Some health professionals might argue that they know little about marketing and thus rely on the agency to propose guidelines for the project. Even so, the organization should have a well-developed description of the service to be marketed, the ultimate goal of the campaign, and potential interfaces with other organizational components to present to prospective agencies.

With requirements in hand, the organization should develop a list of potential agencies. Only in unusual circumstances should the organization consider an agency that does not have experience in healthcare marketing. Healthcare is different from other industries, and healthcare marketing is different from marketing in other industries. Not only is there the danger of a highly visible gaffe if the agency does not know healthcare, but there is also the issue of the time required to explain basic aspects of the organization and its services to an uninformed marketing professional.

Given that relatively few marketing agencies have experience in the healthcare industry and even fewer specialize in healthcare, this list is likely to be short. For the most part, healthcare organizations tend to be followers, and in this situation, an organization might benefit from being a follower rather than a leader. Ideas should be solicited from other healthcare organizations about available agencies and their capabilities. A positive experience with a particular agency on the part of another healthcare organization is probably the best indicator of a good prospect.

Agencies that appear to be qualified in healthcare marketing or are recommended by colleagues should be asked to present their credentials for review, including examples of current or past work, descriptions of staff capabilities, and the company's history. A brief should be presented to the prospect firm that contains the specifics of the proposed campaign, including situational details, objectives, proposed strategy and tactics, target market data, budget and timescales, and information on performance evaluation. As mentioned in Exhibit 13.1, the healthcare organization's marketing sophistication will determine the extent of the brief, but the prospective agency must be given something to which it can respond.

In many industries, standard operating procedure is to consider several agencies before a decision is made. The intent, of course, is to select the best possible agency for the campaign. Given the nature of healthcare and the services being marketed, however, this practice seems like a waste of everyone's time. Nine times out of ten, the healthcare organization does not need the best agency; it needs a good one that can meet its needs. Here again, recommendations from other healthcare organizations ought to assist in the decision.

The agency that the organization chooses must be able to understand the product and the market; have strong research and planning, media planning, and media buying capabilities; be creative; have adequate internal resources; and be able to develop effective campaigns. For health professionals in particular, the agency must be easy to work with. *Easy* in this case means an agency that understands healthcare and the constraints that healthcare organizations face in marketing, understands the time demands made on health professionals, and has an appreciation of the client organization's mission. Because marketing resources are likely to be limited, the sooner the topic of costs can be broached, the better.

Some agency characteristics may be more important in healthcare than in other industries. There is always concern over the extent

(continued)

EXHIBIT 13.2 (*continued*)

to which the agency's culture and management style fits with that of the healthcare client. There is also the issue of potential conflict with existing business handled within the agency network. A healthcare organization that incurs significant costs as a result of treating smoking-induced health problems may not find a comfortable fit with an agency that maintains cigarette firms among its major accounts.

Once an agency has been selected, the organization must negotiate contractual terms. A variety of factors must be considered in developing the project budget, and as already noted, this net should be widely cast. The healthcare organization needs to be aware of any hidden costs, particularly if it is a neophyte in the marketing arena. Agencies without healthcare experience may assume that everyone knows certain expenses will be incurred. The contract should cover not only the amount of remuneration but also the terms and timing of payments, issues of nonperformance and termination, and ultimate decision-making authority. In most cases, some type of confidentiality agreement will also be required as part of the contract.

Clients

The healthcare organization is typically the *client* in the marketing process, and the other entities strive to serve the needs of the client. If the marketing function is internalized, the client is typically another department in the organization. The client should not be considered a passive customer in the marketing process but should play an important role in

- stating the justification for the marketing campaign,
- selecting and briefing the marketing agency,
- providing input into and approving campaign plans,
- integrating promotional planning into marketing planning,
- evaluating and controlling the campaign, and
- financing the campaign.

Media Suppliers

Media suppliers include commercial television companies, commercial radio companies, newspaper and magazine owners, companies that create posters and other artwork, and other organizations that make media available to the campaign. A complex marketing campaign may require the marketing team to coordinate the activities of a variety of media suppliers.

Suppliers of Promotional Materials

A number of other specialist suppliers exist, including printers, producers of promotional gifts, exhibition organizers, and corporate event planners. These specialist services are bought directly by client companies or managed through advertising agencies.

Marketing Consulting Firms

Marketing consulting firms vary with regard to the services they offer. Some offer only one or more specialized services (e.g., market research, media planning, evaluation), and others offer a full range of services. Their input may be broad (e.g., determining the overall strategic plan) or narrow (e.g., providing a targeted mailing list).

Components of a Marketing Department

The following sections describe some of the components that healthcare organizations endeavoring to establish in-house marketing capabilities would need to include in a marketing department. Even if the organization retains external marketing resources, it should be familiar with these components.

Creative Department

The creative department typically houses the "idea people" and deals with words and pictures. This department typically directs activities related to copy, graphics, and art. It creates the visual and/or audio portions of posters, billboards, brochures, television/radio spots, and promotional websites.

Media Planning and Buying Department

The dual job of determining media needs and negotiating for ad placement is an industry in its own right. This area is fairly specialized and may be difficult to comprehensively bring in-house. Media-buying experts know the most suitable type of medium, the best time slots, and the best prices for advertisements. The more central media are to the campaign, the more important this function becomes.

Production Department

The production department is ultimately responsible for producing the promotional material, whatever form it may take. This task may be as simple as translating art from the creative department into printed materials or as complicated as producing a video for television. Like media buying, this function is difficult to fully bring in-house because of the specialized equipment and expertise involved.

Account Management Department

External agencies assign an account manager to each of their clients, and the account management department is the healthcare client's primary contact during the campaign. Likewise, in-house departments assign a dedicated contact to each internal client. Either way, account manager responsibilities include attending all planning meetings, writing activity reports, coordinating tasks, presenting agency (or in-house department) findings, and feeding comments from agency personnel back to the client. The account manager has ultimate responsibility for the client's satisfaction.

Traffic Department

The traffic department is responsible for delivering the artwork or film to the magazine or television station on time. When the promotional campaign involves a number of different media, this process can become complicated.

The Marketing Budget

Budgeting is an essential financial discipline that poses tricky problems in marketing given the difficulty in determining likely demand and likely cost involved in achieving a sales target. Two types of budgets need to be set: annual and campaign specific. The annual budget is the expenditure the organization expects to make on marketing in the coming fiscal year. The organization also must set a budget for each marketing campaign. The cumulative campaign budgets for the year should approximate the annual budget.

Other than for accounting purposes, organizations use their marketing budget to

- set milestones for accomplishment of tasks,
- put all activities in financial terms,
- monitor activities to ensure they are on budget,
- motivate staff to control their spending,
- devolve responsibility and make managers accountable for their actions,
- communicate objectives, and
- increase coordination between all business units, departments, and relevant staff members.

Numerous factors affect the marketing budget. Many of them are obvious, but others are not and may be overlooked by those not familiar with marketing planning. In addition to direct costs, indirect costs and opportunity costs are likely to be incurred. In general, organizations must budget for the following expenses:

- Salaries and benefit costs of marketing personnel
- Market research costs
- Creative costs
- Production costs
- Printing costs (if applicable)
- Postage (if applicable)
- Cost of promotional items (if applicable)
- Media costs
- Evaluation costs

Expenses that are indirectly attributable to the marketing campaign may include the following:

- Administrative expenses or the cost of management and secretarial, accounting, and other administrative services:
  - Salaries of directors, management, and office staff
  - Rent and associated expenses
  - Insurance
  - Telephone and postage
  - Printing and stationery
  - Heating and lighting
- Distribution and selling expenses:
  - Salaries of marketing and sales directors and managers
  - Salaries and commissions of sales staff
  - Traveling and entertainment expenses of salespeople

As noted elsewhere, non-marketing staff will likely have to devote a considerable amount of their time working with marketing personnel to develop the marketing plan or marketing campaign. In addition to incurring direct costs for staff time, an organization may experience considerable disruption in its operations as a result of non-marketing staff involvement in a marketing campaign.

A number of miscellaneous factors may also affect the size of the promotional budget, including

- the geographic market to be covered,
- the type of product (industrial, consumer durable, or consumer convenience items),
- the distribution of consumers, and
- external factors (e.g., competitors' promotional budgets).

Return on Investment

Healthcare administrators have been concerned about the cost and perceived benefit of promotional activities since the inception of healthcare marketing. Of particular concern is return on investment (ROI) of marketing dollars. This concern has been heightened with the financial pressures most healthcare organizations have to confront in the current environment, including smaller profit margins, pressures to cut costs, and increasing marketing costs.

ROI is an indicator of value received in exchange for marketing dollars invested. ROI is typically calculated as a percentage return on the use of specific assets (financial or otherwise). Everyone is familiar with the concept of depositing money in a bank account and receiving interest from the bank. If the annual interest rate paid by the bank is 5 percent, a deposit of $100 will accrue $5 in interest by the end of the year. Thus, ROI is 5 percent.

Of course, the calculation is much more complicated in healthcare. For a straightforward example, consider the calculation of ROI for a direct-mail campaign promoting an urgent care center. ROI would be calculated in terms of the value gained from the direct-mail campaign (e.g., revenue or some proxy for revenue, such as patient volume) reduced by the cost of implementing the campaign. The direct costs in this instance would include expenses associated with developing the campaign, such as advertising agency fees, the printing of promotional material, and postage and handling costs. The revenue directly associated with the campaign would be calculated in terms of any increase in revenue at the urgent care center resulting from the direct-mail campaign. Thus, if the promotional campaign cost $10,000 and $20,000 in new business was generated, ROI would be 100 percent. Remember that, in some cases, the return may be less than the investment, resulting in a negative ROI.

Even this straightforward example involves a great deal of ambiguity. First, the direct costs do not consider the organization's total investment in the campaign. The indirect costs associated with the campaign would include the cost of any market research previously conducted with regard to the urgent care center, the staff time involved in working with the ad agency to design promotional materials and profile the target audience, and staff time spent evaluating the effectiveness (including ROI) of the effort, not to mention the overhead associated with the office space and equipment used for the project. Typically, the fully allocated costs of such a campaign greatly exceed the direct costs.

Second, calculation of the benefits of the campaign is problematic because no time frame has been defined. If the duration of the campaign is six months, should the marketer wait until the end of the campaign to begin measuring changes in revenue, begin measuring during the campaign, or allow for some lag time to determine the ultimate benefit of the campaign? After all, few consumers are likely to have an immediate need for urgent care services, but nine months down the road they may have a need and remember the promotional piece they received.

Third, the effect of a marketing campaign is difficult to isolate in healthcare. If the urgent care center recorded an increase in revenue in the aftermath of the direct-mail campaign, how much of the increase could be attributed to it? Healthcare is unique in that many other factors may influence a consumer's choice of health services provider, and in this case, factors such as changes to health plan provisions, an increase or a decrease in competition, or even demographic changes within the service area may influence the volume of business and hence the revenue.

The indirect benefits of a marketing campaign are additional factors to consider in calculating ROI in healthcare. At first, the urgent care center may concede that, at best, it will break even as a result of the campaign. However, in looking at the big picture, the hospital that owns the urgent care center may be counting on the center to make referrals to the specialists on its staff, which would result in subsequent hospital admissions by these specialists. Thus, a considerable amount of time may pass before the effects of the campaign unfold (see Case Study 13.1).

CASE STUDY 13.1
Measuring ROI for a Marketing Campaign

Southwest Regional Medical Center (SRMC) believed it could boost its orthopedic presence by establishing an orthopedics service line (the Orthopedics Center of Excellence). To support the center, SRMC recruited three new physicians, bought state-of-the-art equipment, renovated a nursing unit, added nurses and technicians, developed and linked a dedicated Web page to its enterprise website, conducted educational programs for referring physicians, made sales calls to primary care physicians, placed articles in local publications, and advertised on

(continued)

CASE STUDY 13.1 (continued)

radio and television and in print media. The total investment in the first year for programmatic changes and marketing was $1.6 million.

To determine ROI for the service line, SRMC compared its increase in income over the Center of Excellence's first year of operation to the incremental revenue it generated. In the year before the service line was established, orthopedics-related services generated $4.5 million in net revenue. In the 12 months after the formal launch date, the center generated $7.9 million in net revenue. On the basis of incremental gain and net revenues, SRMC realized ROI of 76 percent. This ROI figure assumes that the gain resulted from the Center's creation and would not have occurred otherwise.

Some argued that, in addition to direct investment in the service line, indirect contributions (e.g., spillover services provided by other departments) should be figured into the calculation and added to the total cost. SRMC's administrators asked the marketing team to isolate ROI for the programmatic investments and marketing expenditures. The team found this task to be extremely difficult, given the extent to which the different aspects of the service line were intertwined. The marketing team determined that it would need to employ more sophisticated accounting processes to factor out ROI for specific components of the service line.

This case highlights the potential pitfalls of taking ROI analysis too far. Calculating ROI for the entire investment makes sense, but attempting to calculate ROI for every individual element probably does not. SRMC concluded that its evaluation efforts would be better spent developing other indicators of tangible and intangible benefits of the service line initiative, such as top-of-mind awareness of the Center among the public, new referral sources, consumer inquiries, and so forth. Although SRMC was pleased with the overall ROI generated through enhanced operations and the multipronged marketing effort, it was justifiably cautious about carrying ROI analysis too deep into the program.

Discussion Questions
- What factors influenced SRMC to consolidate its orthopedic services under the service line model?
- What programmatic changes were made to establish the Center of Excellence?

> - What marketing options could SRMC have considered, and why do you think it chose the ones it did?
> - Aside from net revenue, were there other tangible and intangible measures that SRMC could have used to evaluate the campaign?
> - What caveats must be observed when trying to isolate ROI for program components?

In summary, the following factors affect the marketer's ability to calculate ROI in healthcare:

- Significant time often elapses between implementation of a marketing campaign and utilization of the service promoted in the campaign.
- Routine checkups aside, most health service utilization is not planned but a spontaneous response to an unanticipated event.
- The accounting systems many healthcare organizations use are not designed to generate the type of data necessary to accurately measure ROI.
- Health professionals, particularly healthcare marketers, typically have limited knowledge about the intricacies of financial management and accounting systems.
- Because of the complexity of healthcare, the impact of marketing on operations and utilization is almost impossible to isolate.
- Healthcare involves so many intangibles that traditional measures of ROI may not be applicable.

Marketing Management

Marketing management is an art and science in its own right and is particularly challenging in healthcare (see, for example, Kotler and Keller 2008b). *Marketing management* can be defined as the analysis, planning, implementation, and control of programs designed to create, build, and maintain beneficial exchanges with target buyers for the purpose of achieving organizational objectives—in short, oversight of the marketing process from start to finish. The last component, control, includes, among other things, measuring and evaluating the results of marketing strategies and plans.

Strong marketing management is particularly important in the healthcare industry. Most healthcare organizations have limited marketing experience. They often have diffuse objectives and a range of customers, and they may have a variety of stakeholders with competing agendas. In any case, there is likely to be considerable skepticism on the part of healthcare administrators with regard to the efficacy of marketing, so strong controls are required.

The negative potential of marketing is also a growing concern in healthcare. Organizations must be careful not to convey the wrong image or appear to be recklessly expending resources on marketing. The damage done by a poorly conceived, targeted, or implemented campaign may be hard to rectify.

There are two aspects to marketing management: (1) managing the process (e.g., forecasting, planning, monitoring, and controlling) and (2) managing the people inside and outside the organization who are involved in the process. The first aspect emphasizes oversight of the structures and resources that support and carry out the functions involved in the marketing effort. The second aspect involves the direct management of the personnel who perform these functions. Neither of these aspects is likely to be in place in most healthcare organizations, but they are both necessary for marketing to be integrated into the corporate structure.

Summary

Many activities are involved in developing a marketing plan or implementing a marketing campaign. The marketing process begins with a decision to embark on a marketing initiative and ends with an evaluation of that initiative. The extent to which the staff of the healthcare organization is involved in the process depends on the extent to which the marketing function is internalized.

In terms of marketing arrangements, a healthcare organization has a number of options, ranging from total outsourcing of the marketing function to developing the full range of marketing capabilities in-house. Each option has different implications for the organization. The organization's circumstances will determine the extent to which these tasks are internalized, and the extent to which the process is incorporated into the operations of the organization will determine the amount of control and responsibility the organization will retain. Even in the case of an outsourced marketing function, staff can expect to spend substantial time interacting with marketing consultants.

The management of the marketing process requires the coordination of a sequence of activities, which include establishing a planning team (and identifying a champion), defining the product, identifying the target audience, specifying marketing objectives, and developing a marketing strategy. Subsequent steps include developing the message and identifying the mechanism for delivering it. Finally, the marketing concept needs to be pretested and modified as appropriate before the marketing campaign is implemented.

Evaluation of the marketing initiative should be top of mind from the outset of the process and, in fact, should be built into it. There are two types of evaluation techniques: process (or formative) analysis and outcome (or summative) analysis. Both have a role to play in the project, although outcome evaluation is particularly important, given that it judges whether the initiative induced the desired change.

Campaign effectiveness can be measured in a number of ways, and most projects will involve more than one means of evaluation—particularly healthcare projects, in which evaluation of the intangible benefits of a marketing initiative is often as important as evaluation of the tangible ones. The ability to measure return on marketing investments has become increasingly important in today's competitive environment. Healthcare marketers must be able to demonstrate the benefits (both tangible and intangible) that result from marketing activities.

The planning process can involve a variety of personnel and departments, depending on the extent of outsourcing involved. Health professionals should become familiar with agencies, marketing consulting firms, media suppliers, and other players in the marketing arena. Every marketing initiative will require interaction with at least some of these entities. If the healthcare organization seeks to internalize the marketing function, it must be sure to include a creative department, a media planning and buying department, a production department, an account management department, and a traffic department.

The marketing budget is used to set annual goals for all marketing activities as well as to guide the implementation of individual marketing initiatives. The budget should consider direct, indirect, and hidden costs. In healthcare, indirect costs are often significant, especially if personnel are pulled away from their core functions to work on the marketing effort and the operation of the healthcare organization is disrupted as a result.

Key Points

- The marketing of any product is not a single activity but involves a complicated set of sequential activities.
- Healthcare organizations have a variety of options with regard to their involvement in marketing—from outsourcing the marketing function completely to bringing the function completely in-house, and everything in between.
- Because the organization's staff will always have to spend some time working with contracted marketing agency experts, marketing activities cannot be completely outsourced.

- A considerable amount of organizational activity is required at the beginning of a marketing campaign (e.g., conceptualizing the product, profiling the target audience).
- During the organizational stage, the steps in the marketing process are laid out (i.e., define the target audience, determine marketing objectives, determine resource requirements, develop the message, and specify the media plan).
- A project plan should be developed to integrate the disparate activities involved in the marketing effort, and an implementation matrix should be created to facilitate it.
- Campaign evaluation is an important but often neglected aspect of the marketing process.
- The process should be evaluated to assess the efficiency of the process, and outcomes should be evaluated to assess the effectiveness of the process.
- The healthcare organization must interface with a variety of entities in the marketing arena, and health professionals should develop a working knowledge of these entities' functions.
- An in-house marketing department would incorporate most of the functions carried out by entities in the marketing arena.
- The marketing budget—whether for the overall marketing effort or for a particular campaign—should be carefully thought out and managed.
- Marketing activities typically involve considerable indirect costs in addition to direct costs.
- Emphasis on return on marketing expenditure (ROI) is increasing in healthcare, and marketers should be familiar with the various methodologies for measuring ROI.
- Marketing management involves managing both the marketing process and the people involved in the marketing effort.

Discussion Questions

- Why is careful planning of a marketing campaign considered so important?
- What is a marketing brief, and why is it so important to the marketing process?
- What role might the marketing agency play in developing and implementing the marketing plan?
- How active a role should the healthcare organization play in the marketing process if the actual marketing is outsourced?

- What component units are usually included in a marketing department, and what functions do they serve?
- What indirect costs must an organization factor into its marketing budget?
- Why is strong marketing management probably more important in healthcare than in other industries?
- In what ways is evaluation in healthcare somewhat different from evaluation in other industries?
- Why should marketers evaluate a marketing project in different ways?
- Why might different approaches be used to evaluate different marketing techniques?
- Why is measuring return on marketing investments more of a challenge in healthcare than in other industries?

MARKETING RESEARCH IN HEALTHCARE

Any marketing effort will inevitably involve marketing research. The term *marketing research*, often used interchangeably with *market research*, encompasses market research, product research, pricing research, promotional research, and distribution research. Marketing research is undertaken to identify the nature of the product or service to be marketed, the characteristics of consumers, the size of the potential market, the nature of competitors, and other essential pieces of the marketing puzzle. This chapter discusses the marketing research process and its role in healthcare.

The Scope of Marketing Research

The scope of healthcare marketing research today is extremely broad. Those who remember the fledging attempts to introduce marketing research into healthcare in the past would be impressed with the breadth of activities now subjected to marketing research. There was a time when an accomplished marketing researcher in healthcare needed to be only somewhat familiar with demographic data and able to conduct a patient satisfaction survey. Now, marketing researchers are confronted with an extensive array of tools and techniques for carrying out an ever-expanding range of research activities.

The scope of marketing research in healthcare reflects the scope of marketing in the industry. As health professionals have expanded their perceptions of marketing from the narrow (and rather naïve) notion of advertising as marketing, the scope of marketing research has also expanded. Researchers are now asked to address issues that would have been considered beyond their expertise and purview in the past. Furthermore, technologically driven innovations of the 1990s, such as database marketing and the Internet, have expanded the options available to marketing researchers.

In terms of scope, the objectives of marketing research may range from answering a focused question, such as "How will consumers react if we raise our monthly fitness program fee from $25 to $40?" to answering a diffuse question, such as "How will the integrated delivery system planned by a competitor affect our market share?" Marketing research is expected to contribute to functions as narrow as measuring patient satisfaction to functions as broad as setting corporate strategy. Examples of marketing research topics include

- determining the appropriate location for an urgent care center,
- identifying employer needs in the area of occupational medicine,
- determining whether a particular market could support an oncology service,
- determining the level of demand among surgeons for robotic surgery equipment,
- measuring enrollee satisfaction with a managed care plan,
- identifying appropriate market niches for a small hospital in a highly competitive market,
- measuring potential business for a national managed care corporation in a certain state,
- determining the types of services desired in a planned community-based clinic, and
- identifying the size and characteristics of the audience amenable to Internet marketing.

This list indicates the scope of marketing research now undertaken in healthcare. Today, there seem to be few aspects of healthcare that cannot benefit from the application of marketing research techniques. See Exhibit 14.1 for vignettes on healthcare marketing research initiatives.

EXHIBIT 14.1
Healthcare Marketing Research Vignettes

The following vignettes are snapshots of the types of marketing research activities undertaken in today's healthcare environment.

Identifying Unmet Healthcare Needs
To plan its services, a faith-based clinic engaged a market researcher to identify segments of the population affected by untreated health problems. The market researcher collected census data and health-related statistics on the service area to identify high-risk populations and their healthcare needs. On the basis of this information, the researcher determined the level of health problems among the sample and the extent to which the problems were being treated.

Evaluating a New Service

A clinical psychologist was interested in establishing an outpatient eating disorders program. She contracted a marketing researcher with expertise in behavioral health to explore the market potential for such a program. The market researcher identified the characteristics of people most likely to be affected by eating disorders, developed an estimate of the number of potential cases in the community, and assessed the strength of competitor programs.

Monitoring Changing Market Characteristics

Physicians in an obstetrics/gynecology practice noticed that they were seeing fewer and fewer obstetrical patients as a result of the aging of the baby boom cohort. At the same time, the number of older women presenting for services was increasing. A market researcher was engaged to assess the situation and found that, because of changing community demographics, the population of older women was slowly but steadily replacing the population of women of childbearing age. The researcher provided the information the physician group needed to determine the feasibility of switching from an obstetrics-oriented practice to a gynecology-oriented practice.

Conducting a Physician Supply/Demand Analysis

Hospital administrators were attracted to a growing suburb located at some distance from the hospital's downtown location. Many of the hospital's medical staff had already relocated to the area to take advantage of the new, emerging market, so administrators began to consider establishing a satellite hospital in that community. The market research department was asked to perform a study to assess the feasibility of this idea. Using software to project demand, the researchers were able to determine the numbers and types of hospital services this population required.

Predicting the Changing Demand for Inpatient Care

Hospital administrators were concerned about the shift away from inpatient care in the community. The patient census had been steadily declining, and some nursing units had already been closed. Although there appeared to be a downward trend in admissions, the administrators wondered whether it would be short term or indefinite. The market research department first reviewed past utilization patterns to determine whether the trend was likely to continue. While the data

(continued)

EXHIBIT 14.1 (*continued*)

indicated a short-term decline in the demand for inpatient care, they also suggested that demand could be expected to pick back up when baby boomers begin joining the ranks of senior citizens.

Determining the Potential of Social Media

A public health agency charged with addressing the epidemic of HIV/ AIDS among the youth in its community wanted to determine the potential for using social media to reach its target population. The agency engaged an expert in market research to determine the extent to which youth in the community were using social media. If it found that use was prevalent, it would explore the types of messages that would resonate with a population regularly involved in texting, blogging, and visiting interactive websites, such as MySpace.

Healthcare marketing research has also been expanding in terms of its set of users. *Users* in this context refer to the organizations that conduct marketing research and the professionals who use the results of this research. Marketing research has historically been limited to large hospitals, national health systems, and some for-profit healthcare entities (e.g., pharmaceutical companies). Only recently have organizations providing direct patient care become heavily involved in marketing research. Today, organizations from home health agencies to urgent care center networks to national managed care organizations use information derived from marketing research.

In healthcare organizations, the demand for market data has soared. Human resources departments need information on the future labor pool; finance departments need demand projections to forecast future revenue; managed care departments need detailed data to negotiate contracts with employers; departments providing patient care need to know anticipated future volumes for planning purposes; facilities planning departments need to know how to allocate floor space commensurate with future demand; physician relations departments need information for medical staff development purposes; and so on.

Strategic planning is yet another area in which the role of healthcare marketing research has widened. Gone are the days when marketing research focused primarily on measuring the corporate image or supporting advertising campaigns. Issues now under consideration at any major healthcare system include human resources analysis, managed care assessment, evaluation of facilities for acquisition, assessment of the impact of competitor activities, justification of the organization's tax-exempt status, and so on. The involvement of the organization's marketing researchers appears to be limited only by the organization's range of services.

The number of target audiences subjected to marketing research has also increased. At one time, patients and the general public were the primary targets of marketing researchers. Today, the subjects of marketing research include patients, consumers, employees, medical staff, employers, and so on. Almost every segment of the population has some relevance for marketing research.

New research techniques are continuously being developed, and old techniques are being adapted to keep up with new circumstances, demands, and technology. These techniques include some of the standard marketing research techniques used in other industries (such as those discussed in Chapter 10), although they are likely to be modified for use in healthcare. The use of advanced geographic information systems has transformed the simple mapping of health-related phenomena into increasingly sophisticated spatial analyses, and the Internet has become a seemingly limitless mechanism for communicating health-related information.

The variety of people participating in marketing research in healthcare has burgeoned as well. More so than in other industries, healthcare demands a multidisciplinary approach to market analysis. Although most market analysts have a good understanding of survey research, the qualitative techniques that are gaining popularity often require a broader range of expertise. As marketing research broadens its scope, there will be an increasing need for people with training in sociology, anthropology, demography, epidemiology, organizational development, and other disciplines.

Marketing Research and Healthcare Decision Making

The most important development in marketing research in healthcare has been its increasing contribution to the decision-making process. Healthcare has become more market driven, and data generated through market research drive marketing. The characteristics of the market can no longer be ignored. More and more, the market's needs are driving the types of healthcare products and services offered.

Today's healthcare environment calls for a more aggressive approach to market research. Marketers must be constantly on the alert for new market opportunities and need to be aware of threats to the organization's market share or financial viability before they have been officially recognized as a problem. In addition, analysts must have monitoring capabilities in place that will flag any out-of-range statistics. For example, if a marketing researcher maintains a database on physicians within the market area, the researcher should be one of the first to identify an area in which a shortage of physicians is emerging.

The growing diversity of American consumers—including healthcare consumers—has also boosted the importance of marketing research. Once the importance of consumers was recognized in healthcare, they came to be subjected to the same segmentation processes as other consumer groups. Despite past predictions of growing homogeneity, Americans have become increasingly racially and ethnically diverse, have maintained and enhanced regional differences, and have adopted lifestyles disparate enough to daunt any marketer (Thomas 2003b). As a result, the characteristics of the American healthcare consumer have changed and health behavior has become less and less predictable.

In many segments of healthcare today, the market is no longer growing. A good example is the slumping demand for inpatient care. The success of inpatient programs, therefore, will rely less on recruiting new customers than on retaining existing ones. Healthcare organizations will have to know more about their existing customers than ever before. On the other hand, anticipating demand on the basis of future customers is also important. For example, the fact that aging baby boomers are beginning to require hospital care at an accelerating rate should be factored into the marketing equation.

Other factors also make market data an essential fixture in healthcare decision making. Organizations can incur tremendous costs if they locate a facility in a problematic site, undertake a marketing initiative at the wrong time, overlook a key niche market, or develop misleading product packaging. The costs involved in building and outfitting a clinic, mounting a marketing campaign, and developing a product are growing, and losses associated with one bad decision may need to be countered with ten good decisions for the organization to recover.

Even more important in an environment of increasingly scarce resources are the opportunity costs of a wrong decision. Situating a clinic in one place means potentially more favorable sites were not selected. Money spent on one promotion cannot be spent on another that may yield higher returns. Product development resources spent on one service could have been spent on another with more potential. By overlooking a critical niche, an organization may have invited a competitor to outposition it in the market.

Decision making in healthcare depends on accurate, timely, detailed, and complete data. Market data must supplement the knowledge base the decision maker has acquired through experience and intuition. Marketing research should be a complement to, rather than a substitute for, a manager's direct contact with the marketplace. Increasingly, the market analyst will be working closely with the administrator to build the knowledge base for decision making.

Finally, marketing research should drive marketing strategy. As discussed in Chapter 9, marketing initiatives should not exist in a vacuum but should support an overarching marketing strategy that in turn supports the organization's long-range plans. The marketing research that the organization has undertaken should drive this strategy. If, for example, research indicates that the organization is a niche player (and the public perceives the organization as such), the marketing strategy should capitalize on this positioning.

Steps in the Marketing Research Process

Any type of information gathering on the marketplace constitutes marketing research; it is not always a formal, expensive process. Although this chapter focuses on the formal aspects of market research, healthcare organizations may take more casual approaches, such as observation and the use of mystery shoppers (see Exhibit 14.2). Much of the time and effort involved in marketing can be attributed to the research activities that lead up to and support the marketing initiative. The type and amount of research undertaken during the marketing process is dictated by a number of factors, including the kind of marketing initiative being formulated, the nature of the organization, available resources, and the intended use of the findings. A critical skill for any marketer is the ability to determine the type and scope of research appropriate for a particular marketing initiative.

EXHIBIT 14.2
Mystery Shoppers in Healthcare

Other industries, being more accustomed to heated competition, frequently use *mystery shoppers* to collect market intelligence. As competition has become more acute in healthcare and the industry has become more consumer driven, healthcare organizations have adopted marketing methods from other industries, including the mystery shopper approach. Although there is still resistance to blatant efforts at acquiring intelligence on competitors, innovative approaches like the use of mystery shoppers are being applied in a number of ways in healthcare.

Mystery shoppers can take a variety of forms, and an organization can use them to collect information about itself or a competing organization. In healthcare, the term *shopper* is probably not appropriate, especially because data can be collected in a number of different

(continued)

EXHIBIT 14.2 (*continued*)

ways. Needing to better understand their processes and level of service, healthcare organizations are admitting pseudo-patients to hospitals or mental institutions, sending would-be patients to the emergency
department to observe procedures, or having potential patients call
the organization's advertised phone number to monitor the type of
responses they experience. These shoppers could be employees of
the organization or, better, external data collectors who have limited
knowledge of the organization.

Using this approach, healthcare organizations can develop an
unprecedented level of appreciation for their own operations, the
knowledge of their personnel, and the level of customer service they
provide. Data collected in this manner can be used to revise procedures, develop training programs, introduce policies and procedures,
and institute personnel changes.

More aggressive organizations may use mystery shoppers to collect information on their competitors, such as operational details, the
volume of services performed, and the sources of their patrons. To
gather this information, mystery shoppers may simply walk the halls of
a competing hospital on the pretense of visiting a patient, call competitors to quiz them on their services, or attend patient education sessions
offered by a competitor. Two mystery shoppers could even masquer-
ade as a couple seeking a nursing home or an assisted living facility for
an aged parent.

This form of qualitative data collection is not likely to provide all
of the hard data necessary for a thorough market analysis. More often,
mystery shoppers provide basic information on which more formal
data collection activities can build. Although the use of mystery shoppers is not widespread among healthcare organizations, this method of
data collection is likely to become increasingly common as healthcare
organizations become more market driven.

In an ideal world, marketing research would be an ongoing organizational function. It is not practical to initiate discrete research projects from
scratch to support each new marketing initiative. By the time most organizations can implement a data collection process, the marketing campaign period
is likely to be over. However, with ongoing monitoring systems in place, they
could, for example, track changes in physician referral patterns, admission
trends, or emerging market niches as they occur.

The marketing research process can be conceptualized as a multistage endeavor. The exact number of stages depends on the project and marketing analyst doing the research, but all research designs include the same basic elements. The process begins with an initial inquiry (e.g., is the management of eating disorders a service worth pursuing?) and ends with an ultimate decision (e.g., a pilot program for eating disorders should be initiated). No two experts completely agree on the steps involved in the research process, and some of the limitations unique to healthcare (e.g., the sanctity of patient records) distinguish the research process in healthcare from the research process in other industries. The following steps model the sequence of activities in a typical research effort, although this order is not set in stone. The steps sometimes interact and often occur simultaneously, and should be modified as appropriate.

Define the Issue

If the marketing issue is not properly defined, the information produced by the research process is unlikely to have much value. In marketing research, issues are usually defined in terms of a process or the problems related to a process. The scope of the research could be broad or narrow, depending on the issues to be investigated.

This first step typically involves developing a general understanding of the organization and its characteristics, the product or service in question, and the market area. A review of the existing literature is an obvious place to start. In traditional research, *the literature* typically refers to the professional journals in which the field's conventional wisdom is codified. Unfortunately, health services marketing has yet to develop a body of professional journals comparable to that of other industries. The literature for health services marketing includes not only standard journals but also newsletters, government reports, technical papers, presentations from professional meetings, annual reports, and the publications of professional associations. Today, marketers can access bibliographic databases, literature reviews, and other sources of relevant information through the Internet. Electronic exchanges among the informal network of health professionals on list serves, bulletin boards, and blogs are also sources of relevant information. The American Marketing Association, for example, sponsors an online special-interest group devoted to healthcare marketing.

Marketing initiatives are typically triggered by some event or situation, and isolating the relevant issues is an important early task in the research process. The introduction of a new service, a move on the part of a competitor, and the identification of a new market for an existing service are all examples of events that may instigate a marketing effort. Development of a precise statement of the issues may reveal a concern altogether different from the one that originally initiated the process.

In this step, the marketer should state some assumptions to drive the process and guide research design. Are certain audiences more important than others? Are there issues or questions that are off limits? What time constraints are involved? Initial assumptions developed at this point should be refined as more information becomes available.

Set Research Objectives

Once the problems have been identified, the research objectives should be set. What questions does the organization want answered? What body of knowledge does the organization want to establish through this process? In turn, these objectives will determine the research design.

The research approach used to accomplish the research objectives is determined by the type of organization and the type of marketing envisioned. In formulating the research design to support the marketing effort, researchers should consider four general categories of research—exploratory, descriptive, causal, and predictive.

The goal of *exploratory research* is to discern the general nature of the problem or opportunity under study and the associated factors of importance. Exploratory research is characterized by a high degree of flexibility and usually relies heavily on reviews of the literature, small-scale surveys, informal interviews and discussions, and subjective evaluation of available data. Exploratory designs are typically used for initial information gathering at the outset of a marketing initiative. The objective of this type of research is to gain insights into the marketing context and to gather information, even if anecdotal, that may determine the usefulness of other categories of marketing research.

Descriptive research involves the development of a factual portrait of the components of the community or organization being examined. These portraits typically do not attempt to explain the "why" of the researcher's observations.

The bulk of marketing-oriented data collection is geared toward descriptive studies.

Market profiles, community assessments, and resource inventories are examples of the products of descriptive research. Any source of information can be used in a descriptive study, although most studies of this nature rely heavily on secondary data sources and survey research. Carefully designed descriptive studies are the bread and butter of marketing research, and they provide the basis for any subsequent analysis.

Causal (or inferential) research attempts to specify the relationship between two or more variables in the situation under study. For example, a study of the relationship between place of medical training and physician referral patterns would probably involve an analysis of cause-and-effect relationships. A study on the market response to a promotional campaign would seek to isolate and identify the ways in which increased advertising, for example, fostered an increase in outpatient visits. Causal research designs typically infer relationships because a direct causal relationship usually cannot be demonstrated.

Little of the marketing-oriented research conducted in healthcare in the past could be characterized as causal research. Although causal research has contributed to an understanding of the motivation for consumer behavior in other industries, health services marketing has a long way to go to arrive at this level of sophistication.

Predictive research uses findings from earlier types of research as a basis for forecasting future events and conditions. Predictive modeling is a form of predictive research that has recently been adopted by healthcare organizations. For example, health plans and managed care organizations can benefit from identifying at-risk enrollees and predicting (and hopefully influencing) their future utilization of services. Predictive modeling used to project the utilization of employee health services on the basis of known characteristics of service users is another example.

Develop the Research Plan

Once the preceding steps have been carried out, a carefully thought-out research plan must be developed. Concepts developed in the early stages (e.g., objectives) need to be operationalized in the research plan. Now that an idea of the type of data required has been established, a plan for data collection and subsequent data analysis can be developed. The categories of data to be considered, the means of collecting the relevant data, the indicators and the analytical techniques to be used, among other attributes, are included in the research plan. The research plan specifies the sequence in which tasks involved in data collection and statistical analysis are to be carried out, the responsible party or parties, the resources required, and the time frames involved.

With regard to data collection supporting the research, decisions will be made with regard to the use of primary data, secondary data, or a combination of the two. If primary research is considered necessary, the data collection technique will have to be determined and the necessary steps with regard to questionnaire design, sampling, interviewer training, and so forth, will have to be implemented.

Because most marketing research is essentially descriptive, the analytical methods used may be fairly straightforward. Data analysis involves converting a series of observations, however obtained, into descriptive statements and/or inferences about relationships. The types of analyses that can be conducted depend on the nature of the sampling process, the measurement instrument, and the data collection method. A variety of analytical approaches can be used to convert raw data into information that supports the marketing process. An effective marketer will be familiar with the techniques used in demographic analyses, the methods developed by epidemiologists, and the various approaches to evaluation analysis.

Estimate Resource Requirements

Time, money, and personnel are required to implement the research plan. If the research is to be conducted in-house, resources can be broken down into direct expenses (e.g., the cost of hiring additional interviewers) and in-kind contributions, such as staff time, office space, and supplies. *Time* refers to the time needed to complete the project and to the time commitment required of personnel. The financial requirement is the monetary equivalent of personnel time, computer time, and materials needed to perform the research. In addition, the opportunity costs incurred by devoting resources to marketing-oriented research rather than to some other endeavor must be calculated to the extent possible. If an outside consultant or resource is implementing the process, costs will be calculated differently.

Project management tools, such as the program evaluation review technique (PERT) and critical path method (CPM), are useful aids for estimating the resources needed for a project and clarifying the manner in which the project will be managed. PERT involves dividing the total research project into its smallest component activities, determining the sequence in which these activities must be performed, attaching a time estimate for each activity, and presenting them in a flowchart. Marketers can use these same time estimates with the CPM method to determine the critical path for accomplishing project objectives. They can then create a chart that indicates the interdependence of the plan's components and the sequence in which they must be carried out.

Collect Data

Data collection involves acquiring the raw data that will be converted into the information needed for the marketing analysis. In selecting the best data collection technique to use for a project, the researcher must weigh the advantages and disadvantages of the different approaches and consider only those that will return reliable and valid data.

The data collection process typically involves both primary data collection and the use of secondary data. Secondary data are almost always collected first because they are likely to be readily available at little additional expense. Primary research is likely to be used to collect data that cannot be acquired through secondary research. For example, in collecting data to support marketing for a new health service, an analyst may examine hospital records for information related to past introductions of similar services (secondary data), conduct interviews to determine current consumer attitudes toward the service (primary survey data), and conduct a pilot study in which consumer reception of the proposed service is measured (primary experimental data).

Because an unlimited amount of data can be collected on an infinite number of topics, the marketer must ensure that any data collected are relevant to the issues at hand. In particular, care must be taken to ensure that the data collected are actionable. In other words, some things may be interesting to know, but if they do not contribute to the achievement of stated objectives, time and money should not be spent collecting information about them. Specifically, the marketer should list the questions that need to be answered by the end of the study and structure the data collection process accordingly. Further, the potential use for any information to be collected should be determined in advance. The use of secondary data in marketing research is discussed in more detail in Chapter 16.

Analyze Data and Draw Conclusions

The main objective in analyzing the data that have been collected is to generate conclusions related to the marketing issues. The conclusions drawn will rely heavily on the analysis outlined in the research design. Properly chosen analytical techniques should generate useful findings, whether the findings concern market share, utilization trends, or changing market characteristics. These conclusions should provide the basis for subsequent marketing activities. Some of them, in fact, become part of the assumptions that have been stated and restated throughout the process. See Case Study 14.1 for an example of market share analysis.

CASE STUDY 14.1
Market Share Analysis

Control of market share is a growing concern in healthcare. This information not only indicates the position of the organization or service in the market but also serves as a basis for evaluating the success of a marketing initiative. This critical piece of information is often difficult to calculate in healthcare.

Southeast Orthopedic Clinic (SOC) had long been the premier orthopedic practice in a middle-sized southern city. Over time, however, competition had become increasingly fierce, and concerns were growing over the perceived erosion of the practice's market share in its community. The physician management team asked the SOC marketing consultant to determine the practice's current market share and, to the extent possible, that of its competitors.

(continued)

CASE STUDY 14.1 *(continued)*

Because the consultant did not routinely calculate market share, the next step was to gather the necessary data for this calculation. The calculation of market share is relatively straightforward *if* the necessary data are available. The formula for calculating market share is

Total volume for the practice ÷ Total volume for the service area
= Market share.

The numerator could be presented in terms of volume (e.g., office visits or hospital admissions), utilization (e.g., number of diagnoses or procedures), or revenue reported for the practice in question. The denominator would be the combined figure of that indicator for all of the providers within the service area. The figure for the practice would be divided by the total to generate the percentage of the market controlled by the practice.

The consultant did not know whether the data needed for the calculation would be readily available. He presumed that SOC would have reasonable data on its own volume, utilization rates, revenue, and so forth. Comparable data on competing practices were not likely to be available, but data on volume for the total service area likely would be.

Fortunately for SOC, data on hospital admissions were reported annually to the state, allowing the consultant to determine the overall volume of orthopedic admissions for the service area, as well as admissions for various types of orthopedic diagnoses. On the basis of data obtained from the state's repository, he was able to determine that 10,000 orthopedic cases were admitted in the previous year. The consultant knew that SOC had admitted 2,000 cases during that time, so SOC's market share of the community's orthopedic patients was calculated to be 20 percent.

For confidentiality reasons, the state would not release data on the hospital admissions recorded by other area orthopedic practices. However, this information was available on individual hospitals and, given that each of the four major orthopedic practices was affiliated primarily with a specific hospital, the consultant was able to develop a reasonable estimate of the market shares of hospital patients for the various players in the orthopedic arena. Had these data not been available, he would have had to assess the relative status of SOC on the basis of the relative size of the various practices (e.g., was the 20 percent market share for SOC commensurate with the size of the practice relative to its competitors?). The consultant was able to further refine the estimate of market share by comparing revenue figures reported to the state by the various practices.

The state data were also useful for refining the market share estimate in terms of the types of patients treated. The hospital data categorized orthopedic admissions by the types of problems seen (e.g., fractures, back pain, torn ligaments). The consultant was able to calculate the practice's market share for each of the major categories. The data indicated that SOC maintained a market share of more than 25 percent for traditional orthopedic services, such as hip replacement and back surgery, but controlled less than 15 percent of the market for newer services, such as arthroscopic surgery, sports injuries, and knee replacement.

As useful as this information was, the consultant was concerned that these data did not capture market share for ambulatory services (i.e., office visits). Office visits for orthopedic services were much more common than hospital admissions, especially because orthopedic care had largely shifted from the inpatient setting to the outpatient setting. In this community, as elsewhere, no repository of data existed for ambulatory services. The consultant was forced to turn to another consultant, who provided software-generated estimates of the utilization of various types of services. Using algorithms developed on the basis of known utilization rates, the consultant was able to indicate the *expected* volume of office visits for the community, along with the breakdown of those visits by diagnosis. When he compared these figures to data on SOC volume, he determined that the SOC share of office visits was 18 percent and, as with the hospital data, the share was higher for traditional services and lower for more contemporary services.

The consultant reported back to the managing physicians at SOC that, overall, their market share for hospital care was consistent with the size of their practice, but their share of ambulatory patients was lower than anticipated. On both the inpatient and outpatient sides, SOC was more prominent with regard to patients with traditional problems but less prominent with regard to more contemporary treatments.

Discussion Questions

- Why do healthcare organizations need to understand market share, and what developments in healthcare are increasing the significance of market share data?

(continued)

CASE STUDY 14.1 *(continued)*

- What are some of the challenges healthcare organizations face in calculating their market share?
- Why is it important to go beyond overall market share for the organization and disaggregate top-of-the-organization data by patient type or procedure?
- How did the SOC market share stack up against its competitors, and in what area was SOC found to be relatively strong? Relatively weak?
- In the absence of actual data, what approach might be used to develop proxy data as a basis for determining market share?
- What did the consultant conclude about the position of SOC in its market?

Recommendation formulation is a relatively new role for market researchers, but one that is likely to grow in importance. Historically, marketing research was seen as a technical support function. The researcher's role was to turn numbers over to administrators, who would make the appropriate decision. As marketing issues have become more complex and research methods more sophisticated, decision makers are increasingly asking marketers to offer recommendations. Instead of providing the decision maker with three objectively compared options for review, the analyst is likely to be asked to indicate the best choice, per the results of the analyses.

Present Marketing Research Results

Marketing research findings are largely useless unless they can be presented in a fashion that allows decision makers to understand them and take appropriate action. If the intended audience cannot benefit from the research findings, the researcher's effort has been wasted. Regardless of the quality of the research process and the accuracy and usefulness of the resulting data, the findings will not be used if they are not communicated effectively to the appropriate decision makers. Furthermore, many executives cannot easily ascertain the quality of a research design, questionnaire, or experiment. They can, however, easily recognize the quality of a report. Therefore, the quality of the report is often used as an indicator of the quality of the research. Exhibit 14.3 describes the use of geographic information systems in the presentation of marketing research data.

EXHIBIT 14.3
Using Geographic Information Systems to
Analyze and Present Marketing Research

The use of geographic information systems (GIS) in marketing research has been common in other industries for decades. Few marketing studies in other industries would be complete without maps illustrating the distribution of markets, consumer segments, usage rates, and other essential data. Further, the use of spatial analysis techniques in developing sales territories and decision making is not uncommon in other industries.

Although mapping applications have been available to healthcare organizations for more than 20 years, most organizations have failed to incorporate mapping and spatial analysis into their operations to the extent found in other industries. Given the importance of the spatial dimension of many aspects of healthcare, it is surprising that GIS is not used more frequently in healthcare. However, considering the relatively recent development of marketing and planning functions and the slow adoption of computer technology in healthcare overall, use of GIS may simply be following suit.

Unlimited opportunities exist for the use of GIS in healthcare. In its most basic form, GIS-generated maps can be used to illustrate any number of health-related phenomena, including distribution of resources (e.g., hospitals, physicians, urgent care centers), patterns of patient flow, demand for health services, market share, and so forth. From a marketing perspective, nothing depicts concentrations of potential customers better than a map.

Beyond mapping, healthcare organizations have other opportunities to apply spatial analysis techniques in marketing research. GIS systems can be used to track trends in population growth and demographic change, determine drive times to various healthcare facilities, compare potential facility sites on the basis of several variables simultaneously, and monitor the progression of disease through the service area. Marketers can also use GIS systems for specialized applications, such as accessibility analysis for managed care plans.

As GIS software becomes more sophisticated but less expensive and easier to use, healthcare marketers are expected to use mapping and spatial analysis capabilities to a greater extent.

Effective communication of research findings to healthcare professionals is a challenge for healthcare market researchers. Typically, marketers present written or oral reports to hospital administrators, physicians, financial analysts, venture capitalists, and a range of other professionals. These individuals are typically well educated, highly positioned executives who are at the height of their careers and at the top of their fields. Even if the audience is only department heads, they are going to have a certain level of technical and/or managerial skills. (In healthcare, most managers are technical professionals [e.g., nurses, x-ray technicians] who have been promoted to management positions but have had no management training in their clinical programs and no previous managerial experience.) On the other hand, few will be able to understand the more arcane aspects of research methodology and statistical analysis. In addition to having different skills, each of these audiences will have different perspectives and biases, all of which a marketer must keep in mind when presenting a report.

Primary Data Collection Methods

Most marketing studies require collection of primary data. There will always be situations, however, when the desired data are not available, particularly in an industry undergoing the rapid and dramatic changes that characterize healthcare today. On a continuous basis, new procedures are performed, new types of insurance plans are introduced, new players enter the market, and so forth, and when new data are released, newer data are already being collected.

The major advantage of primary data is that they are collected for the particular problem or issue under investigation, making them more directly relevant and current than most secondary data. Another major advantage is that primary data collection allows the organization to maintain the proprietary nature of the information collected. Marketers determine the type of information to be elicited through primary research, and the organization "owns" the results; secondary data are derived from questions asked by another party that has different intentions and purposes in mind and maintains control of the data.

There are also disadvantages to primary data collection. It is an expensive and time-consuming process, and administration of the tools used in primary research requires fairly sophisticated skills that an organization's staff may not have. The healthcare terrain is littered with well-intentioned but amateurish attempts at primary data collection.

Before primary research activities can begin, marketers need to determine the means by which they will collect the data. There are many methods available to marketers, and selection of the best method for the project depends on a number of factors. Both quantitative and qualitative research methods are utilized in marketing research. *Quantitative* research (e.g., sample surveys) is considered more objective and readily lends itself to statistical analysis. *Qualitative* research (e.g., focus groups) is more subjective and not amenable to rigorous statistical analysis. Exhibit 14.4 compares quantitative and qualitative approaches to research, and commonly used methods of collecting primary data are described in the sections that follow.

EXHIBIT 14.4
Quantitative and Qualitative Research

For a number of years, the importance of quantitative data eclipsed that of qualitative data in healthcare. Researchers and managers became enamored with surveys and the ability to apply statistical analyses. Because there was a substantial body of knowledge regarding survey research, almost any kind of study that involved interviewing could be conducted with relative ease. Some even argued against the use of qualitative data, claiming that such information was neither scientific nor rigorous.

Indeed, there are advantages to the use of quantitative methods. Survey research lends itself to a wide range of statistical analyses, and the findings from quantitative analyses can be generalized and applied to other populations. The presumed objectivity of survey research and the ease with which quantitative data can be collected and analyzed make this approach popular with marketing researchers. The process generates definitive results (at least within a known range of error) that can be used with confidence in decision making.

In recent years, there has been somewhat of a backlash against the use of quantitative methods, and qualitative approaches have made a comeback. Some, particularly in marketing research, contend that survey research generates misleading results more often than not (Beckwith 2000). Data collected through focus groups, in-depth interviews, and observation provide a richness of detail and a perspective that may not be generated through quantitative analysis. In situations where opinions, choices, and perceptions are involved, qualitative data have come to be preferred. Healthcare providers now conduct focus groups and interviews with "naturally occurring groups" on a regular basis (see the main text for a discussion on these groups). In addition, observation techniques and content analyses are being used to supplement the quantitative approach. Methodologies have been devised to facilitate

(continued)

EXHIBIT 14.4 (*continued*)

the analysis and interpretation of qualitative data, and new software designed for the analysis of qualitative data has furthered these efforts.

Admittedly, there are limitations to the use of qualitative data. They cannot be subjected to statistical analysis, nor can they be generalized and applied to other populations. They are useful in generating broad conclusions and developing hypotheses, but their application should be limited to these activities. In this sense, they provide guidance for the development of quantitative research initiatives.

Contemporary researchers recognize the value of both types of data. In many situations, the two should be collected simultaneously. Surveys are no longer just a set of closed-ended questions with answer boxes to check. Open-ended questions are used, and the answers are analyzed. Even when qualitative and quantitative data are not gathered simultaneously, the value of one type in answering important questions about the other is being emphasized.

Observation

In *observational research*, marketers observe the actions and/or attributes of research subjects through a recording device, such as a video camera. Information is not so much elicited from the subjects as it is captured through structured observation—that is, observation conducted according to specified rules based on stated objectives.

Before observation can be used in marketing research, three conditions must be met. First, the data must be accessible via observation. Motivations, attitudes, opinions, and other internal conditions cannot be readily observed. On the other hand, behavior in a waiting room, for example, can be observed and recorded. Second, the behavior must be repetitive, frequent, or otherwise predictable. Finally, the observation must be of relatively short duration. Thus, researchers are usually restricted to observing activities that can be completed in a relatively short time span, such as clinic visits or segments of activities with a longer time span (e.g., the waiting room component of an emergency department visit).

Observational methods are typically used in marketing research when data cannot be obtained through interviews or secondary sources. This approach is particularly useful in analyzing a process. For example, a hospital might place a trained observer in its waiting area to observe the admissions process. Observers might track individual emergency patients from their initial encounter in the admitting area through their examination. Some organizations use a mystery shopper program (see Exhibit 14.2) to improve the effectiveness of this type of observational research. Sending simulated patients through the admissions process, for example, may generate more information about the process than any other method would yield.

Observational techniques are characterized as participatory or nonparticipatory. In *participatory* observation, the researcher becomes part of the group or activity being observed. Participatory observation allows the observer to analyze the group, situation, or process as an insider. Also, by being part of the group, the researcher minimizes the impact of the observation process on the group's behavior; however, there is always the possibility that the researcher's presence will alter the behavior of those being observed. The drawback to participatory observation is that the researcher typically cannot take notes or otherwise record his or her observations. Thus, the observer must rely on memory to record observations at a later date.

In *nonparticipatory* observation, the researcher is detached from the individuals, situations, or processes he or she is observing. In some cases, the passive observer may view the subjects from afar or, in more controlled environments, through a one-way mirror in an observation booth. The advantage to this approach is that it typically does not affect the behavior of the study subjects because they do not know they are being observed.

Although observational data are useful in documenting what people do, they cannot address *why* people behave in the way they do. Thus, observational research often needs to be supplemented with personal interviews or some other form of data collection to determine the motivations underlying the observed behavior.

In-depth Interviews

In-depth interview, one-on-one interview, and *key informant interview* are terms used synonymously. In-depth interviews typically involve one respondent and one interviewer. The in-depth interview is valuable in situations in which the respondent must be probed for answers. Complicated questions, or questions that do not lend themselves to simple dichotomous responses, are often best asked through personal interviews. The interview does not necessarily follow a defined set of questions that must be asked in a predetermined order; rather, the interviewer uses probing and follow-up questions as necessary to elicit the information he or she is seeking.

In-depth interviews typically last 30 to 45 minutes but can last several hours. The interviewer has the latitude to ask ad hoc questions, follow up on responses that appear worthy of further exploration, and elicit the best information possible through this research framework.

In-depth interviews appear to be most useful when superficial data collection techniques will not work, such as situations in which extensive probing is required; the subject matter is complicated, confidential, or sensitive; or group influence (e.g., in the focus group setting) might be a distraction.

Ostensibly, anyone presumed to have knowledge of the topic under study can be interviewed. However, in healthcare, *key informants* are usually interviewed. Key informants may have a particular set of knowledge (e.g., technical innovators), have a broad perspective on the study issues (e.g., hospital administrators), hold a position in which they have become familiar with the perspectives of a large number of people (e.g., human resources manager), or be opinion leaders (e.g., hospital medical staff members).

It is difficult to imagine undertaking any marketing initiative in a healthcare organization without including in-depth interviews with key informants. As discussed earlier, one of the initial tasks in marketing research is to identify the problems or opportunities the organization is facing. In-depth interviews are an excellent setting for identification of problems/opportunities. In fact, the survey forms used in subsequent quantitative research are typically constructed on the basis of in-depth interviews.

As with all of the techniques discussed thus far, there are some limitations to personal interviewing. It must be carried out by skilled interviewers, and even then there is potential for bias on the part of interviewers or misrepresentation on the part of respondents. Experts may also go off on tangents; a physician-respondent on a soapbox may be difficult to rein in.

Group Interviews

Group interviews have become one of the more popular qualitative research techniques in healthcare. They can be fairly structured, as in the case of focus groups, or more informal, as in the case of naturally occurring groups. *Focus groups* consist of people who are assembled to discuss a topic of interest under the direction of a professional moderator. The objective is to have people express their feelings or views on a range of interests. *Naturally occurring groups* in healthcare might include all people working the same shift in a department or the families and friends of patients admitted to a hospital at the same time.

Information gathered through focus groups can be used for several purposes, such as to help construct a survey instrument. Focus groups are also frequently used to assess needs. For example, a hospital might want to better understand what programs or services referring physicians would like the hospital to offer. In addition, focus groups are often used to test ideas for new programs or services. For example, an orthopedic practice might conduct focus groups among parents of youth between ages 6 and 18 to assess the feasibility of establishing a pediatric sports medicine program. Focus groups are also a valuable way of examining the underlying meaning of survey results. For example, if the results of a quantitative survey showed that 50 percent of emergency department patients thought the service was unsatisfactory, the organization might conduct a follow-up focus group of emergency department users to discover the reasons behind the quantitative findings.

The focus group method should never be used as the primary tool in marketing research, but it does disclose valuable insights that marketers can use to better formulate the issues and develop subsequent research activities. As such, it is a useful supplement to other types of research.

Survey Research

Many, if not most, marketing projects will involve some survey research. Survey research typically takes one of three forms: mail surveys, personal interviews, or telephone interviews. Computerized interviews and fax-based surveys may also be used.

Some healthcare organizations conduct survey research themselves, while others contract with an outside consultant for this purpose. Survey data may also be obtained via a syndicated survey or an omnibus survey. In conducting a *syndicated survey*, a number of organizations band together to share the cost of the research. The participating organizations may have the option of including a few custom questions in the survey, but for the most part, all will receive the same information back. *Omnibus surveys* are ongoing (often panel) surveys in which organizations can participate. The survey firm regularly asks questions of a panel of several thousand respondents, and healthcare organizations can submit questions to be asked of the pool of respondents. The different forms of survey research are described in the sections that follow.

Mail Surveys

Mail surveys are questionnaires sent to a select sample of respondents. Returned survey forms are analyzed according to predetermined analytical techniques. The use of mail surveys is advantageous in that it is a relatively inexpensive way to collect data. Typically, costs involve staff compensation (survey design and data analysis), printing costs, and postage, including return postage. Mail surveys allow respondents to remain anonymous and eliminate the potential for interviewer bias. Mail is also an efficient way to contact people who are dispersed over a large geographical area. For this reason, mail surveys are often used in healthcare to collect patient satisfaction data.

There are also several disadvantages to the use of this method. Response rates to mail surveys are often low and skewed toward certain categories of respondents. The surveys are self-administered, leaving the questions open to the respondent's interpretation. Turnaround time may be lengthy, and the short time frames characteristic of healthcare marketing campaigns may preclude the use of this method.

Personal Interviews

A second method of surveying individuals is through *personal* (or *face-to-face*) *interviews*. An individual interview is a valuable way to collect data when respondents must be probed for answers or when the interviewer is asking complicated questions that may need to be explained. In contrast to the in-depth interview, personal interviews are relatively short, involve a larger number of respondents, and require respondents to be representative of the population being studied. If the survey instrument is well designed, it may be possible to use interviewers who are less knowledgeable about the subject matter. Nevertheless, all interviewers must be trained in basic interviewing skills.

In marketing research, the focus is frequently on specific audiences. For this reason, on-site interviews are often conducted. The waiting rooms of clinics, emergency departments, and other healthcare facilities offer interviewing opportunities.

This survey approach has largely replaced the use of *community surveys* because it offers the advantage of face-to-face interviewing without the expense of door-to-door canvassing. Community surveys were once routinely conducted, but they are much less common today. In a community survey, a sample of households is selected and an interviewer or a team of interviewers contacts individuals in their homes for the interviews. Today, the costs involved in community surveys have become prohibitive. Further, many research organizations are reluctant to use this approach because of the perceived danger of sending interviewers into certain neighborhoods. Potential respondents also are unlikely to be home during the day, and people are becoming increasingly reluctant to open their doors to strangers.

A drawback to the use of personal interviews is the potential for interviewer bias. Poorly trained interviewers may condition responses by their reactions to answers or by their mannerisms, or they may fail to accurately follow the wording of a survey. In terms of cost, the personal interview is the most expensive survey approach. Even for the most basic surveys, training and monitoring expenditures are necessary, and any travel costs must be considered in the budget.

Telephone Interviews

The third common survey technique is *telephone interviewing*. Although consumers are complaining more and more about the intrusiveness of telephone surveys, this methodology still offers many advantages. Telephone interviews are a quick way to acquire information. Interviewers who have a hook (e.g., they are a current patient of the organization) can generally obtain a high response rate. Interviewers can also do a reasonable amount of probing over the phone. On the other hand, a respondent can terminate a telephone interview more easily than a face-to-face interview.

A sampling bias is inherent in this approach because people must have a telephone to be a respondent. Although telephone ownership is high in this country, certain areas or populations may have significantly lower telephone ownership than the national average. Low-income populations and racial and ethnic minority groups, in particular, have lower-than-average levels of telephone installation. Furthermore, cellular phones have replaced landline phones for many segments of the population, and there are prohibitions against accessing cell phones for telemarketing purposes.

Increasingly, people are requesting unlisted telephone numbers, making the phone directory, already a questionable sampling frame, even less useful. To address this problem, software is used to dial random numbers that begin with the prefixes used in the survey area. Other approaches randomly select numbers listed in the telephone directory or other directories. See Dillman (1978) for the seminal reference on the effective administration of mail and telephone surveys.

The use of computer-assisted telephone interviewing (CATI) has become common among survey researchers, and inexpensive software has made this technology available to most interviewers. A CATI system involves a survey workstation in which the telephone interviewer enters answers to survey items directly into the questionnaire programmed into the system. The responses are then automatically entered into the database to be analyzed. The intelligence built into the software application can flag out-of-range answers, adjust subsequent questions on the basis of earlier answers, and lead the interviewer through a series of branching questions.

Computerized Interviews

In *computerized interviewing*, respondents answer questions presented to them on a computer screen. On-site computerized interviewing is being used in more and more healthcare settings. The most frequent use to date is for collecting patient satisfaction data. After a clinic visit, for example, a respondent may be asked to sit down at a workstation and complete the questionnaire shown on the screen. More user-friendly systems allow users to touch the appropriate response on the screen. Others may instruct the interviewee to strike certain keys or tick boxes next to the response they choose.

The on-site approach to data collection is advantageous in many ways. It captures information while it is still fresh in the respondent's mind, and researchers can collect responses from nearly every patient instead of having to rely on a sample. Respondents find it easy to provide the information, and many computer-assisted systems are able to modify the questions during the course of the interview, edit the responses, and even perform analysis. Computerized interviewing saves time and resources and eliminates much of the paper involved in survey research, and results can be tabulated in hours, if not minutes.

There are also disadvantages to this approach. Patients must be willing to cooperate, especially if they are unfamiliar with computers. There is the potential to develop unnecessarily lengthy surveys because implementation is relatively painless. Patients may resent being asked to go to this extra trouble, especially if they are not feeling well or have just paid a large fee. In addition, some analysts believe patient satisfaction responses are not valid unless they have had some time to age; they contend that surveys conducted, for example, two weeks after the visit are more valid than those conducted at the time of the visit.

Some researchers administer surveys via the Internet. Assuming that the target population is wired, data collection via the Internet is convenient and inexpensive. To date, this approach works best in the case of an existing network of customers, an advisory board, or other groupings that may already be linked by e-mail, rather than for general consumers.

Summary

Marketing research encompasses market research, product research, pricing research, promotional research, and distribution research. Health professionals have come to think of marketing in a more positive way, and the accepted scope of marketing research has expanded as a result. The demand for market data has soared, and the requests are coming from an ever-growing variety of data users. Mainly, the opportunity costs of a wrong strategic decision in an increasingly competitive market are prompting this growing demand. Marketing research should be established as an ongoing function of the healthcare organization, not just something considered when an urgent need arises.

Marketing research can take a variety of forms and is not always a formal, expensive process. Any type of information gathering on the marketplace constitutes marketing research. Research can be conceptualized as a multistage process. The exact number of stages varies from marketing analyst to marketing analyst and from problem to problem. The process begins with identification of a problem and ends with a strategic decision. The steps in the marketing research process are similar to those in other industries, although they may need to be modified for use in healthcare. The nature of the research plan is a function of the objectives of the marketing initiative.

Most marketing research projects involve some primary research, and a number of techniques, each with its advantages and disadvantages, can be used. Qualitative techniques include observation, interviews, and focus groups. Quantitative techniques emphasize sample surveys, which may be conducted by mail, over the telephone, in person, or online.

Key Points

- The scope of marketing research in healthcare is expanding as its importance to the marketing process is increasingly recognized.
- Marketing research techniques in healthcare have become increasingly sophisticated as contemporary approaches are borrowed from other industries and healthcare-specific methods are developed.
- As the marketing function matures in healthcare, strategic decisions are becoming increasingly data driven.
- Marketing research in healthcare involves the same steps as in other industries, although they may need to be modified for healthcare.
- Marketing research is likely to involve both primary and secondary data, and the research technique the marketer chooses will be a function of the research topic, available resources, and the data accessible in-house.
- Quantitative techniques, particularly sample surveys, are frequently used in healthcare and can be administered in a variety of ways. There are advantages and disadvantages to the use of each technique.
- Qualitative research has become more common in healthcare as focus groups and in-depth interviews are used to expand on marketing intelligence.
- Marketing research, like other aspects of marketing, is benefiting from the application of contemporary technology.

Discussion Questions

- What developments have made marketing research increasingly important in healthcare?
- In what ways has the scope of marketing research in healthcare broadened, and what accounts for the expanded scope?
- What is the explanation for the growing influence of market research on the decision-making process in healthcare?

- What are the relative advantages and disadvantages to the use of primary research and secondary research?
- Why has most research in healthcare to date been descriptive rather than causal or predictive?
- What are the relative merits of quantitative and qualitative research, and why are both important to marketing researchers in healthcare?
- How has contemporary technology improved the effectiveness of marketing research in healthcare?
- What are the advantages of using more than one technique to research a topic?

Additional Resources

Aday, L. A., and L. J. Cornelius. 2006. *Designing and Conducting Health Surveys: A Comprehensive Guide.* San Francisco: Jossey-Bass.

American Marketing Association Special Interest Groups: www.marketingpower .com/Community/Pages/SIGs.aspx?sq=healthcare+sig.

Berkowitz, E. N., L. G. Pol, and R. K. Thomas. 1997. *Health Care Market Research.* Burr Ridge, IL: Irwin Professional Publishing.

MARKETING PLANNING

Although most healthcare organizations have some level of marketing expertise, organizations engaged in marketing activity are not necessarily skilled in marketing planning. Even today, healthcare marketers are often brought in at the eleventh hour to implement a marketing initiative without a lot of previous involvement in discussion leading up to the campaign.

Marketing planning is the development of a systematic process for promoting an organization, a service, a program, or a product. This straightforward definition masks the wide variety of activities and complexity that characterize marketing planning. Marketing planning may be limited to a short-term promotional project or may be a component of a long-term strategic plan. Because the systematic implementation of a marketing initiative is not possible without a marketing plan, one should be in place before any marketing activities begin, regardless of whether they are to be broad or narrow in scope or of long or short duration. The aim of this chapter is to instill in the reader an appreciation of the importance of the marketing planning process and the role of planning in the marketing endeavor. (For additional information on marketing plans, see Thomas [2003a].)

The Nature of Marketing Planning

Of the types of planning healthcare organizations undertake, marketing planning is most directly related to the customer. Marketing plans are driven by—and single-minded in their focus on—the consumer. The emphasis on promotion in the definition of marketing planning implies that the organization or service is being promoted to someone. Whether the targeted customer is the patient, the referring physician, the employer, the health plan, or another consumer, the marketing plan is built around the needs of someone or something. Although internal factors are often considered (internal marketing is a component of many marketing plans), the marketing plan focuses on the characteristics of the external market with the objective of influencing change in one or more of these characteristics.

Marketing plans geared toward changing the image of an organization are often broad in scope, while marketing plans that focus on a particular product or service are typically narrow in scope. All planning activities should be time delimited, and marketing plans are often rigid in this regard. Clear-cut target dates are almost always included, as the content of a marketing campaign is often time sensitive. A marketing plan that seeks to establish consumer awareness before the opening of a new clinic, for example, does not allow much margin for error in terms of timing.

The approach to marketing planning varies according to the focus of the project and whether the plan is being developed for a new organization or service or for an existing one. In the former case, the intent of the marketing plan is to create awareness, generate initial business, and establish a customer base. The primary emphasis will be on attracting new customers. For an existing organization or service, the intent may be to enhance or improve the organization's image. Objectives may include changing existing customer behavior, such as convincing customers to switch their business to the organization or service from a competitor or encouraging the customer to consume more services. Because information on existing customers is generally available, the planner can capitalize on this knowledge to derive as much additional business as possible. This knowledge can also be used to expand the customer base.

Although marketing planning is often considered a stand-alone activity, it should fit within the context of the organization's overall strategic initiatives. Thus, the objectives of the marketing plan should correspond with those outlined in the strategic plan. A marketing plan should be an inherent component of any formal business plan as well, even if the organization has an established customer base. Potential funders of a healthcare project are not likely to consider a business proposition that does not include a marketing plan.

Levels of Planning

Marketing planning can take place at different levels in an organization. At the highest level, a plan could be developed for a facility or a health system. Thus, a hospital attempting to brand itself might develop a master marketing plan to encompass most aspects of the organization's marketing effort. Such a plan would be comprehensive in its approach and broad in its scope. Its time horizon may be relatively long in marketing terms, involving, say, a two-year implementation period. Plans formulated at this level are likely to be strategic (rather than tactical) in that they attempt to effect large-scale change.

Most marketing plans are geared toward a lower level of operation. The typical marketing plan focuses on a service, a program, or an event. A marketing plan developed to roll out a new service, office site, or piece of equipment;

a promotional plan for a series of patient education seminars; or a plan aimed at increasing patient volume or market share would be fairly narrow in scope and short in duration. A plan of this type is considered tactical (rather than strategic) because it supports relatively specific marketing goals. Its objectives would be more restrictive than those of a facility-wide plan and would be measured, for example, in terms of consumer awareness of the new service, attendance at the patient education sessions, and increases in patient volume.

Although the planning process is similar for both levels of planning—and those in between—it varies slightly for each. These differences are noted in the sections that follow.

The Marketing Planning Process

The steps involved in marketing planning are featured in the following sections. The sequence of steps is also depicted in Exhibit 15.1.

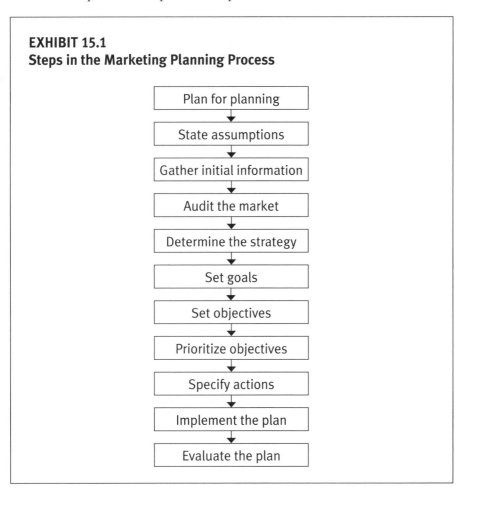

EXHIBIT 15.1
Steps in the Marketing Planning Process

Plan for planning

State assumptions

Gather initial information

Audit the market

Determine the strategy

Set goals

Set objectives

Prioritize objectives

Specify actions

Implement the plan

Evaluate the plan

Plan for Planning

A great deal of preparation is involved in the planning process; planning for planning consumes much of the early effort. The first step in any planning process is to identify the mandate under which the planners are to operate. A marketing campaign may be initiated for any number of reasons. It may be driven by competitors' actions, a political motive, or an immediate financial consideration.

Much of early marketing planning activity is organizational in nature. In addition to specifying the "why" of the initiative, an important task is identifying the key stakeholders, decision makers, and resources involved. If the organization has an established marketing department, much of the initial work (e.g., background research) may already have been completed and the key players may be in place. However, in the case of a newly established marketing function or the marketing of an unfamiliar service, additional organizational effort will likely be required.

Although there is no foolproof combination of team members that will ensure success, certain categories of participants should be involved. The first category includes those familiar with the service or product, the market, and the organization's distribution channels. During the research phase, representatives of the target audience should be involved, whether they be patients, physicians, or employers.

Internal participants in the planning process should be drawn from different functional areas, starting with management. Certainly, the marketing department should play a key role, and if there is a research department, the efforts of the two should be combined. Depending on the issues, other key departments may participate, including the finance, human resources, and clinical departments. The planning process is also unlikely to run smoothly without the cooperation of the information systems department.

During this early stage, the mechanics of the planning process need to be specified. Mechanics include the process format and objectives and such practical issues as the frequency of planning team meetings and the purpose of those meetings (e.g., progress reporting or decision making). Note that the objectives stated at this point refer to what is expected to be achieved during the planning process, not during the marketing campaign.

State Assumptions

Marketers often rush into the development of a marketing plan without carefully considering the assumptions under which they are operating. Assumptions need to be stated not only at the outset of the planning process but also throughout it. For example, marketers might make an assumption about the image the organization wants to convey. There is a big difference between presenting the image of an aggressive, profit-seeking enterprise driven by hard-bitten business principles and the image of a humble, community-based organization intent on serving the needs of the population.

Assumptions should be stated with regard to the potential consequences of the marketing initiative, and healthcare is unique in this regard. In today's reimbursement environment, for example, a healthcare provider does not want to attract all potential consumers for a product or service. The organization wants to attract those who can reasonably be expected to pay. At the same time, the provider does not want to appear as though it is deliberately excluding certain classes of patients.

The assumptions made at the outset reflect the extent to which a product or service has already penetrated the market. The extent to which marketing activities have previously been initiated for the product or service will affect the assumptions under which the planner operates. The approach or appeal to be used in the campaign is another element about which assumptions might be made.

Gather Initial Information

If a healthcare organization has a marketing function in place, the marketing department may already have completed many of the tasks associated with initial information gathering. Typically, the marketing staff will already have examined most aspects of the environment as part of their ongoing market research activities; at most, they will need to update some of their data. A newly formed marketing department or outside marketing consultant, however, may need to undertake a significant data collection effort.

Planners begin the data collection process by gathering general background information on the organization through a review of materials on the organization and the product or service to be marketed. In addition to determining the attributes of the organization and its services, planners need to identify how the organization or service is different from others in terms of salient attributes. Differentiating features should be highlighted. If there are few distinctions between the services and those offered by competitors, differentiation becomes a greater challenge for the marketer.

In a large organization such as a hospital, the marketing staff is not likely to be familiar with all services, especially those that have not been heavily marketed in the past. Hospitals frequently add new services, and some existing services may never have been marketed. Such cases will likely require additional background research.

The initial information-gathering process should also reveal the history of the organization, service, or product being marketed. Planning is futuristic in its outlook, yet the future of an organization, a product, or a service is likely to be inextricably intertwined with its past. Current relationships take the form they do because of historical developments, and past and current experiences and relationships will color future developments. The organization's history is also instructive in developing a plan for its future, and its corporate culture will exert a strong influence on the marketing mind-set.

To minimize duplicate effort, planners typically inventory marketing resources and determine the extent to which current marketing activities relate to the proposed project. Ongoing marketing activities are easy to overlook, especially if they are informal or not "labeled" as marketing. At the same time, planners should determine whether the new initiative would contradict or otherwise conflict with existing marketing activities.

Planners need to note barriers to plan development—both known and potential. First, immutable patterns of behavior in the organization should be identified, particularly if the campaign is to involve internal marketing. Second, problems may crop up if the campaign pits two organizational entities against each other. For example, the director of the emergency department may not react favorably to a marketing campaign that is focused on directing patients away from the emergency department to urgent care centers affiliated with the hospital. Third, regardless of the type of organization, any environmental constraints likely to affect the organization and the provision of its services need to be identified. Some barriers may be surmountable, but others might not be. These understandings can be used to refine the assumptions previously stated.

Planners may benefit from information on similar marketing initiatives in other markets, especially if the initiative involves a product, a market, or an approach with which the marketer has limited familiarity. Planners should be able to incorporate information about marketing approaches that have and have not worked when similar organizations or services were marketed in other contexts.

As the planning process moves forward, more formal data collection is likely to be required. The extent of this data collection effort will depend on the nature of the organization and the type of marketing initiative. A national organization courting a mass market (e.g., a pharmaceutical company promoting an over-the-counter product) probably would perform a market analysis involving substantial detail at the national level. On the other hand, a home health agency licensed to practice in a single county is not likely to need much detail with regard to national home health trends to develop a marketing plan. If appropriate to the initiative, marketers are likely to identify relevant social trends, lifestyle trends, changes in consumer attitudes, health industry trends, and industry or product life cycle information. They may also consider regulatory, political, legal, and technological developments.

Audit the Market

Planners must develop an in-depth understanding of the organization's products and services and the manner in which customers are processed. Typically, they acquire this knowledge through internal and external audits. In an internal audit, planners will be interested in gathering information on some or all of the following factors:

- *Services/products.* What services does the organization provide and/or what products does it produce? What are the characteristics of these services and products?
- *Customer characteristics.* How many customers does the organization have, and what are their characteristics? What demographic characteristics are most pertinent? Where do the organization's patients live, and what is its market area? What is the case mix of current customers? What are the financial circumstances of the patient base?
- *Utilization patterns.* What volume of services and products do the organization's customers consume? How does this volume break down by service line or procedure?
- *Pricing structure.* How does the organization set prices for its services and products? How does this price structure compare to that of competitors or the industry average? How price sensitive are the goods and services offered?
- *Marketing arrangements.* What marketing programs are currently in place, and how is marketing structured? What type and level of resources are available for marketing? Are processes in place for internal marketing?
- *Locations.* To what extent are operations centralized or decentralized? How many satellite locations are in operation, and how were the locations chosen? Are there markets that existing outlets are not serving?
- *Referral relationships.* How are customers referred to the organization? To what extent are there formal referral relationships?

An external audit involves data collection on the environment in which the healthcare organization operates. The following factors are typically reviewed:

- The social, economic, and political environment
- The demographic, psychographic, and socioeconomic characteristics of the target population
- The health status of the target population

- Existing patterns of health service utilization patterns
- Characteristics and offerings of competitors within the market

See Exhibit 9.2 for a summary of the types of data collected through internal and external audits.

Determine the Strategy

The strategy developed during the planning process sets the tone for subsequent planning activities and the parameters within which the planner must operate. Ideally, the strategy used in a marketing initiative will support the organization's mission statement and align with the organization's strategic plan. For example, if the organization's strategy is to position itself as a "caring" organization, marketing initiatives should support this approach.

Likewise, strategic considerations should guide the marketing planning process. The marketing strategy could, for example, be framed as an educational initiative, a public relations rather than an advertising approach, or a soft-sell versus a hard-sell approach, ultimately reflecting the overall corporate strategy.

Set Goals

Goals are accomplishments the organization would like to achieve through the marketing plan. The goal(s) of the marketing plan should reflect the information generated by the background research, align with the organization's mission statement, and be broad in scope and limited in detail—for example, "to establish Hospital X as the most prominent inpatient facility in this market area." Alternatively, for a service-oriented initiative, the goal might be "to dominate the niche for occupational medicine in this market area." Goal setting on the part of healthcare organizations is somewhat problematic given the diffuseness of healthcare goals. Exhibit 15.2 discusses the variety of marketing goals found in healthcare.

EXHIBIT 15.2
The Diffuse Goals of Healthcare Marketing

The mission of a healthcare organization is likely to be different from that of organizations in other industries. A healthcare organization may emphasize its charitable mission or service orientation rather than its profits. Its mission is also likely to be more diffuse. A mission of improving the health status of the community, for example, is a lot different from the profit-maximization goals of corporations in most other industries.

The goals of a healthcare organization are also likely to be much more diverse than those of organizations in other industries. Hospitals, with their myriad functions and interests, are the epitome of the multipurpose organization. A marketing plan for an organization this complex must consider a wide range of perspectives because healthcare services are often established without consideration of the potential profit.

The constituencies of healthcare organizations are different as well. Although a growing number of healthcare organizations must satisfy stockholders, most are more directly accountable to other types of constituencies. For example, a public hospital may have to cater to politicians, consumer interest groups, vested interests in the medical community, and other entities. A church-affiliated hospital may be accountable not only to its board of directors but also to the denomination's leadership.

Furthermore, healthcare organizations are different in that they often provide mandated services. In other industries, an unprofitable product line can simply be eliminated. Hospitals and certain other healthcare organizations, however, may not be able to compete on equal terms unless they are comprehensive in their service offerings. If a hospital drops an unprofitable obstetrics service, other aspects of the organization may be negatively impacted. State regulations may even mandate the existence of the unit, in which case eliminating it would not be an option.

Set Objectives

The next step involves formulating *objectives*—mechanisms that support the attainment of the goal(s) set in the previous step. Goals are general statements, whereas objectives are specific. Objectives should be clearly and concisely stated. They must also be time bound; clear deadlines must be set for their accomplishment. Finally, objectives must be measurable because the marketing plan will typically be evaluated in terms of the extent to which objectives have been achieved. For example, an objective of the goal stated for Hospital X in the previous step might be "The proportion of the general population for whom Hospital X is most prominent will increase from 10 percent to 25 percent within six months." A number of objectives may be specified for each goal, as each is likely to require action on a number of different fronts.

Any barriers to accomplishing the organization's stated objectives should be identified and assessed at this point. A lack of resources or talent is a common barrier to any type of plan. Ethical or legal considerations may be associated with some types of marketing—for example, certain health professionals may be prohibited from using advertising. Issues of appropriateness and taste may also pose problems. For example, the educational level of the target audience might be a barrier to introducing a new high-tech procedure, or public perception of a new procedure as experimental could make potential patients apprehensive about it.

Prioritize Objectives

The objectives specified to support the marketing goal are likely to address different dimensions of the initiative. Although all of the objectives may be considered important or even essential, it may not be feasible to pursue all of the objectives, or at least not all at the same time. Some objectives could even operate at cross-purposes.

As an example of a potential dilemma, imagine a situation in which a project has multiple objectives supporting the establishment of a new facility as the dominant provider in a specified market area. One objective involves increasing public awareness of the facility, and another focuses on increasing patient volume. Although these efforts might overlap, the approach the facility would take to make its name a household word would likely be different from the approach it would take to incent patients to try the new facility. If the facility does not have the resources it needs to pursue these two objectives simultaneously, it may need to prioritize its marketing efforts.

To prioritize the objectives of a marketing plan, planners might envision the initiative in terms of the four Ps: product, price, place, and promotion. For example, they could decide to focus on the product dimension of the marketing mix at the expense of price, place, and promotion. Thus, objectives most related to promoting the characteristics of the product would receive priority. Alternatively, they might capitalize on the price advantage of the product, thereby prioritizing objectives that focus on the pricing dimension.

One last consideration is the possibility of unanticipated consequences resulting from the pursuit of stated objectives. However tedious the job may be, planners need to specify both potential (unintended) consequences and the intended consequences of carrying out each objective. Too often, planners examine intended outcomes in isolation from the potential negative consequences of pursuing the objective.

Specify Actions

The next step in the marketing planning process is specifying the actions to be carried out for each objective. Actions might range from ensuring that postage is available to support a direct-mail initiative to enlisting the services of a celebrity spokesperson. For example, if the objective of a specialty practice is to increase public awareness of its new sports medicine program by 50 percent, actions might include selecting an advertising agency, allocating funds for marketing, packaging the program, and scheduling press conferences. Many actions fall naturally into a sequence, so planners may want to refine the plan by specifying this sequence. Case Study 15.1 presents examples of plan goals, objectives, and actions.

CASE STUDY 15.1
Sample Goals, Objectives, and Actions

Southern Neuroscience Center (SNC) has completed a strategic planning process and set a goal of becoming recognized as the premier neurological specialty group in its region. To support this goal, SNC has developed a marketing plan with the following components:

Marketing Goal
To establish SNC as the premier neurological specialty center in the minds of consumers in its market area

Marketing Objectives
1. Increase awareness of SNC from 40 percent of consumers to 60 percent of consumers within 12 months.
2. Improve patient satisfaction ratings of "excellent" from 80 percent to 90 percent within 12 months.
3. Increase the number of physicians regularly referring to SNC by 25 percent over the next 12 months.

Marketing Actions
For objective 1, actions include

- developing an advertising campaign for local television,
- increasing SNC event sponsorship from two events per year to four events during the next 12 months,
- distributing an SNC newsletter to all relevant members of the medical community, and
- establishing an interactive website featuring consumer-oriented information on neurology and neurosurgery.

Discussion Questions
- What prompted SNC to embark on marketing planning?
- How did SNC use the planning process to address its goal?
- What indicators did SNC use to measure the success of its marketing initiative?
- What potential barriers might SNC encounter in pursuing its marketing objectives?

Implement the Marketing Plan

Planning is ultimately only an exercise, albeit a meaningful one. The payoff comes when the plan is implemented. The planning process creates a road map that the marketer must use to get to the final destination (i.e., goal). To a certain extent, planning is talk, but implementation is action. Fortunately, the handoff from planning to implementation is typically smooth in that the same parties are likely to be involved in both functions.

In addition to a detailed marketing project plan, development of an implementation matrix is essential. The implementation matrix should list every action specified in the previous step and, if appropriate, break each action down into tasks. For each action or task, a number of details need to be specified: the party responsible for the action or task, along with any secondary parties that are to be involved in the activity; resources required to complete the activity (e.g., staff time, money); start and end dates for the activity; and prerequisites that must be fulfilled before the task can be completed. Some type of benchmark should also be stated so the planning team can determine whether the activity was completed successfully. The resource requirements from the implementation matrix should be combined to determine total project resource requirements.

Evaluate the Plan

Evaluation of the plan should be top of mind from the beginning of the planning process. Evaluation should involve ongoing monitoring of the process, including the use of benchmarks and/or milestones to measure progress toward goals and objectives. As discussed in Chapter 13, both process analysis and outcome analysis are used to assess marketing efforts.

Increasingly, marketers are being asked by the administrators who sign their checks to justify marketing initiatives in terms of return on investment (also discussed in Chapter 13). To be able to calculate return, marketers need a carefully constructed marketing plan and must keep detailed records of expenditures and revenues associated with the marketing initiative. Some type of cost–benefit analysis should be conducted before the project is initiated, and every effort should be made to track the benefits that accrue to the organization (in terms of visibility, perception, market share, volume, and revenue) as a result of the campaign. Case Study 15.2 presents a simple marketing plan that includes these elements.

Summary

Most healthcare organizations have some level of marketing expertise today, but that does not necessarily mean they are skilled in marketing planning.

CASE STUDY 15.2
Marketing Planning for a New Program

SouthCoast Institute, a rehabilitation hospital with a historical focus on inpatient services, perceived an opportunity to expand its outpatient capabilities. Among its options was the development of an aquatherapy program to supplement the services SouthCoast was already providing for rehabilitation patients. SouthCoast believed that an aquatherapy program would expand the capabilities of its existing program and make physical therapy available to a wider range of patients than historically served by the inpatient program. SouthCoast staff recognized the need for a marketing plan if they were to successfully introduce this new service.

Plan for Planning

The decision to explore the development of an aquatherapy program was one result of a major strategic planning initiative by SouthCoast. Many of the organizational issues had been addressed within the context of the ongoing strategic plan. A planning team was already in place, and a planning framework had been established.

State Assumptions

The planning team began by stating some assumptions about the aquatherapy service and its relationship to the market:

- There was adequate demand for aquatherapy services within the service area.
- SouthCoast had a "captive audience" for this service among its existing rehabilitation patients.
- Aquatherapy was a new service generally unknown to the public and medical community.
- Considerable outreach would be required to educate the public and raise awareness and acceptance of this new service.
- If properly informed, insurance plans would be willing to reimburse for aquatherapy services.
- There was potential for significant spillover benefits from the introduction of this program (e.g., provide trainers for school swim teams and thereby attract student athletes needing therapy).

Gather Initial Information

The information-gathering process involved collecting background data on existing aquatherapy programs in other markets. In addition,

(continued)

CASE STUDY 15.2 (*continued*)

planners assessed the availability of internal resources and the degree to which the general public and the external medical community were open to the idea of a new program. They also developed a general idea of what was involved in operating an aquatherapy program.

Audit the Market

At the same time, a preliminary internal information-gathering process was implemented that focused on the potential for developing the program within the confines of the existing rehabilitation therapy framework. Data were compiled on the types of procedures and services offered by most programs, the types of patients typically served, reimbursement prospects, and so forth. The analysis examined the existing rehabilitation staff's ability to take on additional responsibility, the potential need to train additional staff in aquatherapy, existing equipment and additional equipment needs, and, perhaps most important, the attitude of the internal medical staff with regard to this proposed service.

The planning team also collected data on the market potential of this service within the institute's target area. It identified potential referral sources and interviewed them to determine their interest in the program. The team contacted local health plans to determine their willingness to reimburse for this service. Finally, the team conducted a competitive analysis and determined that no medically supported aquatherapy program was being offered in the community.

Determine the Strategy

On the basis of the information gathered through the initial research and the internal and external audits, the team felt that a strategy emphasizing education was appropriate for the initiative. Marketing efforts would focus on increasing awareness of and support for the aquatherapy program. At the same time, the strategy would emphasize that SouthCoast was the only organization offering this service in the market area.

Set Goals

With background data indicating significant potential for a successful and profitable service, the planning team set a goal of establishing the institute's program as the premier aquatherapy program in the region.

Set and Prioritize Objectives

In support of this goal, the team established the following objectives:

- Create and implement a comprehensive internal marketing program for aquatherapy within six months.
- Directly contact all of SouthCoast's affiliates and potential referrers outside the institute within six months.
- Within six months, recruit and train a marketing/liaison person to work full time on the aquatherapy program campaign.
- Within six months, identify and contact all community groups that could benefit from the aquatherapy pool.
- Integrate aquatherapy services into the institute's sports medicine and occupational medicine programs within one year.

Specify Actions

Next, the team specified the actions it would need to take to support these objectives:

- Create promotional material to distribute to potential referral agents.
- Set up meetings with relevant internal parties (including medical staff) to explain the program.
- Identify an appropriate person to train as a liaison with the community.
- Identify appropriate external targets for promotional and educational activities.

Implement the Plan

The implementation plan identified the resources needed, the required financial commitment, the parties responsible for the tasks, and timelines for all activities. In keeping with the educational/relationship-building approach, the marketing mix focused on low-key promotional activities and avoided high-profile media advertising. For internal marketing, the plan included a newsletter, articles in other internal publications, flyers in institute employees' pay envelopes, posters, information sessions for staff and referring physicians, and a DVD explaining the purpose of the program for health professionals and insurance plans. For external audiences, the plan included a newsletter, press releases (and other media coverage as appropriate), print advertising (limited to the *Yellow Pages*), limited electronic media (for the grand opening), a DVD, exhibits (e.g., at schools and health fairs), and public presentations (e.g., for support groups, medical societies, and voluntary health associations).

(continued)

CASE STUDY 15.2 *(continued)*

Evaluate the Plan

An evaluation procedure was delineated to assess the progress of the program. Because it was a start-up operation, service utilization would be easy to track. The plan also arranged for a pretest and posttest to be administered to referral agents to determine the extent to which they were made aware of the program (i.e., whether they knew enough about the program to feel confident about referring their patients to it). Satisfaction surveys were developed for patients and referrers. The extent to which the program generated secondary benefits in the community (e.g., with community groups, schools, swim clubs) would also be tracked and periodically reported.

Discussion Questions

- How did broad trends in healthcare marketing influence SouthCoast's thoughts with regard to new product development?
- Why did SouthCoast need to assess the public's openness to the idea of an aquatherapy program before initiating a marketing plan?
- What factors influenced the team's choice of strategic approach? Were there other strategies the team might have considered?
- How did the promotional techniques utilized by SouthCoast reflect its overall strategy?
- In what ways could the success of the marketing initiative be measured?

Systematic implementation of a marketing initiative is not possible without a marketing plan. A marketing plan should be in place before undertaking any marketing effort, large or small.

Although marketing plans geared toward changing the image of an organization are understandably broad, most marketing initiatives focus on a particular good or service. Marketing planning can take place at a variety of organizational levels. At the highest level, plans usually address the planning needs of the entire hospital or health system in relatively broad terms (i.e., strategically).

Most marketing plans, however, are geared toward a lower level of operation. The typical marketing plan focuses on a particular service, program, or event. A marketing plan developed to roll out a new service, office site, or piece of equipment, or a promotional plan for a series of patient education seminars, would be fairly narrow in scope and short in duration (i.e., tactical).

The marketing planning process involves steps that carry the planner from the initial marketing concept to plan implementation. The organization must establish goals, objectives, and a strategy for accomplishing these ends. Objectives must be prioritized, and the unintended consequences of meeting an objective must be considered. Objectives are then broken down into actions, and these actions are laid out in a sequence in an implementation plan. Plan evaluation should be a consideration from the outset of the planning process, and mechanisms for evaluating the marketing effort should be built into the marketing plan.

Key Points

- Marketing planning organizes the marketing effort, whether it involves a major strategic initiative or a narrowly focused campaign.
- The type of marketing initiative envisioned will influence the scope of the marketing plan.
- Planning can occur at different organizational levels, from the top of an organization to a subdivision of a department in that organization.
- The marketing planning process involves a prescribed set of activities that begins with planning for planning and ends with project evaluation.
- The diffuse goals typical of healthcare organizations are a challenge in marketing planning.

Discussion Questions

- In what ways does marketing planning differ from other types of planning in healthcare?
- What determines the organizational level at which planning should occur?
- Why do planners need to lay out assumptions on the front end?
- What types of data are generated through an internal audit?
- Within the planning context, what are the differences between goals, objectives, and activities?
- Given that it may not be possible to pursue all possible marketing objectives, what criteria might planners use to prioritize them?

SOURCES OF MARKETING DATA

Healthcare marketers require a variety of data for planning and implementing marketing activities. They need data to determine market shares, profile potential markets, and initiate direct-to-consumer campaigns, all of which require extensive experience with and knowledge of data sources. This chapter examines the types of data available to healthcare marketers and describes methods of accessing, interpreting, and applying them. The importance of the Internet as a source of marketing information is also explored.

The Data Challenge

Healthcare marketers seeking data have a paradox with which to contend. The healthcare industry generates a wealth of data, but large portions of this bounty are inaccessible to marketers. Unlike other industries, healthcare has never developed national clearinghouses that compile industry data into a central repository. When data are available, they often are deficient. Because health-related information is often internally generated by private healthcare organizations, useful health data sets may be unpublished, proprietary, or difficult to access. The enactment of the Health Insurance Portability and Accountability Act (HIPAA) in 1996 further obstructed marketers' access to health data (see Exhibit 16.1).

EXHIBIT 16.1
HIPAA and Healthcare Marketing

When the Health Insurance Portability and Accountability Act (HIPAA) was enacted in 1996, the intentions were to clarify issues related to the privacy of personal health information (PHI) and guide the behavior of entities (healthcare or otherwise) that had access to

(continued)

EXHIBIT 16.1 (*continued*)

individuals' medical information. Although the medical privacy section was accepted in December 2000 and finalized in 2001, the implications of the legislation for healthcare marketing continue to be debated. The good news is that most marketing activities in which healthcare providers participate are still allowable under the HIPAA provisions.

Covered entities initially expressed confusion over HIPAA's distinction between healthcare communications exempted from the definition of marketing and those considered to be marketing, but permitted. Questions have been raised concerning, for example, disease management communication, prescription refill reminders, and general health-related educational and wellness promotional activities.

Every healthcare provider or entity that communicates with its patients must address the following two issues. First, what is the definition of marketing, and what kinds of communications are allowed without patient authorization? The initial definition of marketing had hospitals and healthcare providers worried that they could no longer use the information in their patient records, classified as PHI, to inform their patients about healthcare services or programs that could directly affect their health. However, most kinds of communication between providers and their patients are allowable under the current marketing exclusions.

Second, the key tenets of a relationship between caregiver and patient—maintaining and improving health—must be considered. This relationship is based on trust, and providers should be able to send information to their patients about recommended screenings and immunizations, new procedures, treatments, and health-related seminars without fear of violating HIPAA regulations.

Officials of the U.S. Department of Health and Human Services (DHHS) concede that when hospitals, physicians, and other care providers offer such information to their patients, they advance the goal of improving their patients' health. Patients expect their physicians, hospitals, and other providers to share medical information that is relevant to activities essential to the provision of healthcare. These concessions by DHHS would permit doctors, hospitals, pharmacists, and health plans to communicate freely with patients about treatment options and other health-related issues, including disease management, case management, and care coordination. Thus, most of the communications programs that healthcare entities are conducting today will not be prohibited by anticipated future changes to the HIPAA Privacy Rule and will not require prior authorization.

Healthcare's increasingly market-driven approach has led to a growing demand for market data, yet the healthcare industry still lags other industries in the collection and dissemination of market-related data. The local orientation and autonomous nature of many healthcare organizations has impeded data sharing. Increasingly, the health marketer's ability (or inability) to access, manipulate, and interpret these data is determining whether marking initiatives succeed or fail.

The primary purpose of this chapter is to outline the categories of data required for marketing activities, describe the ways in which data are generated, and indicate sites where they might be accessed. This chapter is not an exhaustive discussion of this topic; given the growing number of types and sources of health-related data, a comprehensive study would become unwieldy. Rather, the purpose of the following discussion is to inform the reader of the most important types and sources of data for healthcare marketing. This chapter elaborates on many of the information sources introduced earlier in the book by presenting important characteristics of these sources, such as frequency of release, geographic specificity, and methodological limitations.

Initially, a number of the data sets described in the chapter may not seem to be pertinent to healthcare. However, much of what affects the healthcare industry relates to other aspects of society. For example, healthcare marketers have always used demographic data. Beginning in the 1990s, there was an increase in the demand for data on topics once considered unrelated to healthcare, such as employment, housing, and crime.

Data Dimensions

The data useful to healthcare marketers can be categorized along a number of dimensions. Some of the most important dimensions are addressed in the following sections.

Community Versus Organization Data

The act of compiling health data can be approached on two levels: the community level and the organization level. The former involves the analysis of community-wide data, whether the community is a nation, state, county, or market area. These data typically emphasize overall patterns of health service delivery and dominant practice patterns, such as information on patient flow into and out of the service area, levels of overcapacity or undercapacity affecting the area's health facilities, and the availability of different types of biomedical equipment within the service area.

At the organization level, data analysis focuses on the characteristics and concerns of corporate entities, such as hospitals, physician groups, and health plans. These data typically detail an organization's operations in relation to competitors' activities. In organization-level analysis, the overall pattern of health system operation (i.e., community-level data) is important only to the extent that it affects the organization in question. A specialty physician practice, for example, is primarily interested in the details of competing specialty practices (e.g., patient volume, market share, procedures performed) rather than general data on the health service area.

Internal Versus External Data

Marketers require data on both the internal and the external environments. Although healthcare organizations usually turn first to internal information sources, data on the external environment have become increasingly important. Data on the external environment are sometimes difficult to locate and access but, relative to internal data, are more available to the public. See Exhibit 9.2 for examples of internal and external data.

Internally generated data are a ready source of information for marketers. Healthcare organizations routinely produce a large volume of data as a by-product of their normal operations, including information on patient characteristics, utilization patterns, referral streams, financial trends, staffing levels, and other types of information that have implications for marketing.

Internal data are usually compiled through an *internal audit*. The internal audit typically analyzes the organization's structure, processes, customers, and resources. The internal audit may compile data from standard reports generated by the organization's data management systems (e.g., patient activity reports), but additional reports often need to be generated to obtain the necessary data.

Few data management systems in healthcare were set up to generate data for marketing, and many are too inflexible to produce custom data sets. As a result, marketers may have to be creative in manipulating internal databases to obtain the data they require. Financial data are an increasingly important aspect of the internal data with which marketers must be familiar. Marketers must be aware of the profitability of services provided by the organization, the pricing process, and the cost–benefit breakdown associated with the use of different marketing approaches.

Today, most data collection efforts are directed toward external data. As healthcare providers have become more market driven and emphasis has shifted to externally oriented marketing activities, interest in external data of all types has grown. Marketing activities must address the external environment in which they operate. They need to take into consideration national, state, and local trends in healthcare delivery, financing, and regulation. They need to be aware of developments in the local market that will affect their initiatives. They particularly need to have an understanding of the characteristics of other healthcare organizations within the market area, especially competitors.

Primary Versus Secondary Data

Another useful distinction is made between primary data and secondary data. Primary data collection activities involve the use of surveys, focus groups, observational methods, and other techniques. Secondary data collection involves accessing data that were collected for some other purpose but are now used for marketing research. Indeed, most of the data used in marketing research comes from secondary sources. See Exhibit 16.2 for a comparison of primary and secondary data.

EXHIBIT 16.2
Comparison of Primary and Secondary Data

	Primary Data	Secondary Data
Source	Collected by marketer	Collected by someone else
Reason	Collected specifically for this project	Collected for some other unrelated purpose
Usefulness	Directly applicable to the specific project	Must be interpreted to address the project
Ownership	Marketer owns	Someone else owns
Expense involved	Expensive	Free or inexpensive
Skills required	Data collection and analytic skills	Analytic skills
Time required	Significant data collection time required	Immediately available once accessed
Quality	Controlled by marketer	Potentially unknown

Geographic Level

Another notable component of health data is geographic dimension. Data are made available for a number of different geographic units, including administrative units, statistical units, and functional units. *Administrative units* are official entities set up for administrative purposes. States, counties, municipalities, and school districts are some examples of administrative units. Much of the data available to marketers are collected for administrative units.

Statistical units are established primarily for data collection purposes. Primary examples are the units established by the federal government for purposes of data collection during the decennial census, including census regions, metropolitan statistical areas, census tracts, and census blocks. Most demographic data are compiled from these units.

Functional units are established to carry out some practical function and may be unrelated to administrative or statistical units. The best-known examples are the zip code areas designated by the U.S. Postal Service. Their primary function is to support mail delivery. However, because zip codes have become such a common unit for analyzing the spatial distribution of various phenomena, they are frequently used as a geographic unit in marketing research. Another example of a functional unit of particular significance to marketers is *area of dominant influence* (ADI), which was established by the media to indicate the sphere of influence of radio, television, and other forms of media.

Healthcare marketers are likely to operate at different levels of geography, depending on the product being marketed and the type of organization involved. The Centers for Disease Control and Prevention (CDC), for example, focus on national-level data and examine morbidity trends for the entire U.S. population. Pharmaceutical companies with a national market also tend to examine data at that level. A large specialty group is likely to draw patients from a wide geographic area covering several counties; in this case, the county is probably the best unit for data collection. A family practitioner in a solo practice typically serves a fairly defined service area in a county. In this case, the zip code area may be the level at which data would best be collected and analyzed.

The choice of geographic unit for the analysis is important not only because of its implications for the service area under study but also because different types of data are available for different geographic areas. For many types of information, the county may offer the most extensive range of data; generally, the smaller the unit of geography is, the fewer the data available. Although use of the zip code or census tract as the unit of geography may allow for more precise delineation of the service area, access to certain types of data becomes more limited. Thus, there is likely to be a trade-off between the specificity of the service area and the types of data available.

Temporal Dimension

Temporal dimension is another aspect of data that marketers must consider. Health professionals typically think in terms of current data—that is, data that relate to the present time frame or, at least, to the immediate past (e.g., the last set of lab tests). Hence, they are interested in information management systems that can provide real-time access to data.

From a marketing perspective, current data are important but, in some ways, are less important than future data and even historical data. Current data are most valuable as a baseline against which past data can be compared and from which future figures can be projected. Marketing is future oriented, and effective marketing depends on insight into likely future conditions affecting the healthcare environment. Because actual future data do not exist, future conditions relevant to the community or the healthcare organization must be projected. Increasing emphasis is being placed on synthetic projection of the size and characteristics of populations and trends in health service demand and utilization.

Data Generation Methods

The data generation methods discussed in this chapter are divided into four general categories: (1) censuses, (2) registration systems, (3) surveys, and (4) synthetic production. Censuses, registries, and surveys are more traditional sources of data supportive of health marketing activities, although synthetically produced statistics, such as population estimates and projections, have become standard marketing analysis tools.

Censuses

A census of the population involves a complete count of the persons residing in a specific place at a specific time. The U.S. Census Bureau (in the Department of Commerce) conducts a census of population and housing every ten years (the decennial census). The 2010 enumeration will be the twenty-third decennial census.

Although a census theoretically involves a complete count of the population, the decennial census conducted in the United States falls short of a true census in two respects. First, every decade, a segment of the population is missed in the enumeration, resulting in some level of undercount. The undercount is typically less than 3 percent, but its mere existence creates myriad problems. Second, a large portion of the data on population and housing characteristics is obtained from a sample of the nation's households. Only a portion of the population and housing questions is asked of all U.S. households. The remaining questions are asked of approximately one out of every six households. Although the use of sampling significantly reduces the cost of conducting the census, it generates figures that some might incorrectly assume to be complete counts.

The infrequent administration of the census is another source of problems. In a society where rapid change is common, collecting data at ten-year intervals has its shortcomings. With the elapse of time after the census year, the usefulness of the data decreases. Marketers typically need the most current data possible, and even at the time of their release, census data have exceeded their shelf life. (In 1995, the Census Bureau instituted the American Community Survey [ACS], a national annual survey that involves a large sample drawn from the U.S. population. The ACS is expected to eventually replace much of the decennial census.)

The census collects data on the number of people residing in each living unit (e.g., house, duplex, apartment, dormitory) and their characteristics, such as age, race, ethnicity, marital status, income, occupation, education, employment status, and industry of employment. Data on the dwelling unit in which the respondent lives are also collected, including information on the type of dwelling unit (e.g., apartment or duplex), ownership status, value of owned house, monthly rent, age of dwelling unit, and a number of other housing characteristics.

Health-related items are noticeably absent from the census, as few have been mandated by legislative action for collection. Other government agencies, as will be shown later, have a much more significant role in the collection of health-related data than the Census Bureau has.

Marketers value demographic data more than any other data the census collects. These data have direct application to the performance of market analyses and indirect applications as input into models for generating prevalence and demand estimates. Although the census is conducted only every ten years, the Census Bureau maintains the capacity to generate population estimates and projections on an ongoing basis. These figures may not be as detailed as some commercially produced ones—for example, they are calculated down to only the county level—but they are broken down in terms of age, race, income, and other important variables.

Census data may be accessed through a variety of sources. Many libraries, for example, are designated as depositories of U.S. government publications and maintain copies of most Census Bureau reports. The U.S. Government Printing Office also makes some publications available to the public at a reasonable cost. Census data sets in electronic format are sold by the Census Bureau and other data "repackagers." The Census Bureau also offers free and relatively user-friendly online access to its data sets through the American FactFinder feature of its website (www.census.gov).

A lesser-known enumeration of business units, called an *economic census*, is conducted every five years (currently in years ending in 2 and 7). The modern economic census was initiated in 1954 and covers businesses engaged in retail trade, wholesale trade, service activities, mineral industries, transportation, construction, manufacturing, agriculture, and government services. The information collected through the economic census includes data on sales, employment, and payroll, along with more specialized data. These data are available for a variety of geographic units, including states, metropolitan areas, counties, and places with 2,500 or more residents.

The economic census compiles extensive data on healthcare businesses as well. All businesses are assigned a code based on the North American Industry Classification System (NAICS). Aggregated data on businesses in NAICS categories that involve health-related activities (e.g., physician practices, pharmacies, medical laboratories) are available from the Census Bureau. There is no other all-inclusive source that indicates, for example, the number of hospitals, pharmacists, and chiropractors located in a particular area. As with its population and housing data, the Census Bureau is increasingly distributing data from the economic census in electronic form.

Registration Systems

A second method of data generation involves establishing a registration system. Registration systems compile, record, and report a broad range of events, institutions, and individuals in a regular, systematic, and timely fashion. Most of the registration systems relevant to this discussion are sponsored by some branch of government, although other types of registration systems will be discussed as well.

The best-known registries in the United States are the *vital events* (i.e., births and deaths) registries established by the National Center for Health Statistics (NCHS). However, other registries may be valuable, especially when examining changes in the level and types of health services required by a population. Examples include registration systems supported by CDC, the Social Security Administration (SSA), and the Centers for Medicare & Medicaid Services (CMS). Statistics from these agencies are generally available, and many provide raw data from their files.

Various agencies of state government also maintain registration systems of health conditions, reflecting the fact that many health-related activities are regulated at the state level. State health departments typically maintain registries of health conditions (e.g., cancer cases), noteworthy public health problems (e.g., hazardous waste sites), and program participation (e.g., family planning counseling). In addition, state health departments or other designated agencies are responsible for maintaining registries of physicians and other healthcare personnel, hospitals and other health facilities, and other types of health information.

Commercial data vendors also maintain registries of various types, including registries of health personnel (often extending beyond clinical personnel to purchasing agents, chief information officers, and so on) and registries of health facilities, from urgent care centers to ambulatory care centers to hospitals. In some cases, vendors supplement registries maintained by government agencies or professional associations. In others, vendors develop proprietary registries to fill voids in the market.

A variation on registries—the *administrative record*—is being used more and more in health-related research. Administrative record systems are not necessarily intended to be registries of all enrollees or members of an organization or a group but rather of transactions involving these individuals. Thus, a list of all Medicare enrollees would be a registry, but the data generated about Medicare enrollees' encounters with the healthcare system would constitute an administrative system.

Examples of Useful Registries

Health departments at the county (or county equivalent) level are charged with filing certificates for births and deaths and, thus, are the initial repositories of vital statistics data. These data are forwarded to the vital statistics agency within the respective state governments. The appropriate state agency compiles the data for use by the state and transmits the files to NCHS. NCHS is responsible for compiling and publishing vital statistics for the nation and its political subdivisions (see Exhibit 16.3).

EXHIBIT 16.3
The National Center for Health Statistics

Many consider NCHS to be the Census Bureau of healthcare. As a division of CDC, NCHS performs a number of invaluable functions related to health and healthcare. For over 40 years, NCHS has carried out the tasks of data collection, analysis, and dissemination. NCHS also coordinates the state centers for health statistics.

NCHS's responsibilities include compiling, analyzing, and publishing vital statistics for the United States and relevant subareas. The results of this massive task provide the basis for such functions as calculating fertility and mortality rates. In turn, other organizations use these statistics in population estimates and projections. The compilation and analysis of morbidity data are other important functions, and NCHS has developed much of the epidemiologic data available on chronic disease and acquired immunodeficiency syndrome (AIDS) using these registries.

In addition to compiling data from various registration sources, NCHS is the foremost administrator of healthcare surveys in the nation. Its sample surveys are generally large-scale endeavors that take two forms: community-based surveys and facility-based surveys. From

---

a healthcare marketing perspective, NCHS's most important survey is the National Health Interview Survey (NHIS), which it uses to collect data annually from approximately 49,000 households. The NHIS is the nation's primary source of data on the incidence and prevalence of health conditions, health status, the number of injuries and disabilities in the population, health services utilization, and other health-related topics. Surveys that involve a sample of participants from the community include the Medical Expenditure Panel Survey (MEPS), the National Health and Nutrition Examination Survey (NHANES), and the National Survey of Family Growth (NSFG). Another survey, the National Maternal and Infant Health Survey (NMIHS), involves a sampling of birth, fetal death, and infant death certificates.

Important facility-based surveys include the National Hospital Discharge Survey, the National Nursing Home Survey, and the National Ambulatory Medical Care Survey (NAMCS). The NAMCS samples the patient records of 2,500 office-based physicians to obtain data on diagnoses, treatments, medications prescribed, and characteristics of physicians and patients.

The data collected through NCHS studies are disseminated in a variety of ways. NCHS's publications include annual books such as *Health, United States* (the official government compendium of statistics on the nation's health) and publications such as *Vital and Health Statistics*. NCHS sponsors conferences and workshops offering not only the findings from its research but also training in its research methodologies. Some NCHS-generated data are available via the Internet (e.g., www.cdc.gov/nchs/data/hus/hus08.pdf).

By contacting the appropriate NCHS division, health data users can obtain detailed statistics, many unpublished, on all of the topics for which it compiles data. NCHS staff are also available to help with data issues and to provide statistics that the health data analyst might require. In short, NCHS is a service-oriented agency that provides a number of invaluable functions for those who require data on health and healthcare.

CDC has been involved in disease surveillance activities since it was established as the Communicable Disease Center in 1946. Surveillance activities now include programs in human reproduction, environmental health, chronic disease, risk reduction, occupational safety and health, and infectious diseases. These data are compiled into registries that serve as a basis for much of the nation's epidemiologic information.

Data registries are the main source of data on many categories of health personnel. Most health professionals must be registered with the state in which they practice. In addition, most belong to professional associations whose rosters become de facto registries. Like the registration of other types of data, the registration of healthcare personnel involves regular, timely recording of people entering a given profession. Registries of health personnel—either government or professional—must be continuously updated, making them more prone to error than most types of registries.

Commercial data vendors maintain databases of physicians and other personnel, some of which are comparable to the more traditional databases maintained by professional organizations and government agencies. Data vendors may identify emerging professions or marginal practitioners that do not have an association base or are not tracked by the government.

The federal government is a major source of nationwide data on health facilities. The National Master Facility Inventory (NMFI) is a comprehensive file of inpatient facilities maintained by NCHS. The institutions included in this NCHS data collection effort are hospitals, nursing homes and related facilities, and other custodial or remedial care facilities. The federal government keeps the NMFI current by periodically adding the names and addresses of newly established facilities licensed by state boards and other agencies. Annual surveys are used to update information on existing facilities.

Arguably, the nation's most complete hospital registry is maintained by the American Hospital Association (AHA). AHA compiles data annually on the availability of services, utilization patterns, financial information, hospital management, and personnel and continuously updates this database through an ongoing survey of the nation's hospitals. AHA reprints some of the information in secondary sources, such as the *County and City Data Book* and NCHS's *Health, United States*. Certain commercial data vendors have also established hospital databases.

Increasingly, local organizations, such as marketing and regulatory agencies and business coalitions, maintain databases on health facilities. Some private data vendors have begun collecting and disseminating data on non-hospital health facilities as well. Vendors are now selling data on health maintenance organizations, urgent care centers, freestanding surgery centers, and other health-related facilities.

Surveys

Sample surveys are frequently used to supplement data from other sources. A sample survey involves the administration of a survey form or questionnaire to a systematically selected segment of a target population. The sample is designed to include respondents who are representative of the population being examined. Conclusions about the total population are then formed on the basis of the data collected from the sample.

The federal government is a major source of survey research data related to healthcare. Primarily through NCHS, the federal government administers a number of ongoing surveys that deal with hospital, ambulatory care, nursing home, and home health utilization; medical care expenditures; and other relevant topics. The National Institutes of Health and CDC also episodically conduct surveys that generate data of interest to healthcare marketers.

Some professional associations and voluntary organizations conduct notable surveys. The American Medical Association (AMA) regularly surveys its members, as does AHA. Voluntary health associations, such as the American Cancer Society and the American Heart Association, may commission surveys of consumers, patients, or physicians. Foundations may fund projects that involve the collection of data through primary research.

Commercial data vendors sponsor nationwide surveys every year or two that may include as many as 100,000 households. Through these surveys, data are collected on health status, health behavior, and healthcare preferences. Certain market research firms collect health-related data as part of their consumer surveys, and public opinion pollsters may also collect data on health and healthcare. Some of the data collected in this manner are considered proprietary and are available only to clients of these firms. Other vendors sell data to the general public.

Synthetic Data

Synthetic data are figures generated in the absence of actual data through the use of statistical models. Synthetic data are created by merging existing demographic or psychographic data and assumptions about population change to produce estimates, projections, and forecasts. These data are particularly valuable given that census and survey activities are restricted as a result of budgeting and time considerations. Because there is a large and growing demand for information for the years between the official censuses, the production of synthetic data has become a major business. See Case Study 16.1 for an example of synthetic data production.

CASE STUDY 16.1
Generating Population Data for Marketing Planning

In 2005, SunCoast Hospital began exploring the possibility of a satellite hospital in a fast-growing suburban area adjacent to the hospital's existing service area. The hospital's marketing department was given the task of determining the size of the market for hospital services in the targeted area. The decision to proceed with planning for a new

(continued)

CASE STUDY 16.1 (*continued*)

facility would be dependent on identification of a population large enough to support a 50-bed hospital.

Although the question was straightforward, the answer was more difficult to determine. Data collected by the decennial census were considered the most accurate information for a given area, but census data were now five years old. Data from the 2000 census might be accurate enough to use (with appropriate disclaimers) in a relatively stable community, but in this case, the population had been growing so rapidly that five-year-old data were likely to be far from accurate.

The marketing researchers considered techniques they might use to estimate the current (2005) population in the target area. One possibility was to extrapolate trends from known data. This technique assumes that current trends are a continuation of past trends. In this case, the researchers acquired data for the target area from the 1990 and 2000 censuses, assuming that figures from these two points in time would be most realistic. (The researchers could have gone back further, but given the rapid growth in the community, they thought older data would not be appropriate.)

To estimate the population at the time of the study (2005), the researchers used a straight-line method to determine the average annual population increase for the area between 1990 and 2000 and then applied that rate of change to the 2000–2005 period. Thus, the calculation was:

> (2000 population – 1990 population) ÷ 10 years =
> (Average annual population increase × 5) + 2000 population =
> 2005 population estimate.

When the equation was computed, it yielded the following results:

> (20,000 – 10,000 = 10,000) ÷ 10 = 1,000 × 5 = 5,000
> + 20,000 = 25,000.

Thus, the technique generated a 2005 population estimate of 25,000 residents for the service area. This approach assumed a steady population increase of 1,000 each year.

For comparison purposes, the researchers examined the year-to-year percentage increase rather than the increase in absolute numbers. The formula for that calculation was:

[(2000 population − 1990 population) ÷ 1990 population]
÷ 10 years = [(Average annual percentage increase × 5) × 2000
population] + 2000 population = 2005 population estimate.

When the equation was computed, it yielded the following results:

(20,000 − 10,000 = 10,000) ÷ 10,000 = 100% ÷ 10 = 10% per
year × 5 = 50% × 20,000 = 10,000 + 20,000 = 30,000.

This approach yielded an estimate of 30,000 residents rather than
25,000, reflecting that the proportionate increase was relatively greater
than the absolute increase.

Both approaches were equally valid, and both indicated a rapidly
growing population. From the hospital's perspective, a population of
30,000 was better than a population of 25,000. The experience of the
market researcher was brought to bear to determine which estimate
appeared to be the most viable.

Discussion Questions

- Why was a current population estimate unavailable to the
  SunCoast administrators?
- What data did the researchers choose as a basis for calculating
  population estimates and why?
- To use a straight-line estimation method, what assumptions have
  to be made?
- Why did the two techniques yield different estimates when the
  same baseline data were used?
- Given the goal of the hospital, should it have used the more
  conservative figure or the larger estimate?

Both government agencies and commercial data vendors are meeting
today's demand for synthetic data. Within the federal government, population estimates for states, metropolitan statistical areas, and counties are prepared each year as a joint effort of the Census Bureau and the state agency
designated under the Federal-State Cooperative for Population Estimates
(FSCPE). The purpose of the program is to standardize data and procedures
so that generated estimates are of the highest possible quality.

Data generated by commercial vendors are available for small units of
geography (e.g., census block groups), and they often provide greater detail
(e.g., sex and age breakdowns) than government-produced figures. Vendors
may also generate estimates and projections for custom geographic areas

(e.g., a market area). Calculations for smaller geographic areas and population components, however, are less precise than calculations for their larger counterparts, but because these vendor-generated figures are easily accessible and timely, they have become a mainstay of health services marketers.

A major category of synthetic data includes estimates and projections of health services demand. There are few sources of actual data on the use of health services, and projections of future demand are often required, so a number of approaches have been developed to synthetically generate data to fill this void. The general approach involves applying known utilization rates to current or projected population figures. To the extent possible, these figures are adjusted for, at a minimum, the age and sex composition of the target population. Most of these calculations are based on utilization rates generated by NCHS.

Commercial data vendors have led the way in developing demand estimates and projections. Some vendors have developed calculations for the full range of inpatient and outpatient services, although these data are often available only to their established customers. Other vendors provide select data on, for example, the demand for a particular service line. See Case Study 16.2 for an example of the use of synthetic data.

CASE STUDY 16.2
Methodology for Estimating Health Services Demand

For strategic planning purposes, Mountain View Hospital needed to determine the level of morbidity in its service area population and estimate the demand for health services that these conditions would yield. Unfortunately, these types of data were not readily available, and the researcher had to develop estimates and projections of health services demand on the basis of modeled data.

To develop an estimate of the demand for health services in a population, the researcher needed two types of information: utilization rates that could be applied to the defined population and population estimates and/or projections. The utilization rates available reflected the population's age and sex, adjusted for region of the country. The population figures broke down the population into relevant age–sex categories. For each diagnosis-related group, for example, the utilization rate for, say, cardiac catheterization was calculated for each of 19 different age groups and both sexes. These rates were then applied to the respective age–sex groups in the population in question, and the sum of the estimates/projections was calculated.

Utilization rates based on data collected through nationwide surveys were obtained from NCHS. For example, when the rates for each age–sex group for each medical diagnosis for hospital patients were applied to the population estimate (broken into age–sex groups), a reasonably accurate estimation of health services utilization was generated. The following table on cardiac catheterization services illustrates this process.

Calculation of Demand for Cardiac Catheterization

Population		<5	5–9	10–14	15–19	20–24	25–29	30–34	35–39	40–44
Males		1,000	1,050	970	270	2,580	3,530	3,170	3,270	3,230
Females		1,200	1,100	1,030	20	420	1,220	1,550	2,350	3,170

	45–49	50–54	55–59	60–64	65–69	70–74	75–79	80–84	>85
Males	3,110	2,020	1,070	690	280	130	1,050	970	270
Females	2,570	2,560	2,450	1,850	1,530	1,430	1,100	1,030	20

Utilization Rate	<5	5–9	10–14	15–19	20–24	25–29	30–34	35–39	40–44
Males	0.1	0.0	0.0	0.0	0.0	0.1	0.3	1.1	2.5
Females	0.0	0.0	0.0	0.1	0.0	0.0	0.2	0.3	0.7

	45–49	50–54	55–59	60–64	65–69	70–74	75–79	80–84	>85
Males	3.6	9.8	10.4	14.8	18.0	19.8	28.0	24.6	9.4
Females	1.7	2.6	5.2	3.9	9.3	11.7	12.8	8.2	8.9

Demand	<5	5–9	10–14	15–19	20–24	25–29	30–34	35–39	40–44
Males	0	0	0	0	0	0	1	4	8
Females	0	0	0	0	0	0	0	1	2

	45–49	50–54	55–59	60–64	65–69	70–74	75–79	80–84	>85	Total
Males	11	20	11	10	5	3	29	24	3	129
Females	4	7	13	7	14	17	14	8	0	87

Each age–sex category had its own utilization rate for cardiac catheterization. Because this procedure is primarily performed on older adults and senior citizens, relatively few children were affected. As this table demonstrates, the number of cases was calculated separately for each age–sex category, and the results were totaled to determine the overall demand for the population. For example, women in the

(continued)

CASE STUDY 16.2 (*continued*)

40- to 45-year-old age group reported a utilization rate of 0.7 per 1,000, compared with a rate of 2.5 per 1,000 for men in the same age group. Thus, although the populations of men and women in this age group were similar, four times as many cardiac catheterizations were predicted for men than for women in that age group. Each age–sex category was compared in a similar manner.

For this particular population, it appeared that there would be demand for 216 cardiac catheterizations annually, 129 of them for men and 87 of them for women. In the absence of actual data, this model returned a reasonable approximation of the level of demand for this procedure.

Discussion Questions

- Under what circumstances is it necessary to generate synthetic data (estimates and projections) for health services demand?
- What assumptions were made with regard to the utilization rates and population projections used?
- How might the figures look different for a similar table for childbirth or breast cancer?
- What are the dangers involved in making any type of projection with regard to health services utilization, and for how many years out (e.g., 5, 10, 20) should one feel comfortable making a projection?

Sources of Data for Healthcare Marketing

A variety of sources of data are available to healthcare marketers today, and the number continues to grow. These sources are divided into four main categories: government agencies, professional associations, private organizations, and commercial data vendors. The products available from these sources are also divided into two categories: reports that summarize the data and the actual data sets. Although the sources presented in the following sections refer to the agencies and publications responsible for the data set being discussed, there are numerous compendia that marketers may find useful (see Exhibit 16.4).

Government Agencies

Government at all levels generates, compiles, manipulates, and/or disseminates health-related data. The federal government, through the decennial

EXHIBIT 16.4
Federal Compendia of Health Data

Currently, there is no national clearinghouse for data on health and healthcare in the United States, making identifying and acquiring data a challenge for health marketers. There are, however, compendia of health data that might be useful for many purposes. Although no single publication provides all of the data a marketer is likely to need, these compendia offer a reasonable starting point. They not only compile data but also often direct the researcher to the origin of the data and other useful resources.

The best known of the compendia of health-related data is titled *Health, United States*. This work is published annually by NCHS and includes data gathered from NCHS and many other sources. The publication includes data on health status, health behavior, health services utilization, healthcare resources, healthcare expenditures, and insurance coverage. These data are available mostly at the national level, although some state and regional data are available.

A companion publication, *Mental Health, United States*, is published less frequently than *Health, United States* but is the primary source of data on behavioral healthcare. The statistics are based on data collected by the Center for Mental Health Services.

Another more specialized compendium is published by CMS. Simply referred to as *Data Compendium* (followed by the publication year), this book aggregates data on Medicaid and Medicare. The data are drawn primarily from CMS files, although data from sources outside the agency are also included. The data CMS compiles are national-level data. Some state-level data are also reported. No data on sub-state levels of geography are presented.

Because demographic data are so important to healthcare marketers, compendia that focus on this type of data are also useful. The *County and City Data Book* is published every two years by the Census Bureau and includes more than 200 data items for each county and 134 items for each city of 25,000 or more persons. Data of interest to healthcare analysts include population statistics; vital records; hospital, physician, and nursing home statistics; and some insurance data.

The *State and Metropolitan Area Data Book* is published by the Census Bureau every four years and contains 128 data items for each state, 298 variables for each metropolitan statistical area (MSA), and

(continued)

EXHIBIT 16.4 (*continued*)

87 variables for each MSA's central city. *County Business Patterns*, also prepared by the Census Bureau, provides a comprehensive count of the healthcare businesses operating in each U.S. county.

Every year, the Census Bureau publishes the *Statistical Abstract of the United States*. The *Abstract* contains detailed data for the nation as a whole for 31 subject categories (e.g., vital statistics, nutrition), as well as data for states and metropolitan areas. Most states publish a statistical abstract that includes comparable data for the state and its counties and cities.

Source: Adapted from Thomas (2003a).

---

census and related activities, is the world's largest processor of many types of data. Other federal agencies are major managers of data for the related topics of fertility, morbidity, and mortality statistics.

Through NCHS, CDC, the National Institutes of Health, and other organizations, a large share of the nation's health data is generated. The Bureau of Health Resources (Department of Health and Human Services) maintains a master file of much of the health data compiled by the federal government, titled the *Area Resource File (ARF)*. Other federal sources outside of health-related agencies, such as the Bureau of Labor Statistics (e.g., source of data on health occupations) and the Department of Agriculture (e.g., source of nutritional data), create databases of health information. The number and variety of databases generated by federal agencies are impressive, but the variety of agencies involved means databases vary with regard to coverage, content, format, cost, collection frequency, and accessibility.

State and local governments are also major sources of health-related data. In fact, a survey of health data users consistently indicates that state agencies are their primary source of data for marketing research (Thomas 2003a). State governments generate demographic data, and each state has a state data center for demographic projections. Vital statistics data can often be obtained in the timeliest fashion at the state level. University data centers may also be involved in processing health-related data. Local governments may generate demographic data for use in various marketing functions. City or county governments may produce population projections, and county health departments are responsible for collecting and disseminating vital statistics data.

Professional Associations

Associations in the health industry are another source of health-related data, chiefly AMA (and related medical specialty organizations) and AHA. Other professional organizations (e.g., American Dental Association) and facilities maintain databases on their members and on activities related to the organization's membership. These organizations typically develop their databases for internal use but are making them increasingly available to outside parties.

A number of organizations have been formed in recent years that focus specifically on health data, and others have established formal sections that deal with health data within their broader context. The National Association of Health Data Organizations (NAHDO) brings together disparate parties from the public and private sector that have an interest in health data. The National Association of County and City Health Officers (NACCHO) has become active in terms of facilitating access to health data. The Health Information and Management Systems Society (HIMSS) is one of the largest organizations addressing data management issues.

Private Organizations

Many private organizations (mostly not-for-profit) collect or disseminate health-related data. Voluntary healthcare associations often compile, repackage, or disseminate such data. The American Cancer Society, for example, distributes morbidity and mortality data related to cancer. Some private organizations commission and publish special studies on fertility or related issues.

Many organizations repackage data collected elsewhere (e.g., from the Census Bureau or NCHS) and present them in a specialized context. The Population Reference Bureau—a private not-for-profit organization—distributes population statistics in various forms, for example. Other organizations, such as AARP, not only compile and disseminate secondary data but are actively involved in primary data collection and sponsor numerous studies that include some form of data collection.

Commercial Data Vendors

Commercial data vendors are the fourth category of sources of health-related data. As discussed earlier in the chapter, such organizations have emerged to fill perceived gaps in the availability of health data. Commercial data vendors may establish and maintain their own proprietary databases or reprocess/repackage existing data. For example, SMG Marketing maintains databases on nursing homes, urgent care centers, and other types of facilities and makes this information available in a variety of forms. Also included in this group are the major data vendors (e.g., ESRI Business Information, Claritas, Experian) that incorporate health-related databases into their business database systems.

Health Data and the Internet

The Internet has become a force with regard to health data. In addition to consumer-oriented health information, data for use by health professionals are available on the Web, including bibliographical and text files as well as some patient data from various healthcare organizations.

Millions of sites deal with some aspect of healthcare, and some of the most extensive sites have been established by healthcare organizations.

Despite the spate of health-related data available via the Internet, most of it has been of limited usefulness to healthcare marketers until recently. Most health sites offer data geared to healthcare consumers. Today, health-care consumers can find a doctor, diagnose a condition, or order prescription drugs and nutritional supplements via the Internet. More advanced sites may allow users to manipulate site content in basic ways. Even commercial data vendors have attempted to make data more accessible via the Internet.

The federal government has led the charge to make raw data available on the Internet. Agencies such as the Census Bureau, CDC, NCHS, and CMS have expended significant effort posting their data files on the Web. Web-based files can be posted much more expeditiously than data can be published in print form. Data that had to be purchased from agencies in the past are now offered through many of these sites at no charge, and data sets too cumbersome to publish in hard copy are easily distributed via the Internet. As print versions of data reports are steadily eliminated by the federal government and other data generators, the importance of Internet distribution will increase.

Summary

Healthcare marketers need a wide variety of data to research, plan, implement, and evaluate marketing activities. In addition to health-related data, marketers use demographic, psychographic, and economic data, and there is a growing interest in data seemingly unrelated to healthcare (e.g., data on housing, employment, and crime). Health-related data can be categorized as community or organizational data, primary or secondary data, and internal or external data. These data sets can also be categorized in terms of geographic level and period (i.e., past, present, or future). Health-related data are generated through censuses, registries, and surveys. Increasingly, synthetic data are being used for estimates and projections.

Healthcare marketers can access health-related data in a number of ways. Government agencies at all levels are important sources, and the federal government is a major generator and disseminator of many of the types of data that healthcare marketers seek. CDC, NCHS, and CMS are some of the federal agencies that make health-related data available.

Professional associations, such as AMA and AHA, compile data and make statistics and data sets available to the public. Not-for-profit associations, such as the American Cancer Society and the American Heart Association, assemble and distribute data to health professionals and the general public. Educational institutions and research organizations provide a significant amount of data for health professionals. Increasingly, commercial data vendors have entered the field to supplement or, in some cases, supplant the data provided by other organizations.

The Internet allows massive amounts of health-related data to be distributed. The federal government has led the way in posting health data on the Internet, and a variety of public and private entities now provide online data.

Key Points

- Data on healthcare and other topics are essential in researching, planning, implementing, and evaluating marketing activities.
- The healthcare industry generates an incredible amount of data, although many of these data are not easily accessible.
- More restrictions are placed on the use of health-related data than on the use of data related to other industries.
- Most market research is based on secondary data, although primary research must be conducted in some situations.
- Marketers must be familiar with the geographic levels at which data are aggregated to effectively use this information.
- Health-related data are generated via censuses, registration systems, and sample surveys, and marketers need to be familiar with the characteristics of each method.
- In the absence of actual health-related data, synthetic data based on computer models are often generated.
- NCHS is the primary source of health-related data in the United States.

- Other federal agencies are major sources of health-related data and other types of data useful to healthcare marketers.
- Other sources of health-related data include government at other levels (e.g., state level), professional associations, voluntary organizations, and commercial data vendors.
- The Internet is a major source of health-related data, and data sets that are too large to publish in hard copy can be easily distributed online.

Discussion Questions

- Why hasn't the healthcare industry developed data clearinghouses and nationwide sources of market data as other industries have?
- Under what circumstances might primary rather than secondary data need to be collected?
- What disadvantages of the decennial census as a data collection method counter its usefulness in providing almost complete coverage of the population?
- Why are registration systems and administrative records becoming increasingly important sources of data for healthcare marketing?
- What function does NCHS serve, and why is NCHS an important resource for healthcare marketers?
- Under what circumstances do marketers need to access synthetic health-related data generated by government agencies or commercial data vendors?
- Why do healthcare marketers frequently use health-related data generated by agencies of state government?
- What are the advantages of accessing health-related data via the Internet?

Additional Resources

American Hospital Association. 2009. *AHA Guide to the Health Care Field*. Chicago: American Hospital Association.

American Medical Association. 2008. *Physician Characteristics and Distribution in the U.S., 2008*. Chicago: American Medical Association.

———. 2002. *Socioeconomic Characteristics of Medical Practice, 2002*. Chicago: American Medical Association.

Centers for Disease Control and Prevention, U.S. Department of Health and Human Services website: www.cdc.gov.

Morbidity and Mortality Weekly Review, published by the Centers for Disease Control and Prevention.

National Center for Health Statistics (NCHS), U.S. Department of Health and Human Services website: www.cdc.gov/nchs.

NCHS. 2009. *Health, United States, 2008.* Washington, DC: U.S. Government Printing Office. Also available online at www.cdc.gov/nchs/data/hus/hus08.pdf.

U.S. Bureau of Health Professions, U.S. Department of Health and Human Services website: http://bhpr.hrsa.gov.

U.S. Bureau of Primary Healthcare, U.S. Department of Health and Human Services website: http://bhpr.hrsa.gov.

U.S. Census Bureau, U.S. Department of Commerce website: www.census.gov. (See in particular "American FactFinder.")

U.S. Census Bureau. 2004. *County Business Patterns, 2004.* Washington, DC: U.S. Government Printing Office (now available only electronically at www.census .gov/econ/cbp/download).

U.S. Health Resources and Services Administration, U.S. Department of Health and Human Services website: www.hrsa.gov.

THE FUTURE OF HEALTHCARE MARKETING

Part V concludes the book. Chapter 17 summarizes the current status of the field and speculates on the future of healthcare marketing. It also proposes factors likely to influence the future course of marketing in healthcare and identifies hot trends on which healthcare marketers may wish to capitalize.

HEALTHCARE MARKETING IN 2010 AND BEYOND

The field of healthcare marketing is young but rapidly maturing. As it becomes increasingly tailored to the needs of healthcare, substantial changes are anticipated. The highly volatile and unpredictable environment in which healthcare marketers operate makes predicting the future difficult but nevertheless important. This chapter reviews the current status of healthcare marketing and considers the factors that will influence its future direction.

Where Healthcare Marketing Is Today

It is difficult not to be optimistic about the future of marketing in healthcare. Much has been learned from past successes and failures, and better tools are available to healthcare marketers today. Marketers can measure patient satisfaction; they have access to much better consumer data; and new techniques that take advantage of contemporary technology are emerging. Healthcare marketing has matured significantly, and the expertise of marketing professionals in the field has increased dramatically. The data available today, current analytical techniques, and contemporary technology offer capabilities that healthcare marketers would not have envisioned a decade ago. The direct-to-consumer movement is bringing customers back into the spotlight, and their return is good news for healthcare marketers.

During the short history of marketing in healthcare, the field has experienced numerous ups and downs. The appropriateness of the role of marketing in healthcare has always been controversial, and the gains made on behalf of the marketing enterprise during the 1980s and 1990s were hard won. Despite this halting progress, the acceptance of marketing as a legitimate function of the healthcare organization increased significantly in the last years of the twentieth century.

Support for marketing plateaued around 2000 after several years of relatively enthusiastic backing by healthcare administrators. This development was not necessarily negative but demonstrated that the profession was begin-ning to show maturity. Leaving behind some of the excesses of the 1980s and 1990s, healthcare organizations and their marketers adopted a much more realistic approach to promotions.

Because of the increased pressure on all healthcare organizations (and especially not-for-profits) to improve their bottom line, most have come to appreciate the importance of marketing. Given the need to attract patients and increase volume, progressive organizations are placing increased value on marketing in an increasingly competitive environment. Even so, some still see marketing as a cost center and not a contributor to the bottom line.

Although healthcare marketing has been slowed by the economic downturn of 2008 and 2009, healthcare does not appear to be affected to the same degree as other industries in which much more of the corporate budget is devoted to marketing. Healthcare organizations may have backed away from expensive advertising as a result of budget considerations, but as this book goes to press, most are realizing that they cannot wait for a com-plete turnaround to get back to marketing as usual. The budget and staff cutbacks they have made appear to be a reaction to higher operating costs, more expensive personnel, and the overall increased cost of doing business; such modification does not imply that marketing is seen as expendable.

Healthcare marketing has fared best in organizations that have adopted a marketing orientation. In the post-9/11 environment, some healthcare ad-ministrators became so focused on survival, both personal and institutional, that marketing became less of a priority (at a time when it should have been more of a priority). Those with a strategic focus have remained strong sup-porters, whereas organizations that have not incorporated a marketing mind-set are more likely to waiver when confronted with distractions.

Faced with economic challenges, some healthcare organizations have eliminated their in-house marketing departments and reduced long-term in-vestment in marketing staff in favor of short-term commitment to outside consultants. In addition, there has been a growing emphasis on partnering with other organizations for co-marketing, co-branding, and sponsorships.

Other healthcare organizations have taken the Web-based approach to marketing. Those who have developed a significant Web presence—and have adequate capabilities to support it—have found promotion via the Internet to be a successful strategy in the current environment.

Where Healthcare Marketing Is Going

There is every indication that the trend toward more acceptance of marketing in healthcare will continue and that the role of the healthcare marketer will expand. There is growing recognition that marketing is not an optional activity but something every organization must undertake. As more and more organizations couple their marketing function with their business development function, marketing is becoming an inherent part of corporate operations. The question will no longer be "To market or not to market?" but "To what extent will marketing contribute to the success of the organization?"

A growing emphasis on grassroots marketing has become evident. Marketers are developing an ability to attract more and "better" customers and are focusing on improving customer satisfaction. New hires today are likely to receive a marketing orientation regardless of their position, and incentive programs are turning employees into marketers. Marketers are working more closely with the fund development department, fostering customer-friendly facilities, co-marketing with the community relations department, and establishing strong relationships with the target population. These actions are expected to lead to increased business volume, and marketers are in a position to demonstrate that this additional business was generated as a result of their efforts.

Trends Affecting the Future of Healthcare Marketing

The healthcare industry has continued to move in a direction that not only encourages marketing but demands it. Nearly every development in healthcare suggests that the role of marketing will continue to grow dramatically. Consumer choice has emerged as a mantra as baby boomers come to set the tone in healthcare. The diversification of health plan options is expected to add more fuel to this fire, and the expansion of services into new settings (e.g., walk-in clinics at Walgreen's) involves a significant marketing component. If marketers can demonstrate the effectiveness of marketing initiatives, marketing could well become *the* critical function in most healthcare organizations. The trends described in the following sections are expected to influence the direction of healthcare marketing for the foreseeable future.

Shifting Demand for Health Services

The volume and type of demand for future health services are arguably the most important pieces of knowledge a healthcare marketer can possess. In healthcare, however, this information is elusive. The demand for health services is influenced by numerous factors, both inside and outside of healthcare. Some of the emerging demand may be created by the industry as it introduces new products and services; some of it will be a result of changes in reimbursement patterns or the introduction of regulations. Yet other changes in health services demand will reflect broad social trends that have limited direct connection with healthcare. Now, with healthcare reform on the table, the future demand for health services is even more unpredictable.

One might argue that the demand for health services in the United States will be flat for the foreseeable future. Population growth is slow, and a limited number of potential new customers will be added to the pool annually. On the other hand, there is a burgeoning market for elective procedures. Once the economy recovers and healthcare consumers—especially aging baby boomers—regain their financial footing, the demand for elective procedures and vanity products is likely to surge.

Despite the factors that are restraining the use of inpatient care, the demand for inpatient services is beginning to revive, and many hospitals are scrambling to find space to accommodate increasing admissions. This demand can only grow as aging baby boomers come to require more inpatient care. Current demographic trends suggest an increase in the demand for gerontological services, women's services, and specialty care for older adults. This prediction will likely equate to reduced demand for obstetrics and pediatric care but increased demand for care in other areas, such as gynecological services.

Perhaps more than any other factor, the future demand for health services will set the direction of healthcare marketing. For this reason, healthcare marketers need to develop methodologies that will accurately predict the future needs and wants of an increasingly diverse pool of healthcare consumers.

Growing Consumerism

Some observers predicted that the first decade of the twenty-first century would be the decade of the consumer in healthcare, and ample evidence exists to support this contention. The consumer movement has been driven by a number of factors, including a backlash against managed care, the introduction of defined contributions by benefit managers, and the ascendancy of the baby boom cohort as the dominant healthcare consumer group in the United States.

Many see healthcare as increasingly market driven and consumer oriented. They argue that a consumer choice environment is emerging in which healthcare organizations will be required to increasingly cater to the needs and wants of a population that is heterogeneous in terms of demographics, lifestyles, and health behavior.

Competition remains strong, and healthcare organizations will be forced to compete for the attention, business, and loyalty of healthcare consumers at a level unknown in the past. These trends are going to require marketers to understand both existing and prospective customers better than at any previous time. Target marketing will become more important, and mass customization will become common. Direct-to-consumer marketing and customer relationship marketing will also be essential techniques for many healthcare organizations in the future.

Increasing Competition

Healthcare organizations can expect continued and even increased competition for healthcare consumers. The capacity of the system continues to exceed demand in most places, and slow growth in demand coupled with the entry of new players into the healthcare arena can be expected to raise competition to a level not experienced in the past. The emergence of a whole new industry around alternative therapies has added another layer of competition to the healthcare arena as unconventional providers promote goods and services that compete with those of mainstream providers.

The monopolies many healthcare organizations maintained in the past have given way to cutthroat competition, and no component of the industry remains unaffected. Hospitals face competition from other hospitals, from physicians and other clinicians, and from entrepreneurs entering healthcare from other industries. Physicians face competition from other physicians, from hospitals and urgent care facilities, and, increasingly, from alternative therapists. Health plans face heated competition for customers, and the survival of managed care plans depends on their ability to sway enrollees. Even the pharmaceutical industry has become more competitive as more products compete for a patient pool that is not growing all that quickly.

New products and services continue to be introduced, and healthcare consumers need to be educated on these issues—and convinced to purchase a particular brand. An industry experiencing such a profusion of new products and services cannot help but be highly competitive. In many instances, existing products and services have become increasingly standardized, challenging marketers to find creative ways to differentiate their organizations from competitors.

The Dominance of Technology

Regardless of the trends that develop in healthcare, the industry will continue to be heavily vested in technology. Despite those who decry the impersonality of a technology-based system of care, this dimension of health services is becoming more and more dominant. Technology not only will play an increasing role in the provision of care but will also be a major factor in the development of new products and services. The growing acceptance of electronic patient records and the ultimate conversion of clinicians to computer enthusiasts will ensure that the industry is permeated with technology at all levels.

These developments mean that healthcare marketers must be knowledgeable about the technology underlying the provision of care. Marketers must be able to explain cutting-edge technology to consumers and sell them on the use of these techniques. They will be asked to differentiate these techniques from traditional techniques and convey those differences to prospective patients.

Healthcare marketing will similarly be affected by the ubiquity of technology. Traditional approaches to marketing are being supplanted by more complex methodologies that capitalize on contemporary technology. Database marketing, customer relationship marketing, and predictive modeling are all based on information technology. Even traditional marketing approaches, such as direct-to-consumer approaches, will take advantage of information technology as they become more sophisticated.

Increasing Costs

After a brief period of moderated costs in the healthcare industry, most experts predict rising costs for the foreseeable future. Some increases are already evident. A number of factors are contributing to the higher costs of providing health services and the consequent higher prices charged to consumers. Although consumers in the past have been insulated from the costs of healthcare, the changing insurance environment and the emergence of a large elective surgery industry are making cost issues central to the concerns of consumers, employers, and anyone else who is paying for health services.

A lack of price-based competition and the extraordinary role of third-party payers limited the relevance of the pricing component of the four Ps in the past (see Exhibit 3.4), but in the future, pricing will become a more salient issue. Health plans, providers of elective procedures, and other entities are increasingly likely to compete on the basis of price, and healthcare marketers must be in a position to support this marketing angle. Further, marketers must be able to explain to consumers why prices are increasing or why their provider's prices are higher than a competitor's.

Emphasis on Outcomes

Many observers suggested that during the first decade of the twenty-first century the focus would shift to outcomes in healthcare. In response to concerns over the effectiveness of the healthcare delivery system and persistent disclosures of the level of medical errors in the system, their prediction has come true. Healthcare providers must not only defend adverse outcomes they report but capitalize on favorable outcomes. As more payers turn to a pay-for-performance system, the importance of positive outcomes will further increase. Patient safety issues will continue to be paramount, and a considerable groundswell of support for more controls over patient care has emerged.

Marketers will have to be front and center on the outcomes issue. They will need to develop promotional campaigns based on high surgical success rates or low mortality rates. They may have to rationalize low success rates or high mortality rates. In any case, marketers are likely to be the go-between for providers and the public, the regulators, and the policy setters.

Growing Labor Force Concerns

Despite the weak labor market, healthcare providers continue to face shortages of key personnel. Although there have been cyclical labor shortages in the past, the current shortfall is more extreme than previous ones, and there is little chance for short-term amelioration of the problem. While the most highly publicized shortages are for nurses, there are shortages of many other clinicians and technical staff, and now even some predictions of a future physician shortage. Even though the recession has reduced the demand for many health services and, hence, the need for health professionals, shortages remain because the areas in which they are evident are generally essential services.

To fill these vacancies, providers are attempting to attract staff from other providers. As a result, much of healthcare marketers' energy has been shifted away from attracting consumers to attracting skilled personnel. Gone are the days when nurses and other personnel automatically showed up in response to job postings. Marketers must develop aggressive recruitment plans that differentiate their organizations from others competing for the same pool of workers, especially now that prospective employees have conceded that salary is only one factor—and may not be the most important factor—driving their decision to accept a position. Some healthcare marketers are having to extend their recruitment energies even further to develop a new set of skills to address the growing number of foreign nationals working in the U.S. healthcare industry and the trend toward attracting healthcare workers from overseas.

Healthcare marketers are also faced with the challenge of retaining skilled staff. This challenge requires marketers to have internal marketing skills and an ability to support administrative efforts aimed at developing an environment that fosters loyalty among nurses and other personnel. Better than anyone, marketers should know what drives customers, even if they are internal customers.

Globalization

The globalization trend affecting other industries is also affecting healthcare. More immigrants of increasingly diverse backgrounds are requiring health services, and the employment of foreign-trained medical personnel is growing. Some health systems are actively seeking patients from other countries and adapting their marketing techniques to cater to these new audiences. Other providers are opening health facilities overseas to export U.S. medical expertise to populations that cannot support the sophisticated specialty services Americans take for granted. Health systems in other countries are aggressively soliciting U.S. citizens to travel abroad as patients to India, Thailand, Singapore, and other countries, offering significantly lower prices and, often, a luxury vacation. U.S. insurance companies that recognize the cost savings resulting from the use of overseas health facilities are slowly but surely abetting this movement.

Globalization is like many other phenomena: Once it starts, it is not likely to stop. Healthcare marketers who spent the past decade learning to appeal to an increasingly diverse U.S. market are now faced with an even greater challenge as their organizations seek customers from overseas. Those charged with marketing an organization's new facility in Singapore, for example, not only have to adapt marketing techniques to a new situation but also have to become knowledgeable about a different culture and business environment.

Healthcare Marketing: Seizing the Opportunity

Healthcare marketers have a better opportunity to seize the moment in healthcare than ever before. They need to continue to demonstrate the contribution marketing can make to the bottom line and its value in developing and promoting new services. Marketers need to be involved early in the strategic planning process so they can influence the development of services and programs and make the organization more customer oriented. They need to demonstrate the potential contribution marketing can make to new ventures and identify trends on which the organization may want to capitalize (e.g., patient safety, consumer empowerment). They must ensure that all initiatives have a marketing component and that clinicians appreciate the significance of marketing.

The most important action marketers can take is to demonstrate their role in developing, enhancing, and packaging services that meet the needs of the market. The ability to match products to customer needs is a unique contribution marketers can make. Marketers need to have the ability to persuade decision makers of the important role of marketing and to provide evidence of the success of marketing initiatives. To do so, marketers must shift their perspective to that of the decision maker. In short, marketing professionals must go beyond the basics of successful marketing and bring a value-added dimension to the table.

During periods of financial retrenchment, healthcare administrators are always looking for costs they can cut, and the marketing function is often at the top of that list. In this environment, healthcare marketers must develop an appreciation for the relative costs of different marketing techniques and media. As distasteful as it might be to some, marketers must develop enough knowledge of financial analysis to be able to calculate the return on the marketing investment.

Today, healthcare marketers have a unique opportunity to shape the future of the field. They are well positioned to contribute to the success of their organizations, to ensure the health and satisfaction of healthcare consumers, and to enhance the overall health status of the community. See Exhibit 17.1 for a discussion of attractive future opportunities.

EXHIBIT 17.1
The Next Hot Marketing Areas

The following areas are likely to be targeted by healthcare marketers for the foreseeable future. Given the unpredictability of healthcare, these "hot spots" are likely to change rapidly and should be considered examples of the types of trends on which marketers might wish to capitalize.

Elder Care

The aging of the U.S. population guarantees that elder care will be a growing concern for healthcare marketers for the foreseeable future. Although the health of U.S. seniors has improved over the health of elders of previous generations, the numbers alone ensure that geriatric care will be a major industry well into the twenty-first century. Healthcare providers are already beginning to experience increases in the demand for senior services. This trend will be exacerbated as the baby boom cohort enters old age. Marketers should be cognizant of the lifestyle differences among the elderly and take these differences into consideration in marketing planning. Furthermore, future developments with regard to Medicare reimbursement are likely to have a major effect on service utilization by the senior population.

Older Adult Services

A category of services that is competing with elder care for attention is older adult care. Although those aged 45 to 64 do not require the same intensity of services as the elderly, they are at an age during which chronic conditions arise and symptoms of physical deterioration appear. Physical impairment is not the only manifestation; people in this age group are prone to suffer from conditions related to stress and psychological dysfunction. Midlife crises, menopause, empty nests, and other factors create anxiety for Americans in this age group. These services have become particularly critical now that the huge baby boom cohort has begun to enter its 60s. There is burgeoning demand for specialists who treat chronic conditions, and the elective surgery component of the system can be expected to expand dramatically as baby boomers seek services aimed at slowing aging and preserving youthfulness.

(continued)

EXHIBIT 17.1 (*continued*)

Fitness and Sports Medicine

Although the fitness craze of the last couple of decades of the twentieth century appears to have leveled off in terms of growth, the wellness, fitness, and sports medicine industry is not going to go away. Despite reports of an increasingly sedentary population, the demand for fitness programs and equipment, sports medicine, and nutraceuticals remains high. The huge baby boom cohort is emphasizing products and services that purport to be healthy or natural. Interestingly, the "green" movement appears to be having the spillover effect of encouraging more healthy lifestyles. More fitness activities mean more sports-related injuries among people who are not used to strenuous exercise. As a result, demand for the services of orthopedic surgeons, physiatrists, rehabilitation counselors, and other health professionals in the sports medicine field can be expected to increase.

Ethnic and Minority Healthcare

Since the 1980s there has been an explosion in the number and variety of racial and ethnic groups in the U.S. population. Burgeoning ethnic groups, such as Hispanic Americans; growing racial groups, such as Asian Americans; new immigrants; and the significant African American population are groups that health services providers have left largely untapped. An increasingly diverse population will call for culturally sensitive programs and creative marketing. Healthcare marketers are beginning to see the opportunities rather than the challenges engendered by this growing racial and ethnic diversity, and many organizations are beginning to adapt their services to cater to these new target audiences. The demand for health services will grow significantly among many ethnic groups (not to mention the pool of potential overseas customers), and healthcare organizations must position themselves to take advantage of these emerging opportunities.

Vanity Services

The growth in cosmetic surgery, laser eye surgery, and other elective procedures has been dramatic over the past two decades, and now the baby boomers promise to fuel even greater demand for health services that make them look and feel better. Consumers must pay out of pocket for most of these services, and the discretionary income of baby boomers should contribute to rapid expansion of the elective component of health services. Many of these procedures are practical responses to the physical deterioration that affects everyone, as witnessed by the demand for laser eye surgery and arthroscopic procedures. Other procedures, such as face-lifts, tummy tucks, and hair transplant procedures are clearly elective. Although the demand for many of these procedures was driven by older women in the past, statistics now indicate that an increasingly younger population is demanding vanity services and that just as many men as women are seeking these services. Although the current economic downturn has suppressed demand for elective procedures, this area will likely experience a surge of pent-up demand once the economy recovers.

Skin Care

Recent developments in skin care procedures are just in time to meet exploding demand. The growth of the senior segment of the population will increase the demand for therapeutic skin care (e.g., for skin cancer), while the burgeoning baby boom population will demand cosmeceuticals that reduce age spots and keep their skin looking young. From rejuvenating creams to laser skin therapy, demand for all types of skin care should increase dramatically. The demand for skin care will reinforce the demand for vanity services and fitness programs already noted.

Alternative Therapies

Although the demand for alternative therapies has been increasing steadily since the 1980s, no one realized the size of this industry until the 1990s. By that time, U.S. consumers were spending more on alternative therapies than they were on conventional therapies, and the burgeoning industry supporting alternative therapies had become well entrenched. Once limited to certain ethnic groups and subsegments of the population, the use of chiropractic services, acupuncture, naturopathy, and massage therapy now cuts across most segments of the U.S. population. As the underlying orientation of U.S. healthcare has changed and the U.S. public has become more open to unconventional approaches, the demand for alternative therapies has exploded. The use of alternative therapies has become so widespread as to be considered mainstream. The correspondence between the emerging preferences of baby boomers and other segments of the population and the attributes of holistic care and other alternative therapies ensures that this industry will experience major growth for the foreseeable future.

(continued)

EXHIBIT 17.1 *(continued)*

International Healthcare

American healthcare organizations are facing an increasingly diverse patient population as the number of immigrants grows and the variety of ethnic groups increases. They are also experiencing an increase in the number of foreign nationals traveling to the United States for medical care. At the same time, some American institutions are expanding their operations overseas, and medical supply and equipment companies are becoming multinational. The trend toward "medical tourism" is creating an entirely new market for health services as overseas facilities cater to Americans and other foreign nationals looking for treatment at lower costs.

These developments suggest growing opportunities for marketers who are able to capitalize on the growth of international healthcare. With the growing ethnic market, all healthcare organizations are going to have to become more culturally sensitive and be able to develop marketing initiatives that resonate with desirable ethnic markets. There is also likely to be growing competition for affluent foreign nationals who seek medical treatment in the United States but are not familiar with U.S. institutions. Marketers will need to develop increasingly sophisticated marketing skills if they are to contend with worldwide competition among providers of medical supplies and equipment, and pharmaceutical companies seeking to conduct clinical trials overseas must be able to "sell" their programs to patients. As medical tourism becomes more common, healthcare facilities all over the world will need a wide range of marketing capabilities.

Summary

As the field of healthcare marketing matures, substantial changes can be anticipated. Although healthcare marketing has encountered some fits and starts during its first 30 years, it now appears to be in relatively good shape.

There is every indication that the trend toward more acceptance of marketing in healthcare will continue and that its role in healthcare will expand. The industry is coming to recognize that marketing is not an optional activity but a function every organization must perform. As more and more organizations couple their marketing function with their business development function, marketing is becoming an inherent part of corporate operations. The data available today, current analytical techniques, and contemporary technology offer capabilities that healthcare marketers of an earlier day could not have imagined. The future demand for health services will set the direction of healthcare marketing, and marketers must develop adequate methodologies for predicting the future needs and wants of healthcare consumers.

Nearly every development in healthcare suggests dramatic growth for the future role of marketing. Factors likely to affect the direction of healthcare marketing in the United States include growing consumerism, heightened competition, continued technological advances, increasing costs, emphasis on outcomes, labor shortages, and the globalization of the industry.

Today, healthcare marketers have a unique opportunity to shape the future of the field. They are well positioned to contribute to the success of their organizations, to ensure the health and satisfaction of healthcare consumers, and to enhance the overall health status of their communities.

Key Points

- After various fits and starts, healthcare marketing is maturing as a field and becoming increasingly accepted in the medical community.
- Marketing has moved from the fringes of healthcare to a central position in the boardroom.
- The fate of marketing remains somewhat dependent on the economic environment, although progressive healthcare organizations are building marketing costs into their core budgets.
- Healthcare marketing will continue to evolve in response to developments in the healthcare industry.
- Current trends in healthcare appear to suggest a greater need for marketing.
- Emerging developments, such as consumer engagement, new forms of competition, and globalization, all point to a larger role for healthcare marketers in the future.
- Healthcare marketers have an unprecedented opportunity to shape the future of their field and demonstrate the value of marketing to their organizations.

Discussion Questions

- What indications do we have that the roller coaster ride that has characterized healthcare marketing since the 1980s is leveling off?
- What are some of the major trends currently characterizing healthcare, and what are their implications for marketing?

- How is marketing uniquely positioned to address some of the more challenging aspects of contemporary healthcare?
- What developments indicate that marketing is becoming more of a core function in healthcare organizations?
- What responsibilities do marketers have in promoting the field of marketing to "internal customers" in their organizations?
- What educational role should marketers perform for healthcare consumers?
- What healthcare "hot spots" are projected for the future, and how can marketers respond to these opportunities?

Additional Resources

Society for Healthcare Strategy and Market Development. 2008. *Futurescan: Healthcare Trends and Implications 2008–2013.* Chicago: American Hospital Association.

Thomas, R. K. 2008. "How to Be a Healthcare Marketing Hero." *Marketing Health Services* 27 (4): 44.

Glossary

A

account management—The mechanism by which a marketing agency interfaces with a client regarding a marketing campaign

administrative records—A form of registration system that maintains a record of transactions involving individuals included in the registry

administrative unit—A bounded geographic area formally defined for administrative purposes, such as a state, county, municipality, or school district

advertising—Any paid form of nonpersonal presentation and promotion of ideas, goods, or services by an identifiable sponsor transmitted via mass media for purposes of achieving marketing objectives

agency—An internal or external entity that supports some or all aspects of an organization's marketing effort

alternative therapy—An umbrella term that refers to a variety of therapeutic modalities used as alternatives to conventional allopathic medicine; also referred to as *complementary therapy*

American Marketing Association (AMA)—The primary U.S. organization devoted to the promotion of the field of marketing, a section of which is devoted to healthcare marketing

area of dominant influence (ADI)—The geographic territory covered by a particular form of media (e.g., newspaper circulation area, radio broadcast area)

attitude—A position a person has adopted in response to a theory, belief, object, event, or another person

audience—A set of people, households, or organizations that read, view, hear, or are otherwise exposed to a promotional message

awareness—The extent to which a consumer is cognizant of or familiar with a product; the initial goal of a promotional effort

B

banner ad—A small promotional graphic that appears in a newspaper or on a Web page

benefit segmentation—A method of dividing the target audience according to the benefits it seeks from a good or service (e.g., value, quality, convenience)

brand—A concept involving a name, symbol, or other identifier used to identify a seller's goods and/or services and differentiate them from similar goods and/or services offered by competitors

branding—The process of creating a brand for a company, service, or product

business-to-business marketing—The process of building profitable, value-oriented relationships among businesses

C

call center—A centralized communication hub established by a healthcare organization for purposes of capturing incoming customer inquiries and generating outgoing marketing messages

call to action—A statement, usually at the end of a marketing piece, encouraging members of the audience to take initiative with regard to the good or service being promoted

campaign spokesperson—An individual—typically a well-known person—who is presented as a representative of an organization conducting a marketing campaign

causal research—A form of research that attempts to specify the nature of the functional relationship between two or more variables in the situation under study

Centers for Disease Control and Prevention (CDC)—The federal agency charged with monitoring morbidity and mortality in the United States

census—A complete count of the people residing in a specific place at a specific time

Census Bureau—The agency within the U.S. Department of Commerce responsible for the decennial census and other data collection activities

channel—The mechanism used to distribute a promotional message, goods, or services

channel management—A formal program for reaching and servicing customers in a particular marketing channel

client—A customer that consumes services rather than goods; in advertising, the entity being served by the advertising agency

coding system—Any of several classification systems used in healthcare to record diagnoses, procedures, and other healthcare events

co-marketing—An approach to marketing in which two or more organizations combine their efforts in the joint pursuit of their respective objectives

commercial data vendor—A private organization established for purposes of collecting, compiling, analyzing, and/or disseminating data

communication—The process used to convey information in print or electronic form to internal and/or external audiences

community outreach—A form of marketing that presents an organization's programs to the community to establish relationships with external entities

competition—The effort of two or more organizations acting independently to secure the business of the same customers

composition—Characteristics that make up a population, such as demographics, lifestyle patterns, and payer category

computerized survey—Survey conducted via the Internet or other computerized medium

concierge services—Customized health services offered to a select number of customers who pay a premium for the personal attention

consumer—In healthcare, any individual or organization in the population that is a potential purchaser of healthcare goods and services

consumer behavior—Patterns of consumption of goods and services

consumer engagement—Identifying and profiling consumers and subsequently involving them in desired behaviors through two-way interaction

consumer product—Healthcare good distributed through traditional retail outlets (e.g., drug stores) and directly purchased by the customer

consumerism—A movement in healthcare in which healthcare consumers take a more aggressive role in defining their healthcare needs and the manner in which those needs should be met

cosmeceutical—A health or beauty product that combines the attributes of a cosmetic and a drug (e.g., anti-aging creams)

cost-benefit analysis—An evaluation technique that compares the cost of a project (in terms of dollars or other resources expended) with its anticipated benefits

CPT-4—Current Procedural Terminology, the coding system used to classify medical procedures for record-keeping purposes; CPT-4 is the most recent version

creative department—The component of the marketing department responsible for copy, graphics, and other artistic content

cross-selling—A marketing approach through which existing customers are encouraged to buy additional products and services related to the initial purchase

culture—A society's way of life and worldview; the tangible and intangible aspects of society that reflect its beliefs, values, and norms

customer—The purchaser of a good or service; the end user of a good or service

customer relationship management—A business strategy designed to optimize profitability, revenue, and customer satisfaction by focusing on customer relationships rather than transactions

customer satisfaction—The degree to which customers' wants and needs are fulfilled; customers' level of contentment with a good or service

D

database marketing—The use of a data set of past and current customers and future prospects to promote an organization's products

deferred contribution—A form of employee benefit that involves the allocation of "credits" to the employee's account to be used in a manner designated by the employee

demand—The extent to which a target population needs and/or wants a particular product or service

demographics—The range of biosocial and sociocultural attributes of a population that can be used to determine market potential

decision making—The process a consumer follows to determine a need for a product, evaluate the available options, and make a choice

decline stage—In life cycle analysis, the stage at which a product or industry decreases in importance and is typically supplanted by another product or industry

descriptive research—The development of a profile of a community or population that describes the characteristics of that community or population but does not explain the causes of those characteristics

direct marketing—A form of marketing that targets specific groups or individuals with specific characteristics and transmits promotional messages directly to them

direct-to-consumer marketing—A marketing approach that targets the end user rather than referral agents or intermediaries

discretionary purchase—A purchase that is elective (e.g., laser eye surgery, hair transplant) rather than non-elective (e.g., bypass surgery)

display advertising—A promotional approach that makes use of posters, billboards, and other signs to present a product to the public

diagnosis-related groups (DRGs)—A coding system used to classify inpatient diagnoses and procedures

DSM-IV—Diagnostic and Statistical Manual; the primary coding system used to classify behavioral health problems; DSM-IV is the most recent version

durable good—A tangible product that is used over an extended period (e.g., a hospital bed)

E

early adopter—An individual or group that is willing to try new products and services before they are accepted by the general public

effective market—The portion of the potential business within a market area that an organization believes it can capture

elasticity—The tendency for the demand for services to rise and fall in response to factors both inside and outside of healthcare

elective procedure—A clinical procedure that is not considered medically necessary and is carried out at the discretion of the customer

electronic media—Media that transmits content electronically, including radio, television, and the Internet

emergent care—Emergency treatment necessitated by a significant, urgent medical problem

encoding—The conversion of information into a message that will resonate with a target audience

end user—The person or organization that ultimately consumes a good or service, regardless of who makes the purchase decision or pays for the product

enrollee—An individual who is enrolled in a health plan

environmental assessment—A systematic process of data collection and analysis for purposes of profiling and evaluating an organization's external environment

epidemiologic transition—A change in a population's predominant characteristics (e.g., a predominance of acute health problems in a population shifts to a predominance of chronic health problems as a result of increasing average age in that population)

estimate—The calculation of a figure (e.g., size, number) existing in a current or past period using some statistical method (e.g., calculation of the size of a population between censuses)

ethical evaluation—An assessment that emphasizes the marketer's responsibility and accountability to the target audience

ethics—A code of behavior that specifies appropriate moral stances, particularly in professional dealings

ethnicity—A demographic attribute reflecting common racial, national, tribal, religious, linguistic, or cultural origin or background among members of a population

evaluation—The systematic assessment of the efficiency and effectiveness of an initiative

exploratory research—A form of research aimed at discerning the general nature of a problem or opportunity under study and identifying associated factors of importance

external audit—The process of examining the environment in which an organization operates; an environmental assessment

F

flanking strategy—A marketing tactic that seeks to avoid confrontation with better positioned competitors by bypassing their captive audiences and cultivating neglected target audiences

focus group—A data collection technique that involves eliciting opinions and perspectives from a panel of individuals who interact under the direction of a leader

forecast—A form of projection that attempts to identify likely future developments

functional unit—A bounded geographic area formally defined for the execution of some practical function, such as mail delivery

G

gatekeeper—In healthcare, an individual or organization that makes decisions on behalf of an end user or otherwise controls the purchase of goods and services

geographic information system (GIS)—Computerized application that uses geographically linked data for purposes of spatial analysis and map generation

geographic segmentation—A method of dividing a target audience on the basis of its geographic location (as opposed to other attributes)

geographic unit—A physical area demarcated by defined boundaries and used in spatial analysis

globalization—The increasing interconnectedness of organizations around the world; the expansion of organizations across national borders

goal—A generalized statement indicating a position an organization wants to attain at some point in the future; an ideal state that an organization strives to achieve

good—A tangible product typically purchased in an impersonal setting on a one-at-a-time basis

government relations—A process through which healthcare organizations maintain liaison with the government agencies that regulate them, determine reimbursement levels, provide funding, or otherwise restrict their status

growth stage—In life cycle analysis, the phase in which a product or industry begins to take off and establish its dominance in the market

guest relations—An approach to marketing that emphasizes customer service, patterned after the hospitality industry

H

health—From a traditional (medical model) perspective, a state reflecting the absence of biological pathology; from a contemporary (healthcare model) perspective, a state of overall physical, social, and psychological well-being

health plan—Public or private medical insurance available to individuals or groups

health professional—Generally refers to anyone involved in healthcare in a clinical (e.g., physician), administrative (e.g., hospital vice president), or technical (e.g., information technology director) capacity

health (or healthcare) system—The entirety of personnel, facilities, and other resources composing a healthcare entity

healthcare—Any activity, whether formal or informal, performed with the intention of restoring, maintaining, or enhancing the well-being of an individual or population

healthcare model—A paradigm for viewing health and illness that takes a holistic view incorporating biological, social, and psychological dimensions

hierarchy of needs—The prioritization of personal needs ranging from basic survival needs to self-actualization needs

Health Insurance Portability and Accountability Act (HIPAA)—Legislation that limits access to individuals' protected health information

I

ICD-9/ICD-10—International Classification of Disease, the standard coding system medical practitioners use to classify diseases; the current version, ICD-9, is to be officially replaced by ICD-10 in 2013

image—A conception that a company wants to project about itself, its products, and/or its services that emphasizes subjective rather than objective attributes (e.g., a caring hospital rather than a well-staffed hospital)

image advertising—A promotional approach that focuses on the overall attributes of an organization as opposed to specific services or programs

impact evaluation—An assessment of the changes brought about through the marketing effort

implementation plan—A component of the marketing plan that lays out the process for accomplishing the objectives specified in the plan

incentives—Enticements offered to customers or potential customers in an effort to procure a sale

incidence—The number of new cases of a disease, disability, or other health-related phenomenon in a population during a specified period

in-depth interview—A data collection technique that involves one respondent and one interviewer who uses probing questions to elicit detailed information from the respondent

industrial product—Goods used to produce or support the production of other goods

inpatient care—Medical care provided by a hospital to patients who are admitted for a least one night

institution—A pattern of behavior that evolves to meet a societal need; the social and cultural components that constitute the social structure

institutional advertising—Promotion of an organization rather than the organization's products

integrated marketing—An approach to marketing that emphasizes consistency within the promotional strategy and achieves synergy between its component parts

internal audit—The use of an organization's internal data for purposes of assessing organizational efficiency and effectiveness

internal marketing—Efforts by a service provider to effectively train and motivate its customer service employees and all support personnel to work as a team to generate customer satisfaction

Internet marketing—Use of the Internet to promote an idea, organization, service, or good

Internet survey—A data collection technique that involves the administration of a questionnaire via the Web

introduction stage—In life cycle analysis, the phase in which a new product or industry is introduced

L

life cycle—The maturation of a population, product, or industry from birth to death

lifestyle—The entirety of attitudes, preferences, and behaviors of an individual, group, or culture; the basis for psychographic segmentation

long-term care—Generic term applied to non-acute care provided for an extended period and, in some cases, until death (e.g., nursing home care)

low-intensity marketing—Promotional activities that involve low-cost, relatively unobtrusive marketing techniques (e.g., banner ads)

M

mail interview—A data collection technique that involves the distribution of a survey instrument via the mail to a predetermined set of respondents who subsequently return the completed questionnaires via the mail

managed care—Health insurance plans that contract with providers and healthcare organizations to provide care for members at negotiated rates

market—A real or virtual setting in which potential buyers and potential sellers of a good or service come together for the purpose of exchange

market area—The actual or desired area (usually defined in terms of geography) from which organizations (usually for-profit organizations) draw or intend to draw customers; often used interchangeably with *service area*

market penetration strategy—An approach to marketing that emphasizes extracting more product sales and/or greater service utilization from an existing customer base

market segmentation—A process used to group individuals or households with characteristics in common for purposes of target marketing

market share—The percentage of the total market for a product/service category that has been captured by a particular product/service or by a company that offers multiple products/services in that category

marketing—The process of planning and executing the conception, pricing, promotion, and distribution of ideas, goods, and services to create exchanges that satisfy individual and organizational objectives (American Marketing Association definition)

marketing brief—A short document developed for use by a marketing agency or consultant that presents the specifics of the campaign to the extent that they are known

marketing budget—The itemization of the resources allocated for a global marketing effort or a specific marketing campaign

marketing campaign—A formal, organized effort to promote a product to a target audience

marketing consulting firm—An external agency that provides any of a variety of services to support an organization's marketing function

marketing management—The analysis, planning, implementation, and control of programs designed to create, build, and maintain beneficial exchanges with targeted buyers for the purpose of achieving organizational objectives

marketing mix—The proportionate roles that product, price, place, and promotion play in marketing a good or service

marketing planning—The development of a systematic process for promoting an organization, a good, or a service

marketing research—The collection of information for purposes of identifying and defining marketing opportunities and problems; generating, refining, and evaluating marketing actions; monitoring marketing performance; and clarifying the marketing process

mass marketing—A marketing approach that targets the total population as if it were one undifferentiated conglomeration of consumers, typically through broad-based approaches such as network television or newspapers

maturation stage—In life cycle analysis, the phase in which a product or industry reaches its apex and ceases to grow

media—See *medium*

media buying—The marketing function that involves researching, selecting, and negotiating media exposure to support the marketing effort

media plan—A document developed for a marketing initiative that outlines the objectives of the promotional campaign, the target audience, and the media vehicles that will be used to reach that audience

media supplier—Commercial television companies, commercial radio companies, newspapers and magazine owners, poster companies, and other organizations that provide communication channels for marketing campaigns

medical model—The traditional paradigm of Western medicine, which is based on germ theory and emphasizes a biomedical approach to health and illness

medical tourism—Travel to a foreign country for purposes of obtaining medical care; international medical travel

medicalization—A trend in which a growing number of problems are defined as health problems, an increasing portion of the population is brought under medical management, and the healthcare institution accrues increasing amounts of influence over society

Medicaid—The joint federal-state health insurance program that provides coverage for low-income individuals

Medicare—The federal health insurance program that provides coverage for older Americans

medium—A print or electronic mechanism for delivering a promotional message

message—The information that the marketer is trying to convey; the content of a promotional piece

micro-marketing—An approach to marketing that breaks the market down to the household or even the individual level to target those most likely to consume a product

mission—The overarching goal of an organization; the reason an organization exists

monopoly—A situation in which one organization controls the total market for a good or service

mystery shopper—An individual hired to pose as a potential customer for a healthcare good or service to covertly collect information on an organization or operation

N

National Center for Health Statistics (NCHS)—The nation's leading source of health-related data

need—A condition that requires a health service; an objective determination that medical care is necessary

networking—Efforts at establishing and nurturing relationships with individuals and organizations with which mutually beneficial transactions might be carried out

new product strategy—An approach to marketing that attempts to introduce a new product into an existing market

newsletter—A form of print or electronic communication used to inform internal or external customers

niche—A segment of a market that can be carved out because of the uniqueness of the target population, the geographical area, or the product being promoted

nondurable good—A good or tangible product that is used once or a small number of times and then disposed of (e.g., disposable medical supplies)

non-elective procedure—A clinical service that is considered medically necessary

not-for-profit—An organization that has been granted tax exempt status by the Internal Revenue Service

O

objective—A specific, concise, time-bound, formally designated achievement to be accomplished in support of a goal

observation—A data collection technique in which the actions and/or attributes of those being studied are recorded either by an individual or through a mechanical device, such as a video camera

oligopoly—A situation in which a small number of organizations dominate a market or an industry

outcome—The consequences of a clinical episode (e.g., cure, death)

outcome evaluation—An assessment of how effectively a marketing initiative reached its objectives

outpatient care—Medical care provided outside a hospital or other inpatient facility; ambulatory care

P

packaging—The presentation of a good or service in terms of physical attributes or positioning

patient—An individual who has been officially diagnosed with a health condition and is receiving formal medical care

payer—In healthcare, the individual or organization responsible for medical expenses

payer mix—The combination of payment sources characterizing a population of patients or consumers; the basis for payer segmentation

personal interview—A data collection technique that involves the administration of a survey through face-to-face interaction between an interviewer and a respondent

personal sales—An oral presentation of promotional material in a conversation with one or more prospective purchasers for the purpose of generating sales

place—The point of distribution of a healthcare good or service

positioning—The placement of an idea, organization, or product in the minds of the market population, relative to its competition

predictive modeling—A statistical method for identifying and quantifying the likely future need for health services on the basis of known utilization patterns for a defined population

predictive research—A form of research that uses known characteristics of a phenomenon to predict future characteristics or actions

prevalence—The total number of cases of a disease, disability or other health-related condition at a particular point in time

price—The amount of money charged for a product (e.g., doctor's fee, insurance premium)

primary care—The provision of basic, routine health services, including preventive care

primary data—Data generated through surveys, focus groups, observational methods, and other techniques

primary research—The direct collection of data for a specific use

print media—Any mechanism for delivering an advertising message that uses the printed word, such as newspapers, magazines, journals, and newsletters

process evaluation—Assessment of the efficiency with which the marketing campaign was carried out

product—A good, a service, or an idea; the object of the marketer's promotional activities

product advertising—Promotion of an organization's goods and services rather than of the organization overall

production—An industry focus on the generation of goods rather than their distribution, which deemphasizes the use of marketing

production goods—Goods (e.g., raw materials) used to produce other goods

professional advertising—Promotion that targets members of a profession, such as law, medicine, engineering, or architecture

projection—The use of one of a number of statistical techniques to calculate a future estimate (e.g., a population)

promotion—Any means of informing the marketplace that the organization has developed a response to meet its needs

promotional mix—The combination of marketing techniques used to execute a marketing campaign

prospect—A consumer who might be interested in a particular good or service; a potential buyer

protected health information—Under HIPAA regulations, medical data that could be linked to a patient and should therefore not be shared or transmitted except under prescribed circumstances

provider—Generic term for a health professional or organization that provides direct patient care or related support services

psychographics—Lifestyle characteristics of a population, such as attitudes, consumer purchase patterns, and leisure activities, that can be used to determine market potential

public relations—A form of communication management that uses publicity and other forms of promotion and information to influence feelings, opinions, or beliefs about an organization and its offerings

public service announcement—A free advertisement displayed via print or electronic media in support of a community program, as part of the media's responsibility to the public

publicity—Any promotion that draws attention to an organization in a general way without targeting a particular audience

purchase decision—The ultimate goal of a marketing campaign; a consumer's commitment to buy a good or use a service

Q

qualitative research—Research conducted using subjective means, such as observation, interviews, and focus groups

quantitative research—Research conducted using objective means, such as experiments and sample surveys

quaternary care—Super-specialized care provided in large medical centers for the treatment of complex cases (e.g., organ transplantation, trauma care)

R

referral—Designation made by a primary provider that directs the customer to another provider for services

referral relationship—An understanding between two healthcare entities that one or both will direct clients to the other for specified services

registration system—A mechanism that systematically compiles, records, and reports a broad range of events, institutions, or individuals; may serve as a source of consumer data (e.g., Medicare enrollment)

reimbursement—Method of repayment in healthcare; compensation paid by a third-party payer to a provider or patient for the cost of services rendered/received

relationship management—An approach to marketing that focuses on the long-term relationship between the buyer and seller and not on a onetime sale; also called *relationship marketing*

report card—A mechanism based on standardized assessments and established criteria that is used to compare healthcare providers and health plans

retail healthcare—Health services designed to attract discretionary consumption as opposed to medically required consumption (e.g., health spas, cosmeceuticals)

return on investment (ROI)—The benefit—however measured—an organization realizes as a result of its investment in marketing

S

sales—An approach to business that emphasizes transactions between a buyer and a seller rather than the distribution of promotional information

sales promotion—An activity or material that highlights the value of a product in an effort to induce consumers or resellers to purchase it

sample survey—A data collection method that involves the administration of a questionnaire to a segment of a target population that has been systematically selected

second-fiddle strategy—An approach to marketing that concedes a subsidiary position in the market and focuses on being an effective runner-up

secondary care—A level of health services that involves moderate complexity of care and a moderate level of resources and skills

secondary data—Data that were collected through primary data collection methods and are now being used for some other purpose, such as market research

secondary research—The analysis of data originally collected for some other purpose than their desired use

segment—A component of a population or market defined on the basis of some characteristic relevant to marketers

segmentation—The process through which a population is divided into meaningful segments for purposes of market analysis and strategic development

sender—In communication theory, an entity that generates a message to be disseminated to a target audience

service—An activity or process (or sets thereof), carried out by a service provider, that meets the needs of a consumer

service area—The actual or desired region (usually defined in terms of geography) from which an organization draws or intends to draw its customers; often used interchangeably with *market area* but more commonly used by not-for-profit organizations

service line—The bundling of healthcare services into unique products by aligning the functions and disciplines of a healthcare organization with the healthcare needs of distinct populations to facilitate service management and marketing efforts

shopping good—A product that consumers research to compare competing brands on such attributes as price, style, or features

Society for Healthcare Strategy and Market Development (SHSMD)—A section of the American Hospital Association that serves marketing and planning professionals in healthcare

social marketing—An approach to effecting behavioral change in the general population through the use of marketing techniques, such as public relations and advertising

social media—An umbrella term for a variety of communication modes that use technology to support innovative forms of interaction (e.g., texting and instant messaging, blogs, podcasts, Twitter)

specialty advertising—The use of product- or organization-specific items (e.g., pens, T-shirts) to promote a product or organization

specialty good or product—A consumer product, often a sought-after, big-ticket item that carries a particular brand name

spokesperson—A person, usually a celebrity, chosen to speak publicly on behalf of a healthcare organization or its services

sponsorship—Promotion through organizational support (financial or other) of an event or program

statistical unit—A bounded geographic area formally defined for data collection purposes, such as the geographic units developed by the Census Bureau

strategic plan—A comprehensive guide to action developed by an organization for purposes of achieving an objective

strategy—A general approach to be taken to meet market challenges

support services—Nonclinical, operational activities, such as the procurement of medical supplies, billing and collections, and information management

survey research—A category of data collection techniques that involve the use of a questionnaire administered in any one of a number of ways

SWOT analysis—An approach to assessing an organization that examines its strengths and weaknesses as well as the opportunities and threats that confront it

synthetic data—Estimates, projections, and forecasts generated statistically, as opposed to actual data

T

target marketing—Promotional initiatives that focus on a market segment to which an organization desires to offer goods or services

telemarketing—Sales via telephone, through either outbound or inbound calls

telephone interview—A data collection technique that involves the administration of a survey instrument by an interviewer to a respondent via the telephone

tertiary care—Health services for the treatment of serious health conditions that require specialized clinicians, equipment, and facilities

test market—A group or population on which a marketing theme or concept is tried out

third-party payer—An entity other than the provider (seller) and patient (buyer) that pays for the cost of goods or services, usually an insurance company or government-sponsored health plan

trade show—A convention in which vendors can present their products to interested parties

traffic department—The component of a marketing agency responsible for providing copy, film, and so forth to the entities involved in the media

U

up-selling—Convincing a buyer to choose a more extensive (and inevitably higher priced) product over the more downscale option

urgent care—A need for medical care for a relatively minor condition that requires immediate attention but is not significant enough to require emergency room care

usage segmentation—A method of dividing a target audience on the basis of its historical utilization of a product or organization

utilization—A measure of the extent/level of health services use

V

value—Anything that a society considers important; usually an intangible concept, such as youth, economic success, education, or freedom

vanity services—Health services, usually elective, provided in response to consumers' desires to improve their physical appearance or functioning (e.g., cosmetic surgery, spa therapy)

visibility—A marketing campaign goal that involves raising the public's awareness of a product or organization and increasing top-of-mind recall

W

want—A consumer's desire for a health service rather than a medically identified need; a health service want may or may not correlate with a health service need

word-of-mouth—Positive (or negative) communication among consumers about an organization, product, or service

References

American Academy of Family Physicians (AAFP). 2009. "National Survey of Family Doctors Shows Recession Takes Startling Toll on Patients." Press release, May 19. www.aafp.org/online/en/home/media/releases/ newsreleases-statements-2009/nationalsurvey-familydoctors-recession.html.

Are, C. 2009. "Global Expansion of U.S. Health Care System and Organizations." [Online article; retrieved 9/25/09.] www.medscape.com/viewarticle/587903.

Assael, H. 1992. *Consumer Behavior and Marketing Action.* Mason, OH: Southwestern.

Association of Academic Health Centers (AAHC). 2006. "Health Workforce." [Online information; retrieved 11/18/09.] www.aahcdc.org/policy/workforce .php.

Barber, F., R. K. Thomas, and M. Huang. 2001. "Developing a Profile of LASIK Surgery Customers." *Marketing Health Services* 21 (2): 32–35.

Bashe, G., and N. J. Hicks, eds. 2000. *Branding Health Services: Defining Yourself in the Marketplace.* Jones & Bartlett. Gaithersburg, MD: Aspen.

Becker, B. W., and D. O. Kaldenberg. 2000. "Factors Influencing the Recommendation of Nursing Homes." *Marketing Health Services* 20 (4): 22–28.

Beckwith, H. 2000. *The Invisible Touch.* New York: Warner Books.

Benjamins, M. R. 2003. "Religion and Preventive Health Service Use Among Older Adults." [Paper presented at the annual meeting of the American Sociological Association, Atlanta, GA; retrieved 11/23/09.] www.allacademic.com//meta/p_ mla_apa_research_citation/1/0/7/8/9/pages107890/p107890-1.php.

Bennett, P. D. (ed.). 1995. *Dictionary of Marketing Terms,* 2nd edition. Chicago: American Marketing Association.

Berkowitz, E. N. 2006. *Essentials of Health Care Marketing,* 3rd edition. Gaithersburg, MD: Aspen.

Berkowitz, E. N., and S. G. Hillestad. 2004. *Healthcare Marketing Plans: From Strategy to Action,* 3rd edition. Boston: Jones and Bartlett.

Campbell, G. S., D. Sherry, and D. J. Sternberg. 2002. "Effective Web Integration: A Hospital Case Study." *Marketing Health Services* 22 (2): 40–42.

Centers for Medicare & Medicaid Services (CMS). 2008. "NHE Summary Including Share of GDP, CY 1960–2007." [Online information; retrieved 11/18/09.]

www.cms.hhs.gov/NationalHealthExpendData/02_NationalHealthAc-
countsHistorical.asp#TopOfPage.

Craig, R. P. 1998. "The Patient as a Partner in Prescribing: Direct-to-Consumer Advertising." *Journal of Managed Care Pharmacy* 4 (1): 15–24.

Demchak, E. 2007. "The Elusive Health Care Consumer: What Will It Take to Activate Patients?" [Online article; retrieved 4/20/09.] www.rwjf.org/newsroom/
product.jsp?id=23072.

Dillman, D. A. 1978. *Mail and Telephone Survey: The Total Design.* New York: John
Wiley & Sons.

Engel, G. L. 1977. "The Need for a New Medical Model: A Challenge for Biomedi-
cine." *Science* 196: 129–36.

Fell, D. 2002. "Taking U.S. Health Services Overseas." *Marketing Health Services* 22
(2): 21–23.

Fisher, E. S. 2008. *The Dartmouth Atlas of Health Care: 2008.* Hanover, NH: The
Dartmouth Institute for Health Policy and Clinical Practice.

Friedman, S. A. 2009. "Common Exhibit Marketing Mistakes and Ten Tips on How
to Avoid Them." [Online article; retrieved 4/17/09.] http://marketing.about
.com/od/eventandseminarmarketing/a/exhibitmkrtg.htm.

Gagnon, M. A., and J. Lechin. 2008. "The Cost of Pushing Pills: A New Estimate of
Pharmaceutical Promotion Expenditures in the United States." [Online article; retrieved 7/27/09.] www.plosmedicine.org/article/info%3Adoi%2F10
.1371%2Fjournal.pmed.0050001.

Gardner, A. 2009. "Many Clinical Trials Moving Overseas." [Online article; retrieved
10/2/09.] http://health.usnews.com/articles/health/healthday/2009/02/
18/many-clinical-trials-moving-overseas.html.

Gombeski, W. R., J. Taylor, K. Krauss, and C. Medeiros. 2003. "Cost-Effective
Advertising Through TV and Newspaper 'Banner' Ads." *Health Marketing
Quarterly* 20 (3): 37–54.

Hathaway, M., and K. Seltman. 2001. "International Market Research at the Mayo
Clinic." *Marketing Health Services* 21 (4): 18–23.

HCPro. 2007. "Marketing to Women: Proven Techniques to Reach Key Healthcare Decision-Makers." [Online information; retrieved 11/23/09.] www.
hcmarketplace.com/prod-5800/Marketing-to-Women-Proven-techniques-
to-reach-key-healthcare-decisionmakers.html.

Iacobucci, D., B. J. Calder, E. Malthouse, and A. Duhachek. 2002. *Marketing Health
Services* 22 (3): 16–20.

IMS. 2009. "2008 U.S. Sales and Prescription Information." [Online information;
retrieved 7/27/09.] www.imshealth.com/portal/site/imshealth/menuitem
.a46c6d4df3db4b3d88f611019418c22a/?vgnextoid=85f4a56216a10210Vgn
VCM100000ed152ca2RCRD&cpsextcurrchannel=1.

Ireland, R. C. 2003. "Service Line Management Primer." [Online article; retrieved
6/30/09.] www.snowinst.com/articles/sll-primer.htm.

Johnson, T. D. 2008. "Census Bureau: Number of U.S. Uninsured Rises to 47 Million."
[Online article; retrieved 10/2/09.] www.medscape.com/viewarticle/ 567737.

Kaiser Family Foundation. 2008. "Prescription Drug Trends." [Online information; retrieved 7/27/09.] www.kff.org/rxdrugs/upload/3057_07.pdf.

———. 2003. "Immigrants' Health Care Coverage and Access." [Online information; retrieved 9/25/09.] www.kff.org/uninsured/upload/Immigrants-Health-Care-Coverage-and-Access-fact-sheet.pdf.

Kotler, P. 1999. *Marketing Management: Analysis, Planning, Implementation, and Control.* Upper Saddle River, NJ: Prentice Hall.

———. 1975. *Marketing for Nonprofit Organizations.* Upper Saddle River, NJ: Prentice Hall.

Kotler, P., and K. Keller. 2008. *Marketing Management,* 13th edition. Upper Saddle River, NJ: Prentice Hall.

Lake, L. 2009. "Branding from the Inside Out." [Online article; retrieved 9/10/09.] http://marketing.about.com/od/marketingyourbrand/a/internalbrand.htm.

Litch, B. K. 2007. "The Re-emergence of Clinical Service Line Management." *Healthcare Executive* 22 (4): 14–18.

MacStravic, R. E. S. 1977. *Marketing Health Care.* Gaithersburg, MD: Aspen.

Mangini, M. K. 2002. "Branding 101." *Marketing Health Services* 22 (3): 20–23.

Maslow, A. 1970. *Motivation and Personality,* 2nd edition. New York: Harper & Row.

McGee, M. K. 2008. "Hospital Takes Its Grand Opening to Second Life." [Online article; retrieved 9/30/09.] www.informationweek.com/news/internet/ebusiness/showArticle.jhtml?articleID=206801783.

Medical Tourism Association. 2009. "Medical Tourism Sample Surgery Cost Chart." [Online information; retrieved 9/25/09.] www.medicaltourismassociation.com/procedures.html.

Merchant Medicine. 2009. "Retail Clinics by Metro Area." *Merchant Medicine News* 2 (4): 1–3.

Moynihan, R., I. Heath, and D. Henry. 2002. "Selling Sickness: The Pharmaceutical Industry and Disease Mongering." *British Medical Journal* 324 (7342): 886–91.

National Center for Health Statistics (NCHS). 2009. "Health United States, 2008." [Online information; retrieved 7/24/09.] www.cdc.gov/nchs/data/hus/hus08.pdf.

Noonan, M. D., and R. Savolaine. 2001. "A Neighborhood of Nations." *Marketing Health Services* 21 (4): 40–43.

Pol, L. G., and R. K. Thomas. 2001. *The Demography of Health and Healthcare,* 2nd edition. New York: Kluwer Academic/Plenum Publishers.

Powers, T. L., and M. R. Bowers. 1992. "Challeneges and Opportunities for Personal Selling." *Journal of Healthcare Marketing* 12 (4): 26–32.

Prochaska, J. O., J. C. Norcross, and C. C. DiClemente. 1995. *Changing for Good.* Reprint, New York: HarperCollins, 2006.

Pyrek, K. M. 2002. "Retail Medicine: Hype or Hope for the 'Worried Well.'" [Online article; retrieved 6/15/09.] www.surgistrategies.com/articles/2c1feat2.html.

Reuters. 2008. "Study Reveals Wellness Program Enrollment Rates Vary by Industry." [Online article: retrieved 7/28/09.] www.reuters.com/article/press Release/idUS140661+04-Sep-2008+BW20080904.

Rogers, E. M. 2003. *Diffusion of Innovations*, 5th edition. New York: Free Press.

Sarasohn-Kahn, J. 2008. *The Wisdom of Patients: Health Care Meets Online Social Media*. Oakland, CA: California Health Care Foundation.

Scott, D. M. 2009. *The New Rules of Marketing and PR*. Hoboken, NJ: John Wiley & Sons.

Smart Money. 2007. "As Health Costs Soar, More Find Care Overseas." [Online article; retrieved 10/2/09.] www.smartmoney.com/spending/deals/as-health-costs-soar-more-find-care-overseas-20918.

Society for Healthcare Strategy and Market Development (SHSMD). 2009. *Salary, Compensation, & Work Satisfaction Study*. Chicago: American Hospital Association.

———. 2008. *By the Numbers*. Chicago: American Hospital Association.

Take Care Health Services. 2009a. "Take Care Clinic." [Online article; retrieved 7/15/09.] www.takecarehealth.com/about.

———. 2009b. "Take Care Health Employer Solutions." [Online article; retrieved 7/15/09.] www.takecareemployersolutions.com.

Thomas, R. K. 2008. Unpublished proprietary study.

———. 2005. Unpublished feasibility study.

———. 2003a. *Health Services Planning*, 2nd edition. New York: Kluwer.

———. 2003b. *Society and Health: Sociology for Health Professionals*. New York: Springer.

Thomas, R. K., and M. Calhoun. 2007. *Marketing Matters: A Guide for Healthcare Executives*. Chicago: Health Administration Press.

Tracy, B. 2008. "The 7 Ps of Marketing." [Online article; retrieved 4/15/09.] www.healthcaresuccess.com/articles/the-7-ps-of-marketing.html.

U.S. Census Bureau. 2009. "American FactFinder." [Online information; retrieved 4/15/09.] http://factfinder.census.gov/home/saff/main.html?_lang=en.

———. 2000. "American FactFinder: Census 2000 Summary File 3, Matrix P53." [Online information; retrieved 3/15/09.] http://factfinder.census.gov/home/saff/main.html?_lang=en.

U.S. Department of Commerce. 2009. "Trade Data and Analysis." [Online information; retrieved 10/21/09.] www.export.gov/tradedata/index.asp.

Van Dusen, A. 2008. "U.S. Hospitals Worth the Trip." [Online article; retrieved 9/25/09.] www.forbes.com/2008/05/25/health-hospitals-care-forbeslife-cx_avd_outsourcing08_0529healthoutsourcing.html.

Wennberg, J., J. L. Freeman, and W. J. Culp. 1987. "Are Hospital Services Rationed in New Haven or Over-utilised in Boston?" *Lancet* May 23; 1 (8543): 1185–89.

Woods, J. 2007. "What's Driving the Trend Towards Retail Medicine?" [Online article; retrieved 7/30/09.] http://seekingalpha.com/article/38887-what-s-driving-the-trend-towards-retail-medicine.

INDEX

About the Author

Richard K. Thomas, PhD, is vice president of Health and Performance Resources in Memphis, Tennessee, and has been involved in healthcare market research and consultation with hospitals, clinics, health plans, and other healthcare organizations in both the public and private sectors for more than 30 years.

Dr. Thomas holds MAs in sociology and geography from the University of Memphis and a PhD in medical sociology from Vanderbilt University. He holds faculty appointments at The University of Tennessee Health Science Center and the University of Mississippi, where he is also a fellow of the Center for Population Studies.

Dr. Thomas is active in publishing and has authored or co-authored 20 books on health-related topics, most notably health services planning, healthcare market research, and the demography of health and healthcare. He has authored dozens of articles on healthcare and given numerous presentations, seminars, and workshops on related subjects. He previously served as the editor of *Marketing Health Services*, the healthcare journal of the American Marketing Association. He now sits on the board of directors of the American Health Planning Association.